Dr. Wright's Book of Nutritional Therapy

Dr. Wright's Book of Nutritional Therapy

Real-Life Lessons in Medicine without Drugs

by Jonathan V. Wright, M.D.

Rodale Press Emmaus, Pennsylvania

Book design by Barbara Field

Printed in the United States of America on recycled paper,
containing a high percentage of de-inked fiber.

Library of Congress Cataloging in Publication Data
Wright, Jonathan V
    Dr. Wright's book of nutritional therapy.

    Bibliography: p.
    Includes index.
    1. Diet therapy.   2. Nutrition.   I. Title.
II. Title: Book of nutritional therapy.   [DNLM:
1. Diet therapy—Popular works.   2. Nutrition—Popular
works.   WB400.3 W951d]
RM216.W86   615'.854   79-17018
ISBN 0-87857-270-8   hardcover

          10   hardcover

        Printed in 1982

To Berkeley, my wife.

And to all of those with whom I've worked, both successfully and unsuccessfully, to regain and maintain health, and insofar as possible, to prevent disease.

Contents

Prologue

The hunter stalked his prey through the awakening forest. As the early rays of the sun filtered through the branches overhead, he moved noiselessly from tree to tree. Finally halting, he quickly but carefully fitted an arrow to his bowstring, aimed, and let fly. This time he hit his mark; he was glad, because he had not eaten since the previous day. He walked to where his arrow had fallen, carefully removed the chocolate-covered jelly doughnut, and walked away, eating his breakfast.

The four women had wandered far to find food for the midday meal. Finally the oldest, wise in the ways of their tribe, saw a familiar plant. She'd seen it only once as a girl, but had remembered it. From it they gathered the cans of spaghetti and meatballs, and started home.

The children, thirsty again, ran to the tree they knew well. At this time of year, it provided the most delicious orange-flavored fruit drink, with 50 percent more vitamin C than the competing tree on the other side of their village.

Does all that sound a bit ridiculous? I'm sure you'll agree it does, but there's an extremely serious point: we probably have the same bodies, physically and biochemically, that the primitive hunter, the prehistoric women, and their children had thousands, tens of thousands, a million years ago. Certainly there are individual differences, but the overall human plan has been the same, as far as scientists can tell, for roughly three to four million years.

For all but the last 10 to 12 thousand of those years, or 99 ½ percent of the known time that man has been on earth, the food eaten by our ancestors has been what they could hunt, fish, gather, or dig. Even agriculture and large-scale domestication of cows, pigs, chickens, and other food animals is (relatively speaking) in its infancy in the whole history of man, having been practiced for only ½ percent of the time span of our race.

The instant in time occupied by widespread use of refined flours, refined sugars, and synthetic food chemicals is barely one hundred years long.

Simply put, your body and mind are suited to (scientists sometimes say adapted to) the types of foods that people have eaten for hundreds of thousands of years. It isn't suited to the radical dietary changes of the last one hundred years. No wonder so much of the illness of our century is due to what we eat. Our bodies are trying to tell us something is wrong.

The changes produced in the way we live by science and its technology are at once a blessing and a curse. Some of these changes are highly desirable; other changes, particularly in our food, are like trying to fit a horse and buggy with rockets and send it to the moon.

In the long run, it won't fly. It's time to return to the food our bodies are best suited to.

Now let's look at one more scene. This time, we see a conscientious mother, trying to care for her family by preparing for them the best foods she knows how. She's serving a good cut of beef, vegetables fresh from the store, milk for the children, whole-grain bread, and fruit. She's proud of herself; what could be a better balanced meal?

Actually, she's done well, and better nutritionally than many. Many dietitians would be pleased; governmental authorities would proclaim that such healthful fare needs no supplementation: "Everything needed is in the food."

But the beef has antibiotic residues, and is much more fatty that it should be, as the animals were force-fed grains, and inactive.

Some of the vegetables were grown in zinc-deficient soil, in one of the 32 states reported deficient by the United States Department of Agriculture in 1961. Others are lacking manganese and selenium. They're all minus considerable B vitamins and vitamin C, lost in transportation and storage. Naturally, they all have small quantities of pesticide residue.

The milk, high in calcium and protein, is also high in cadmium and lead, as the cows were pastured near a busy freeway, a few miles downwind from a large industrial factory. The factory's met antipollution requirements, mostly, for the last 3 years . . . but what it dispersed into the soils from the air over the previous 30 years won't ever be fully known.

The unblemished fruit was kept that way with the help of insecticides, which also penetrated into the fruit itself to a small degree, after helping to kill the bugs. Of course since the fruit was grown thousands of miles away, some of it was picked green, and gas-ripened.

No, this isn't a scare story. It's a for-real description of many an average meal. If it hasn't made you want to stop eating, it hopefully will help you to understand why, in our century, even the best diet isn't good enough, if we want to stay as healthy as we can.

As you proceed through this book, keep in mind the long history of our species, and the changes of our century. I hope this perspective will help you to understand the "how" and—more important—the "why" of nutritional therapy, preventive medicine, and nutritional biochemistry.

Acknowledgments

The author would like to thank:

Mark Bricklin for his invaluable editorial guidance and suggestions.

Carol Baldwin for her research assistance and for the entire listing and description of health organizations, as well as much of the book list.

Caroline Davis for her research assistance.

J. I. Rodale and Robert Rodale for providing a pioneering voice and forum for natural, preventive, and holistic health care.

Introduction:
Nutritional Medicine and You

"What are you doing with all those weird vitamins and minerals? . . . What do you call what you're doing, anyway? . . . Are you some kind of health-food doctor, treating disease with diets? . . . Don't you believe in drugs? . . . Isn't what you're doing radical experimentation?"

Preventive medicine, nutrition, nutritional biochemistry. These are all terms used to describe a type of medical practice that's becoming increasingly common. While certainly not yet adopted by the majority of medical practitioners, it's destined to become a very important part of the medical practice of the next few decades.

Public awareness of preventive medicine and nutritional biochemistry is slowly growing, but understanding of what it means, and particularly what it can mean personally, is quite variable. More often than not, these terms evoke images of alfalfa sprouts, vegetarian diets, and downing enormous quantities of vitamin C at the first sign of a cold.

While these practices come up from time to time in preventive medicine and nutritional biochemistry, they're only minor parts of an overall pattern, an integrated philosophy of health care practice whose roots go deep in time, and whose branches spread wide in the light of present-day knowledge.

Preventive medicine studies the history of the human species over the last three to four million years, particularly as events of that long span have affected human health and disease. True, there are large gaps in that knowledge, some of which will never be filled in. But it is the firm belief of all practitioners of preventive medicine that gleaning as much knowledge as possible about the history of the human species is vitally important in discovering both how to prevent and how to treat disease in any presently living individual. Of course, not only our human species must be studied, but all factors in our environment, past and present, that have a bearing on health.

Does that sound like an enormous, impossible job? It's certainly overwhelming for any one individual, and may never be perfectly accomplished. But many individual researchers and practitioners in preventive medicine have made a good start on this task; it's their distilled wisdom and insight which makes up the core of present-day preventive medicine.

The nutritional part of preventive medicine should become clear as you go through the rest of this volume. I'll just say now that the dietary rules of preventive medicine aren't just the latest fad, put together lightly without much consideration of the long-term implications. Not at all: they're based on principles as old as nature itself. They'll remain the same as long as there are humans to follow (or ignore) them.

The preventive medicine part of this type of medical practice covers—as much as possible—everything that's known about staying healthy, keeping disease from happening in the first place. This being a less-than-perfect world, illness is going to happen from time to time (although not as often if we follow the concepts of preventive medicine). The cure or control of disease and its symptoms is largely the area of nutritional biochemistry.

The human body is composed of water, proteins, fats, carbohydrates, vitamins, minerals, hormones, and various other naturally occurring molecules. The fundamental premise of nutritional biochemistry is that bodily disease should be entirely treatable with the same elements of which the body is composed, if we can just figure out which ones, when to use them, and the right quantities and proportions.

This premise is simple logic. If your automobile breaks, what do you fix it with? Parts identical to the ones broken, not airplane parts, or parts from other cars that don't fit or belong to your car. Likewise with anything else broken; we usually try to find a part identical to the one in need of replacement for the best repair.

Obviously, the human body is by far more complex than any machine man has yet devised, but the principle remains the same.

Before going further, I want to note that no practitioner of nutritional biochemistry makes the claim that all illness is of biochemical origin. Quite obviously, there's traumatic injury; there's certainly psychosomatic disease. It's the large part of disease, generally labeled physical, with which I'm concerned.

Also, in talking about replacing identical parts, large-scale surgery such as heart transplant is not at all what's meant. The parts that nutritional biochemistry is concerned with are the molecules of the human body. The aim is to cure or control disease with substances natural to the body before the illness proceeds to the point where surgery is required.

It's not an impossible dream. In fact, that's exactly what practitioners of nutritional biochemistry are doing with all those "weird vitamins and minerals," as well as other natural substances. The aim is to supply missing parts so that the bodily system can repair itself.

In addition to supplying missing parts, it's sometimes necessary to remove excesses of both natural and unnatural substances that are causing problems. Sometimes vitamins, minerals, or other natural substances act as levers capable of regulating or modulating whole systems of enzymes or hormones, even though used in small quantities.

Where does all this come from? Isn't it some kind of unproven experimentation?

As mentioned, the roots of this pattern of health care go very deep in time. But the modern branches, expressed as nutritional biochemistry, extend broadly through that most modern and up-to-date part of medical science, biochemical research, both fundamental and applied.

There's been an explosion in biochemical research over the past few decades. One expert in human biochemistry, Jeffrey

Bland, Ph.D., of the University of Puget Sound, points out that the "doubling time" for new biochemical research findings is now down to seven years, and falling. This means that there's been new information and research work published over the last seven years equivalent to the whole total that previously existed.

It's difficult enough for practitioners and others directly concerned with nutritional biochemistry to try to keep up with research work and new information; practitioners in other areas of medicine sometimes aren't even aware that it exists.

Unfortunately, many of the major medical journals read by physicians don't contain this type of information. They're still concerned almost exclusively with drug therapy or surgical procedures. Fundamental biochemical research is thought to be not of any practical interest. Much applied biochemical work involves the use of vitamins or minerals, and frequently isn't published for just that reason. (Fortunately, this situation is starting to change, but has a long way to go.)

So where do practitioners of nutritional biochemistry obtain their information? Usually, from the many more obscure journals, not just of medicine, but also biochemistry, chemical engineering, agriculture, environmental science, biophysics, and other related fields. Frequently, the information is from foreign medical and scientific journals, particularly British, but also German, French, and Japanese. Last, but certainly not least, there are books published by researchers and practitioners. Many of these books are published because the research presented is not acceptable to regular medical journals. But much of the information is valuable, all the same.

The point is, information exists, much more than is sometimes suspected, about the use of diet, vitamins, minerals, and other natural substances in the treatment of illness. Practitioners of nutritional biochemistry collect as much of this information as they can. The bibliography in chapter 54 and the references given with many of the subsequent cases give an indication of some of the information available.

The applicability of nutritional biochemistry is wide. My own medical practice and postgraduate training is family medicine, another relatively new specialized area. Like many other family practitioners, I have what might be called a nonsurgical general practice of medicine. As can be seen from the cases which follow, nutritional biochemistry applies across the wide range of problems seen in a general or family practice: heart disease, diabetes, high blood pressure, arthritis, eczema, bursitis, depression. . . . In a way, it's a "general" specialty, not one with a very narrow focus.

Preventive medicine and nutritional biochemistry together actually constitute a specialty area of their own. Certainly, this field is not as yet recognized as an official specialized area by most of what might be called organized medicine. However, its approach is unique, and the body of information is sufficiently large, requiring just as much study as other medical specialties—which is one good reason for not blaming your doctor for not applying a vitamin-and-mineral approach to his practice. Most busy physicians simply don't have the time to learn what in effect is a whole new specialty field, even if they wanted to.

Returning to nutritional biochemistry specifically, I'd like to mention that, although its goal is to treat physical disease only with substances natural to the body, this goal is not as yet 100 percent successful. Most practitioners of nutritional biochemistry aren't fanatical or dogmatic about the natural approach. It's taken whenever possible, whenever it works. But always kept in mind is the purpose of any type of medical practice: to help keep people healthy, and to help those ill to return to health, insofar as possible, in the quickest and safest manner possible. When necessary, I can write just as illegible a drug prescription as any the pharmacist has ever seen. I'll always do so, if that's what it takes to help a situation. Or if surgical referral is needed, that'll be done, too. Not everything can be done in a natural way.

However, by using the approach of preventive medicine and nutritional biochemistry, I've been able to cut down the number of drug prescriptions and drug use in-office by 80 percent since my first year in practice.

Nutritional therapy is in fact a very conservative approach. More orthodox medical practitioners, particularly those who don't understand preventive medicine and nutritional biochemistry, sometimes tend to be quite critical, saying that it's "radical" and "dangerous."

Very little could be further from the truth. Actually, drugs, surgery, radiation, chemotherapy . . . many of the more orthodox tools are in fact radical departures in the history of medical practice. Most of the routine treatments of modern medicine have been in existence for only a few decades, at the very most. Since for many of us, these techniques have been around for most of our lives, they seem very usual, while a return to more natural means appears unusual. Looked at in the longer perspective of time, though, the exact opposite is true.

Drug therapy and surgical therapy are demonstrably more dangerous than the use of diets, vitamins, minerals, and other natural substances in the treatment of illness. Many, many more people are injured by drug side effects than by the side effects of nutrients used in therapy, both in absolute numbers and as a percentage of persons treated. When side effects do happen from nutritional therapy, they're likely to be lesser in degree than drug side effects.

The criticism is sometimes raised that nutritional therapy is dangerous because a condition otherwise treatable by regular medical means will be too far gone by the time the patient gives up on it and goes on to regular treatment. That criticism is almost beneath answering: any practitioner who has the best interests of his/her patients at heart will do everything possible to make sure this doesn't happen. Patients should be kept informed of alternatives, and no competent practitioner in any field becomes offended if another opinion is sought.

Another issue is brought forward by this criticism: each individual's personal responsibility for his or her own health. Practitioners in preventive medicine and nutritional biochemistry are very firm believers in this concept. That is partly because of the preventive orientation, which inevitably involves considerable patient education in the principles and practices needed to maintain health. Once these principles are explained or in some way taught, it's each person's responsibility to follow them. Obviously, no physician is going to follow you around to make sure you do so.

As a physician, I'm there to offer information and advice, not authoritarian direction. I'm not infallible; I try to be as accurate as possible as much of the time as possible. I think I come as close as anyone can. In fact, that's the best any physician (or any professional in any field) can do. But I know I can't help 100 percent of all those I see, 100 percent of the time.

Recognizing these facts, anyone who doesn't take an active role in their own health care is putting themselves at possibly unnecessary risk, with any physician of any sort. To return to my point of take-off: if a condition isn't getting better by a certain approach—natural, drugs, or whatever—it's the individual's responsibility, as well as the physician's, to recognize it, and try to do something else about it.

Treatment with nutritional biochemistry is inherently no more likely to let something go too far than any other system of treatment, given competent, caring physicians, and patients who take some of the responsibility for their own care.

Ever since the first teachers of medicine and the first students, a fundamental principle has been to proceed from the mildest, safest measures, gradually through stronger and more dangerous measures in the treatment of illness. Very clearly, the ways and means of preventive medicine and nutritional biochemistry, the more conservative approach, should be tried before proceeding to drug, surgical, or other more radical treatment.

The cases which follow illustrate some of the treatments used in nutritional biochemistry and preventive medicine, as well as outlining some of the principles involved. Even though the overall philosophy and pattern of practice in these cases is the same, you may note that dietary recommendations for some persons go a lot further than for others, or are quite different when it might seem they'd be similar. Occasionally, some of the other measures will vary when it appears they should be similar. Even though the reasons are explained in each case, the differences might be puzzling.

Dissimilarities originate both from the nature of nutritional therapy, and from the differences between each of us as individuals.

Preventive medicine and nutritional biochemistry for some

are just like a foreign language. Even though the individual has decided that this type of health care should be tried, it's sometimes impossible to go very fast at first. Can you imagine trying to speak Serbo-Croatian in one week, or one month, even with the best of lessons?

The situation of the nutrition-oriented physician is in some places and times little better. While people do come in voluntarily, willing to learn a more healthful way, the degree of conscious and unconscious resistance to any great change from usual eating and living patterns is often quite large. (I don't know how many times I've repeated, for what seems like the twenty-seventh time to the same individual, "Yes, I really do mean getting rid of 100 percent of all the refined sugar and white flour. Not just most of it; all of it, please.") The practitioner quickly learns how far to go and how fast.

Each individual is very different. A few persons have decided they're going to do absolutely everything in the way of dietary change and other natural treatments in an effort to become healthy and stay that way. In a relatively short time, they've practically cleared the pantry of everything they shouldn't eat, and more important, filled it with things they should. They've taken each supplemental substance faithfully, cooperating fully.

With others, there's just so far they'll go. I hear from time to time, "I'd rather die young than give up my coffee (or cigarettes, sugar, or allergenic food)." That's certainly each individual's right; the responsibility of care for one's own health cannot help but include the right not to take care of it. (What puzzles me is why individuals who've chosen such a route ever come back to see me, or any other physician—but that's another story.)

The physician in nutritional practice also learns quickly which persons are adaptable to change. Within reason, I try to work with persons of widely varying adaptability, recognizing that not everyone can, or wants to, proceed at the same pace.

A nutritionally oriented doctor's problems do not end with patient relations. Some physicians see such a threat in an unorthodox colleague that they'll "boil him alive" at the first opportunity.

By coincidence, just as I was composing this section, I came across a letter to the *Medical Tribune*, February 7, 1979, that gives one physician's frustrating experience with this "missionary-and-cannibal" syndrome.

Multivitamins and Other Unorthodox Therapies*

Like most physicians I believed that most people get the vitamins they needed from their food—until about a year ago. Then, through the proddings of my wife, I started to read Pauling, Williams, Irwin Stone, and Carlton Fredericks. I even started reading on laetrile because of the almost miraculous recovery of a friend from terminal bilateral cystadenocarcinoma of the ovaries after using laetrile and other nutritional treatments. I started giving vitamin supplements to my patients with various forms of joint pains, peripheral vascular disease, angina pectoris with very good results with most of them. One patient with unstable angina, whom I was ready to send to the surgeons for a bypass, improved so much on multivitamins—vitamin C, vitamin E, and lecithin—that he can now run around the block a few times without experiencing angina.

Of course, I didn't keep all this to myself. I told my colleagues here at the Center and most of them started thinking of me as a quack. In one of our conferences, I presented to them various evidences on the benefits of vitamin C in various diseases. Because most of the evidence presented was not based on controlled, double-blind studies, and also because up until that time the only reports they had read about on vitamins (from orthodox sources) were mainly negative, their reception of my discussion was very cold, although polite. I realize that they feel this way because they follow the lead of the AMA, the FDA, and the respected leaders in the medical profession. The general attitude is: If the medical establishment doesn't know it, then it's either wrong or not worth knowing. This attitude, I feel, is one of the reasons why after many years and billions of dollars worth of research we haven't made any significant dent in the treatment and

°Reprinted with permission of *Medical Tribune.*

prevention, especially prevention, of cancer and *other* degenerative diseases such as cardiovascular disease and arthritis. . . .

Juan N. Dizon, M.D.
Dr. Martin Luther King Jr. Health Center
Bronx, N.Y.

Dr. Dizon's treatment (at least to this point) by his colleagues has actually been fairly mild. Physicians have been called up before their county or state medical societies, cut off professionally, forced to resign from hospitals, and even had their licenses suspended for practicing nutritional therapies.

I'm not saying at all that bad doctors of whatever persuasion shouldn't be made accountable. But the problem in many of these cases has not been bad doctoring: it's been practicing medicine in other than the usual and customary manner, which automatically makes it bad, regardless of whether it works. In my limited experience, I've encountered many examples of bad practice in the regular manner; but often very little is done about it. In the words of a fellow practitioner of nutritional therapy: "A fair result in an unusual treatment is considered much worse than a terrible outcome achieved in the usual and customary manner." Unfortunately, that is often all too true.

Given the hostility of some segments of organized medicine, why do nutrition-oriented physicians persist? Very basically, because we believe it's the best available health care for our patients. Combined with the best elements of regular medicine, the combination is the best there is. Why should we as physicians or patients settle for less?

Part I

A Casebook
of Nutritional
and
Natural Therapy

Often, an apparently simple problem has complex origins and requires a variety of treatments. In this case, the opposite is true: a woman with a number of symptoms centered around her menstrual periods was helped with a single nutrient: pyridoxine, or vitamin B_6. . . . With a discussion of the drug approaches which are usually used rather than B_6, and a special note on estrogen and B_6.

1

A Case of Menstrual Upset with Acne and Depression

Sally Kraft came in with a defeatist approach. "I'm 26 now," she said, "and have been going to doctors about my problems since I was in the sixth grade. They've given me a lot of treatments, and the best has only worked a little bit. I really don't think you can help me either."

This type of beginning remark happens from time to time, but the fact that the person has come into my office belies an absolute belief in it. So I asked Mrs. Kraft (as I usually do when someone starts this way) why then had she come in.

"Well," she replied, after a long pause, "some of my friends have been helped with things they've had for a long time. I've heard a lot about diet and vitamins, so I thought I'd give it another try."

So far we hadn't gotten to talking about the problem. Mrs. Kraft appeared reluctant to start. So I asked what I could try to help her with.

She looked very surprised. "My face, of course," she said, implying how could I have missed it. It was certainly true—her face was, honestly speaking, a mess. It was reddened over the cheeks and nose, and slightly puffy. The skin appeared coarse, a little like a "pigskin" football, and the redness was deepened in patches. There were pimples scattered all over, and many cysts and deeply infected areas, called pustules. Her forehead was nearly as bad as her cheeks, the redness extended into her hairline, and seemed to terminate in a slightly greasy dandruff.

Overall it appeared like an especially bad case of acne, but somehow, worse.

After I inquired what the problem was, Mrs. Kraft appeared to become notably discouraged. So I thought it best to explain that frequently a problem was not simply the most obvious symptom. There might be associated symptoms or clues of seemingly minor significance which could be a key to an entire problem. So, we had to go into her health background as well. Since the condition of her face bothered her most, I asked her to start there.

Her trouble began about a year or so before her menstrual periods had begun. Initially, it seemed "like a regular case of acne" with small pimples and cysts scattered about her face. But once her menses started, "it really hit bad." She noted that before her first few periods her face "blossomed" with pimples and cysts all over. For a while, the condition settled down for one to three weeks between cycles, but at age 15 or 16, it became constant: "bad all the time, but awful before periods." Since that time, it had remained as it now appeared.

Since her facial problem worsened before her menstrual periods, I asked if she had other premenstrual problems, also.

"Sure," Mrs. Kraft replied. "But so many of my girl friends have them, too, that I don't really think they're connected. I have fluid retention, and I get really cranky a few days before my periods, too."

I agreed that many women had these problems, but mentioned that they're really metabolic abnormalities that can be corrected, *not* just a "normal part of menstrual cycles" or "just nerves." This was likely with her, also. But I needed more details.

Mrs. Kraft then told me that she sometimes "put on 10 or 15 pounds of water" premenstrually. "It just comes on me suddenly." But she never considered it that much of a problem: "I just naturally retain fluid," she said. She pointed out that her mother had the same "water trouble" all her life, as did her sister. "I figure I always have 7 or 8 pounds of water," she said.

I asked again about the premenstrual nervousness.

"Well," she said, pausing once more for a long time, "I guess it's more than just a little nervousness. Sometimes I catch myself screaming at the children over nothing, and just can't stop. My husband says it's impossible to live with me before some periods."

It seemed obvious that this was difficult for her to discuss, so I decided to go on to other areas. I asked if she had ever taken birth-control pills, and if she had to stop them.

Mrs. Kraft looked surprised. "Yes," she said, "but how did you know? I tried two or three kinds, but they all caused the same problems. I got depressed and anxious all at once. I got headaches, breast tenderness, and nausea. My fluid retention became much worse. So I finally stopped taking them."

When I asked if she had any other health problems, she said no. As her other symptoms indicated a potential for trouble with pregnancies, I asked her about this, too.

"I forgot about that," Mrs. Kraft said. "I had toxemia with pregnancy twice. Once it got so serious I had to be hospitalized. My blood pressure was up, but I didn't have convulsions or anything."

As I felt this completed the picture of metabolic abnormality, I asked about treatments she'd had.

For her skin, she'd used a variety of medications, mostly containing cortisone or one of its synthetic relatives. These "did better than anything but still not much." So she stopped them.

For the infectious part of her skin condition, she'd been put on a variety of antibiotics, including tetracycline, erythromycin, and different types of penicillin. These had also only helped a little, and she'd stopped when she began to get frequent yeast infections. "After that, I gave up on dermatologists," she said. "Nothing seemed to help."

Diuretics, "water pills," had been prescribed for the chronic fluid retention. They'd gotten rid of much of the edema fluid, but left her feeling "all weak and washed out." She stopped taking these, too, when the weakness got too bad. Presently, she only took them before menstrual periods when the edema was acute. Her mother told her that the reason she felt badly with "water pills" was that they made her body lose potassium and other minerals, and this had made her a little scared. She tried potassium replacement, which helped a little, but she still didn't like the idea.

One treatment that she still was taking regularly was tranquilizer medications before menstrual periods. They made her a little foggy, and "they don't cure anything," Mrs. Kraft observed, "but I had to do something. When I realized how I was treating my children and husband, I decided I'd rather be foggy than go on like that. So I take them regularly before periods."

Mrs. Kraft stopped. "What's all this got to do with my face problem?" she asked. "If I could just get rid of that, I could probably stand all the rest."

It doesn't happen often, but occasionally a seemingly diverse collection of symptoms will wrap itself up into a neat bundle responding to a single-vitamin treatment. I hardly ever expect this to happen, since our living biochemical systems are so complex that many alterations are needed to progress from disease to health. But it had occurred to me that Mrs. Kraft might have one of those unusual "single-agent" problems, and the more she told me, the more likely it seemed.

The key to her problems was in their regular fluctuation with her menstrual cycle. This applied not only to her common problems of fluid retention and nervous tension but also to her unusually severe, persistent facial rash. This same "key" fit her problems with the birth-control pills, and her toxemia of pregnancy. It even made sense that some of her problems seemed to run in her family. In fact, all of her problems we'd discussed pointed to a need for an increased intake of pyridoxine, or vitamin B_6.

So much research has in fact been done on the relationship of vitamin B_6 to cyclic women's health problems that it can and has filled volumes. Why it is not more widely applied, I don't know, but I listed for Mrs. Kraft some of the research that applied directly to her:

· Dermatologists have reported that vitamin B_6 alleviates "flares" of acne before menstrual periods (see Snider and Dieteman).

· Research done at the University of Cincinnati showed that externally applied vitamin B_6 cured skin conditions very much like hers, although not as bad (see Schreiner).

· British medical journals have reported that vitamin B_6 can relieve depression and anxiety associated with estrogen therapy. While this estrogen was synthetic, and given for therapeutic reasons, its biochemical effects are similar to those of internal estrogen (see Adams).

· A report from New York Medical College points out that pyridoxine corrects estrogen-caused biochemical abnormalities (see Luhby).

· Work done by John M. Ellis, M.D., a private practitioner in Mount Pleasant, Texas, has shown that vitamin B_6 is one of the key factors in prevention and control of toxemia of pregnancy. It is especially important in abolishing edema during pregnancy, without salt restriction or diuretics.

My own clinical work has shown that vitamin B_6 eliminates nearly all cases of premenstrual fluid retention, as well as many other symptoms not listed above that recur regularly before menstrual cycles. It also will help some cases of chronic noncyclical fluid retention in nonmenopausal women.

The list could go on and on, but I felt this was sufficient. I asked Mrs. Kraft to take 100 milligrams of pyridoxine, 4 times a day. Since the University of Cincinnati research had shown that sometimes B_6 was only effective if applied externally, I asked her pharmacist to compound a cream with 100 milligrams pyridoxine per gram of ointment. To "cover all the bases," I asked the nurse to give Mrs. Kraft 300 milligrams of pyridoxine by injection.

Mrs. Kraft was skeptical; but when she had made certain that all of this was harmless, she agreed to give it a try. She thought for a minute. "Sounds like I should take baths in B_6, too," she said. I replied I might just ask her to do that, if it would help, but not just yet. More seriously, I asked her to check back in three weeks.

When she returned, the report was very encouraging. The 400 milligrams of pyridoxine daily, by mouth, had gotten rid of her fluid retention completely, and hadn't left her "drained." In fact, her energy levels were better. More important, her facial condition was nearly cleared up on the left side, but only slightly better on the right.

Of course, I suspected that she'd been putting the B_6 cream on just one-half of her face, to see if it really worked. But she said no, she'd put it all over, and her whole face had improved. However, three days before, she'd gotten an infection beneath her right earlobe, and it had rapidly spread, flaring up the right side of her face once more. But she was much happier and not discouraged, as she thought it would go away again once she got rid of the infection.

I agreed that this was probably so, and gave her an antibiotic prescription (of course warning her to take *Lactobacillus acidophilus* during and after the antibiotic therapy). Also, I emphasized once more that vitamin B_6 as far as is known is harmless, so she should adjust the dosage to what seemed to work the best for her. She said she would, and promised to come back in another month.

Another month passed; when Mrs. Kraft checked back in this time, she was much more talkative. "I never would have believed it," she confided, "but that vitamin B_6 has cleared up so many of my problems that I feel like a new person."

She looked like a new person, too. Once her infection was gone, she found that by taking 400 to 600 milligrams of pyridoxine daily, she could keep her face completely free of the rash. She even proved it to herself by not taking the vitamin for 48 hours, whereupon the rash started to reappear. She immediately began taking it again, and the rash cleared. "I won't stop again. I'm convinced," she said. She'd also found that in her case, the vitamin B_6 cream wasn't necessary. The tablets "took care of everything."

But that wasn't all. Her fluid retention was completely gone

("I've lost 11 pounds"). She'd had two menstrual periods while taking pyridoxine, and not only didn't need tranquilizers, but felt "calm as I've ever been." Her husband had been amazed. "He couldn't even tell my menstrual period was coming on, and he always could before.

"I only screamed at the kids when they deserved it, and I didn't get out of control," she reported. In fact, she felt an "inner calm" present, which she'd never had before. She'd noticed, though, that before her periods she'd had to double the dose of pyridoxine to keep the fluid and nerves under control. I assured her it was all right to do so.

Still, she had some questions. One was about her family. "I figured this must run in my family, since Mother and my sister have some of the same problems. So I told them. They tried it, and they're both better. Then I read up on it, and found out it was harmless, like you said, so I gave it to my kids. They're little and don't have fluid or acne, but I just wanted to see what it would do."

She waited, as if she'd perhaps done something wrong. I just waited too; I wanted her to finish.

"So," she said, "my husband and I were really surprised again. All three of them are lots less nervous. And they're all sleeping all night now, for the first time since any of them were born." (The oldest is six.) "Is that OK?"

I indicated it was, and before I had a chance to explain, she was on to her real worry.

"I looked up the Recommended Dietary Allowance [RDA] for vitamin B_6, and was shocked to find that it was only 2 milligrams. I'm taking 400 to 800 milligrams a day, and get worse if I don't. Is it really OK?"

I asked if she hadn't just answered her own question. What would happen to her if she took only 2 milligrams a day of vitamin B_6?

"I'd be back where I started, with my awful face, fluid retention, and nerve troubles," she replied. "Why do I need so much more than the Recommended Dietary Allowance, though?"

This question comes up so often that I get tired of answering it; but as she'd never had the explanation before, I gave it again.

"First," I said, "is the simple fact that everyone is different. This is so obvious it shouldn't need to be stated, but the U.S. Food and Drug Administration [FDA], like many other government agencies, tries to fit everyone to an 'average' when it is entirely nonsensical to do so. The RDAs are an example of this kind of nonlogical thinking. The FDA would make the best use of the RDAs by abolishing the list entirely.

"Nutrient requirements for good health vary so widely that drawing an average is impossible. What's barely enough for one person might be way too much for another. Each of us has a nutritional pattern as individual as our fingerprints. What if the FBI had to work with the 'Average Criminal Fingerprint'? It would be just as reasonable as the RDA, and just as reliable, too."

Climbing down from my soapbox, I returned to Mrs. Kraft's personal question. I reminded her that she had read on her own that vitamin B_6 was harmless. Further, she should trust her own perceptions of how she felt, and keep feeling well in her own individual way.

She agreed that this made good common sense, and was "pretty much what I'd decided to do anyway, but won't all that B_6 get out of balance with my other B vitamins?"

I replied that when a person needs large quantities of any single nutrient, and not the rest (to stay healthy), there frequently exists a metabolic problem (sometimes hereditary) that can only be corrected by that vitamin. As B vitamins are frequently partners with our body's intracellular enzymes in helping them to make chemical transformations, it was likely in her case that one (or more) of her enzymes was "weak" and needed much more of its partners' help to work properly. In summary, she needed more of one vitamin to stay in chemical balance, and wouldn't be requiring as much of the rest.

Our appointment time was running out, so I changed the subject. I pointed out that it makes little sense to take vitamins, and neglect the basic quality of the everyday diet. I advised Mrs. Kraft (as I do all my patients) that just for general good health, the food she ate should be whole, natural, unrefined, and processed and cooked as little as possible. This especially meant excluding refined cereal products, sugar, and all artificial colors, flavors, and preservatives.

Pyridoxine (B₆) and Menstruation

One of the rules of scientific research in medicine says that if a single treatment can be found for several related symptoms, then that treatment is preferable to a separate treatment for each symptom, and is probably closer to the underlying cause of all of the symptoms.

Premenstrual fluid retention is usually treated with diuretics ("water pills"), if treated at all. Pyridoxine works better.

Premenstrual anxiety, nervousness, and tension are usually treated with tranquilizers, such as Valium. Pyridoxine is more effective.

Premenstrual acne (identified by worsening before menstrual periods, improvement at other times) is usually treated with antibiotics, or acne scrubs and creams. Pyridoxine is more helpful.

Valium and other tranquilizers are generally thought to be harmless. For most people, they don't cause serious problems. But possible side effects include drowsiness, incoordination, confusion, constipation, depression, and possible dependence. That is only a partial list, taken from a standard prescribing reference.

Antibiotics can provoke allergy; they also cause numerous upsets in body ecology. In women, they frequently lead to yeast infections. Pyridoxine is nontoxic.

Given the choice of diuretics, tranquilizers, and antibiotics versus pyridoxine therapy, the logical choice would seem to be vitamin B_6.

A final note about the treatment of premenstrual problems: at present, a new category of drugs, bromocriptines, are starting to be touted as an exciting new development in treatment of premenstrual problems. They do in fact work, and probably better than any of the other drugs mentioned above.

A review of the biochemistry of the bromocriptine drugs shows that pyridoxine can do all the same jobs they do, and once again with fewer potential side effects.

Mrs. Kraft's premenstrual acne, anxiety, and fluid retention was much worse than most women suffer who have these problems. Her problems were at least partly genetic. Her mother, sister, and children all benefitted from extra vitamin B_6. But even where menstrual problems are milder, pyridoxine works extremely well.

Although Mrs. Kraft gave her children vitamin B_6 on her own, having been told it was nontoxic, it's far preferable to give children therapeutic doses of vitamins and minerals only under the guidance of a physician experienced in their use. Special care must be taken with supplements such as iron, vitamins A, D, and B_3 (niacin), copper, and selenium, among others. Generally, vitamin C and other B vitamins, and calcium, as well as vitamin E, are safe, but it's still best to check with an experienced practitioner about anything more than short-term use.

In summary, it can be said that estrogen inhibits many pyridoxine-dependent enzymes, particularly those that help transform the amino acid tryptophan to niacin. Since these substances are very important to mental health, it's no surprise that women are subject to estrogen-related fluctuations in mood.

Extra pyridoxine reverses this simply by helping the enzymes of the tryptophan-to-niacin "pathway" work better, as well as other pyridoxine-related enzymes, despite estrogen's inhibiting influence.

That is not the entire explanation, but it is probably the best researched, and an excellent "model" of how pyridoxine works in countering the effects of estrogen.

FURTHER READING

Adams, P. W. et al. "Effect of Pyridoxine Hydrochloride (Vitamin B_6) upon Depression Associated with Oral Contraception." *The Lancet*, April 28, 1973, pp. 897–904.

Ellis, John M., and Presley, James. *Vitamin B_6: The Doctor's Report* (New York: Harper & Row, 1973).

Fredericks, Carlton. *Breast Cancer: A Nutritional Approach* (New York: Grosset & Dunlap, 1977).

Kotake, Y., and Murakami, E. "A Possible Diabetogenic Role

for Tryptophan Metabolites and Effects of Xanthurenic Acid on Insulin." *The American Journal of Clinical Nutrition*, July 1971, pp. 826-29.

Luhby, A. Leonard et al. "Vitamin B_6 Metabolism in Users of Oral Contraceptive Agents. 1. Abnormal Urinary Xanthurenic Acid Excretion and Its Correction By Pyridoxine." *The American Journal of Clinical Nutrition*, vol. 24, June 1971, pp 684-93.

Mudd, S. Harvey. "Pyridoxine-Responsive Genetic Disease." *Federation Proceedings*, vol. 30, no. 3, May/June 1971, pp. 970-76.

Schreiner, A. W. et al. "Seborrheic Dermatitis: A Local Metabolic Defect Involving Pyridoxine." *The Journal of Laboratory and Clinical Medicine*, vol. 40, 1952, pp. 121-29.

Schreiner, A. W.; Rockwell, Evelyn; and Vilter, Richard W. "A Local Defect in the Metabolism of Pyridoxine in the Skin of Persons with Seborrheic Dermatitis of the 'Sicca' Type." *The Journal of Investigative Dermatology*, vol. 19, 1952, pp. 95-96.

Snider, B. Leonard, and Dieteman, David F., research reported in "Teenage Girls' Premenstrual Acne Flare Cut with Vitamin B_6." *Ob. Gyn. News*, May 1, 1974, p. 5.

A widower is bothered by intermittent cramping of his calves on walking any distance. The pain subsides when he rests. The condition results from impaired circulation in the lower legs, denying sufficient oxygen to the muscles being used. This case is fairly advanced, and surgery is a possibility, but over a period of months most of the discomfort subsides when the patient follows a program of better diet, exercise, and multiple supplements.

A Case of Leg-Cramping (Intermittent Claudication)

2

Ben Davis was obviously a farmer. His leathery-appearing, well-tanned, and wrinkled neck and facial skin, and calloused hands testified to a lifetime of hard outdoor work. Completing the image, he wore overalls, well worn but clean, a faded plaid shirt, and a battered hat. Even his manner was typical; blunt, right to the point.

"Fix my legs or I'm moving to a rest home," he said.

"What's the problem?"

"Hurt. Can't walk to the barn without setting."

"Where do they hurt?"

"There." He indicated his calf muscles.

"Do they hurt when you don't walk?"

"Can't set still and tend the cows."

"Do the muscles cramp?"

"Yep."

"Do your legs get numb?"

"Right one does."

"How long do you have to sit?"

"Depends. Five to 15 minutes. Lots worse lately."

"How long has this been going on?"

"Three to four years."

"Have you seen a doctor about it?"

"That's why I'm here."

"Before now, I mean."

"Nope. Just got bad."

"When did it get bad?"

"Two to three months ago. Figured it'd go away. It didn't."

"Please come over here to the examination room."

Mr. Davis removed his overalls and got on the examination table. I started by checking his legs.

His leg color was normal. His right calf and foot seemed cooler than the left. Both lower legs had lost most of their hair.

No pulses could be found in either foot or ankle. Likewise, no pulse was detectable behind either knee. By contrast, there were fair-to-good pulses in his groin; once again the left side was better than the right. Listening with a stethoscope, I couldn't hear any abnormal noises.

His arm and neck pulses were normal. His heart sounded strong; his blood pressure wasn't elevated.

"You have blockage in the blood flow to both legs," I said. "The right appears worse than the left. Since the blood isn't getting through very well, you don't get enough oxygen delivered to your leg muscles when you exercise them. So, they cramp and hurt. Technically, the condition you have is called intermittent claudication."

"Figured all that, except the fancy name you hung on it. What I want to know is what to do about it. Can I get it cut on and over with?"

"Sometimes relatively simple surgery will clear out a blocked artery. I'll refer you to a vascular surgeon for an evaluation. But your problem doesn't look that simple. You might need replacement of a long stretch of blood vessel down both legs."

"That bad." He got up and put his clothes on. "Nothing else I can do?"

"I didn't say that. Like many other health problems, there

frequently is more than one solution. If one doesn't work, another might."

"So, what else?"

"Some doctors use chelation. This often works well. The treatment is done by giving a medication intravenously that is said to remove excess calcium from artery walls, helping to break up obstructions. Some people have had before-and-after x-rays showing improvements."

"Take many treatments?"

"Twenty or more, usually."

"Time?"

"Three to four hours each time."

"You do that?"

"Occasionally."

"How come only occasionally?"

"Because very often dietary changes and vitamin and mineral supplements will do the same job."

"Cheaper, too, I bet. How much does that chelation cost?"

"It's relatively expensive, but not as expensive as surgery."

"Figured that. I'll try the diet and pills first; if that don't work, maybe I'll try something else."

"That's what I'd recommend. But I'd still recommend you see the vascular surgeon for an evaluation at least. Maybe I'm wrong, and simple surgery might help a lot."

"OK. Now, what pills do I take?"

"Before starting that, I want you to get a few tests done."

"Tests? What for?"

"To see if you have any associated problems that might contribute to your blood vessel disease; and to help determine which vitamins and minerals might help."

"What other problems?"

"Diabetes, high cholesterol, and mineral deficiencies, for example."

"Where do I go?"

I marked a slip for his lab tests, and sent him to see the nurse. Also, I gave him the names of two vascular surgeons, and asked him to make an appointment with one of them.

Mr. Davis returned in a month. He'd seen the surgeon, whose report was already in his record. After looking it over again, I said: "It appears that if you do have surgery, it would have to be quite extensive. The tests Dr. Anderson did show blockage all up and down your arteries, both sides from your thighs on down."

"That's what the man said."

"Your glucose tolerance test showed a borderline diabetes— right on the edge between normal and high. Your cholesterol test is within normal, but on the high side, 249. Normal is 150 to about 250. The rest of your blood tests were OK."

"What about that piece of hair you took?"

"That was used to check for minerals. Your test is better than I expected—you're low in only chromium, selenium, and manganese. Unfortunately, all of these may be important in vascular disease. Your chromium level is so low, the laboratory could hardly find it. That probably has a lot to do with your borderline diabetes."

"Before you go prescribing a whole stack of vitamin pills, I'm going to tell you right now there's only so many I'm going to take. I can't see swallowing 50 pills a day."

"Even maximum vitamin and diet therapy doesn't always work in cases of claudication, though usually it does. But if you limit what you'll take, you give yourself less of a chance."

Mr. Davis thought a minute. "I'll take a few for awhile. That don't work, maybe I'll take a few more. Rather have surgery than pop dozens of pills all the time."

"I'll put down the most important ones first."

"OK."

"Before I do that, we need to talk about diet."

"What diet? Same things every day, since the wife died five years ago."

"I'm sorry to hear that."

"Not your fault. Cancer, just like her sister."

"What do you eat?"

"Mornings: toast and milk. Lunch: cheese sandwich, milk. Dinner: meat, potatoes, gravy, milk."

"You must really like milk."

"Got cows."

"No vegetables or fruits?"

"Just apples. Haven't got time. . . . Never could cook anyway. Only get to town once a week."

"What kind of bread?"

"Regular white bread."

"With that kind of diet, it's not a surprise you have health problems."

"Haven't got time for a lot of cooking and fussing."

"Don't you have a garden?"

"Gave it up after the wife died."

"It's very important you make some dietary changes if you're going to give yourself the best chance of improvement. It's not necessary to do a lot of cooking to eat nutritious foods. The most nutritious foods are usually fresh and uncooked; they can just be cleaned and eaten.

"I'd like you to eat several raw vegetables every day. Switch around a lot; use different ones. Get different kinds of nuts and seeds, and fresh fruits. You still should be able to go to town only once a week. Please switch from white to whole-grain bread. Do you use pasteurized milk?"

"My cows are clean. Boiled milk's only good for city folks."

"Fine. Now, about vitamins and minerals. . ."

"Remember, I'm not taking many."

"First, vitamin E. I want you to take 2,000 units daily. . . ."

"Two thousand units?"

"That's only two pills if you get the big ones."

"What's it do?"

"Several researchers have found it helps intermittent claudication, especially the type you have. Next, zinc. . ."

"You didn't say low zinc."

"Researchers at the University of Missouri found that zinc has a beneficial effect in severe vascular disease even when deficiency doesn't exist. Please get chelated zinc, 50 milligrams, and use it 3 times a day.

"Chromium is very important since you're so low in it. It'll help your blood sugar control; some doctors believe it helps blood vessel disease also. That should be 1 milligram, twice daily. Also, you'll need selenium, to help the vitamin E work. One hundred micrograms, twice a day for now.

"Next, vitamin C. Back in the 1950s, a doctor showed with angiographic studies—that's dye in the blood vessels—that vitamin C could help reverse atherosclerosis in some patients. Unfortunately, that wasn't ever followed up by other researchers. I want you to start with 1 gram—1,000 milligrams—of vitamin C 3 times a day, and raise the dose by a gram a day until it gives you gas or diarrhea, then cut back a little, and stay at that dose, whatever it is."

"That could be ten pills a day or more!"

"Hold on. I didn't say pills . . . vitamin C also comes in a powder. About 4 grams a teaspoon, and less expensive, too."

"Can I mix it with milk?"

"If you want. I'm not sure how it'll taste."

"It'll taste fine. Is that all?"

"You were deficient in manganese . . . but, since you don't want to take many pills to start . . . I want you to try some calcium pangamate."

"What's that?"

"Most of the research on calcium pangamate [sometimes called vitamin B_{15} or pangamic acid] has been done overseas, especially in Russia. It seems to be particularly helpful in cardiovascular diseases . . . some of my patients wouldn't be without it. They say they're much less tired when they take it. Researchers say it helps in improving oxygen metabolism to the tissues: since that's a large part of the problem that gives you leg pain, I want you to try 50 milligrams, 3 times a day."

I completed the list for Mr. Davis. He studied it for a few minutes.

"Twelve pills a day, and a lot of vitamin C powder. More than enough."

"Actually, that's not everything that might help."

"Enough for now. If I need it, I'll try the rest later." He got up. "Got to go buy some carrots," he grumbled, as he left.

Mr. Davis had very little improvement for 2½ months. I encouraged him to continue, as improvement sometimes takes longer than that. At 3 months, he told me he could definitely go farther; "to the barn and back, anyway." By 9 months, he was "only feeling twinges."

After some experimentation, he's found that 8 grams of vitamin C, 800 units of vitamin E, 50 milligrams of zinc, and 100 milligrams of calcium pangamate, "that Russian vitamin," keep him feeling fine with only an occasional pain after an especially heavy day. If he doesn't take his calcium pangamate, he says his legs "just feel more tired." Without his zinc, vitamin C, or vitamin E, his pains start to return. With some urging, he's stayed on what he calls his "health food diet." I can't be sure he'll never need surgery, but there's an excellent chance that he won't; at least he's put it off for several years.

Even though the exact cause of atherosclerotic disease is said to be unknown, it's fairly obvious where a large part of Mr. Davis's problem originated. In the five years after his wife's death, his diet was rather unbalanced: milk, meat, cheese, white bread, potatoes, gravy, and apples, with apparently very little variation. He ate practically no vegetables or fruits, fresh or otherwise. The list of potential vitamin and mineral deficiencies from such a diet is, of course, a long one.

Of course, there's probably a genetic factor, too. In another person the same dietary pattern might have produced a different sort of illness. As always, disease is usually the result of a disharmonic interplay between environment and heredity. But no matter what the heredity, Mr. Davis's diet pattern could be depended upon to produce some health problem.

Many sources, including major medical journals, have called vitamin E "a vitamin in search of a disease." Unfortunately, these same authorities weren't too enthusiastic about looking very hard.

However, it has been grudgingly admitted that intermittent claudication such as Mr. Davis had is one disease where vitamin E may have a specific place. (Nutritional/biochemical practitioners have many other uses for vitamin E; I'm speaking of orthodox medical use here.)

Intermittent claudication is just "fancy language" (as Mr. Davis termed it) for on-and-off cramping. However, it's not just the usual type of leg cramps; the term medically denotes the type of cramping caused by use of legs which have insufficient blood flow, except at rest. Exercise brings on cramps; resting, relief: therefore, intermittent claudication.

Several researchers have shown vitamin E to be helpful in relieving this problem. Exactly how it does so isn't known. Looking over Mr. Davis's diet, it's apparent that the best sources of vitamin E—whole grains, nuts, seeds, liver—all were missing.

Zinc at present is enjoying considerable popularity among researchers. It seems a new zinc finding pops up every few months from university centers. Now the word *zinc* can be spoken almost without embarrassment among medical practitioners. However, among the many currently mentioned uses for zinc, its potential place in atherosclerotic vascular disease isn't much noted.

On the other hand, both chromium and calcium pangamate are still under much official suspicion. Although 1 milligram of chromium appears to be the most useful dosage strength, and the number of chromium-toxicity cases from taking supplement pills has been very low, the Food and Drug Administration (FDA) at time of writing has decided to limit the maximum dosage to 200 micrograms. So, to achieve a useful effect, 5 tablets must be used at a time, often 2 or 3 times daily.

Chromium taken in excess, especially by children, can be harmful. But then, so can iron and aspirin, not to mention drain cleaner. . . .

The status of calcium pangamate is even worse. Despite the fact that it's nontoxic, considerable effort has been expended on the part of federal authorities to "protect" us from it. Finding it in stores is highly variable, depending on the vigilance of whichever authority is doing nothing better at the moment.

My own patients, as noted above, are sometimes very enthusiastic and convinced about the effects of calcium pangamate. Several of them have conducted (on their own, without my prompting) self-experiments going on and off it, and noting the effects. The comments I hear most frequently are "my muscles felt less tired" or "my heartbeat was more regular" or "I just felt stronger" (particularly from cardiac patients).

I've heard these comments often enough that I'm convinced it isn't a mass delusion. Overseas research backs up these "uncontrolled" observations.

Some 25 years ago, in 1954, G. C. Willis, M.D., and colleagues showed that small doses of vitamin C were sometimes effective in clearing atheroma-blocked arteries. He proved this with before-and-after angiographic studies. That sort of study is still one of the standard means of studying blood vessels.

It might be expected that such a finding, that atherosclerotic blockage in blood vessels is reversible, would have created a sensation.

Well, it didn't. In fact, no researcher (as far as I'm aware) even bothered to follow up on Dr. Willis's finding. It sank without a trace. I've found vitamin C, especially given in high doses intravenously, to be very effective, as well as safe, in helping to "clear out" blocked arteries.

Of course, like any other nutritional/biochemical treatment, I never give it alone. It's always combined with good diet, other needed nutrients, and exercise.

No one should get the notion, and I hope I'm not giving the impression, that this or any other treatment is foolproof. I remember with sadness sending an occasional patient off to surgery when all nutritional/biochemical treatment I know of has failed. But more often, especially when treatment is applied soon enough, the outcome is more like Mr. Davis's.

Of course, even successful treatment is not the best course. As always, prevention is.

FURTHER READING

Calcium Pangamate (Vitamin B₁₅ or Pangamic Acid)
The McNaughton Foundation. *Vitamin B₁₅ (Pangamic Acid): Properties, Functions and Use* (Montreal: McNaughton Foundation, 1965).

Chromium
Schroeder, Henry A. "Frontiers in Trace Element Research." Paper presented at the international symposium Trace Elements and Brain Function, October 1973, Princeton, N.J.

Vitamin C
Willis, G. C. "The Reversibility of Atherosclerosis." *Canadian Medical Association Journal*, vol. 77, July 15, 1957, pp. 106–9.
Willis, G. C.; Light, A. W.; and Gow, W. S. "Serial Arteriography in Atherosclerosis." *Canadian Medical Association Journal*, vol. 71, December 1954, pp. 562–68.

Vitamin E
Boyd, A. M., and Marks, J. "Treatment of Intermittent Claudication." *Angiology*, vol. 14, 1963, pp. 198–208.
Haeger, Knut. "The Treatment of Peripheral Occlusive Arterial Disease with a-Tocopherol as Compared with Vasodilator Agents and Antiprothrombin (Dicumarol)." *Vascular Diseases*, vol. 5, 1968, pp. 199–213.
Reilly, C. P. "Are Vitamin E Supplements Beneficial?" *The Medical Journal of Australia*, vol. 2, no. 21, November 23, 1974, p. 795.
Williams, H. T. G.; Fenna, D.; and Macbeth, R. A. "Alpha Tocopherol in the Treatment of Intermittent Claudication." *Surgery, Gynecology & Obstetrics*, April 1971, pp. 662–66.

Zinc
Henzel, J. H. et al. "Trace Elements in Atherosclerosis, Effi-

cacy of Zinc Medication as a Therapeutic Modality." *Proceedings of the Second Annual Conference on Trace Substances in Environmental Health,* 1968, pp. 83–99.

A 35-year-old woman comes in for a checkup because of a family history of heart disease. While her circulatory system does not seem to be in poor shape, she does have extremely dry skin, with red, shiny areas around the nose and mouth. That symptom, along with excessive thirst and excessive earwax, suggests a deficiency of essential fatty acids. Dietary correction clears this up, but in the process, probably also helps the problem she originally came in for—her heart.

3   A Case of Dry Skin

Pat McMillan was in for a checkup. We'd gone over her health history, which was fairly good. She'd had her tonsils out, broken her arm when she was 13, and had two children, both healthy.

Pat was 35. Both her parents were alive; Pat's mother had had a heart attack the year before. She'd recovered well, but this had motivated Pat to think about getting a checkup.

"I always thought the men were supposed to get the heart attacks," she said. "We women have other problems—hysterectomies, or breast problems." She laughed.

"I've always been like my mother. Same height, body build, I even look very much like her. I had a little high blood pressure when I was pregnant, nothing serious, but just like she did."

"Did she have high blood pressure any other time? Before her heart attack?"

"Yes, the doctors had her on 'water pills' for three or four years before. She said she had a mild case of high blood pressure.

"One other thing. It's not very important, but it's an awful nuisance. I have this terribly dry skin. I put different creams and lotions on it, which does help, but it seems I have to use them every day. Even then, I get a little dry. My mother has the same problem, and so does my daughter. It seems to run in our family.

"Other than that, I really have no health problems. I'd just like to do anything I can to keep from having a heart problem, if it's possible."

We finished her health history. She didn't smoke, and drank alcohol only occasionally. She'd recently read *Psychodietetics: Food as the Key to Emotional Health* by Emanuel Cheraskin, M.D., D.M.D., and Marshall Ringsdorf, Jr., D.M.D. and was gradually working toward a good healthful diet, and "away from all that junk food." She'd started taking vitamins C and E, as "It seems like everybody needs them," but had decided to wait until after her checkup before she took anything else.

Her only other symptom of note was very slight swelling of her breasts before menstrual periods. She'd not mentioned that as she hadn't thought of it as a symptom: "I thought everyone had that," she remarked.

Once we were done with her health history, she went to get ready for her examination.

The most immediately obvious abnormality was, as she had said, her extremely dry skin. She'd purposely not used any skin moisturizers for a week, and it showed. There were dry flakes everywhere. Her legs were especially bad, shedding showers when touched. Her arms and back were also quite flaky. Her whole skin surface was very dry, except her face. ("I had to put some cream on my face, or I wouldn't go out in public!") Where her skin was especially dry and flaky, it seemed just a little shiny.

"Are you thirsty a lot?" I asked.

"How did you know? My husband says that for the amount of water I drink, he's surprised I don't spend most of my time in the bathroom. That's always surprised me, too: I seem to drink a lot more water than I put out. And with all that water, I can't understand why my skin is so dry. You'd think I'd be water-logged."

She also had a slight redness in the creases of skin on both sides of her nose, where it joined her cheeks and upper lip.

"Has this redness been worse, or spread down towards the corners of your lips?"

"It did when I was younger, but not in the past few years. But my daughter—she's 15—has a terrific case. Red from both sides of her nose down to her mouth, and even some on her chin. It's so embarrassing for her. I was that way when I was a teenager, too."

The rest of her examination appeared normal, except for a large amount of rather hard earwax. I mentioned this to Mrs. McMillan.

"I've always had that," she laughed. "My mother was forever telling me to wash my ears. I wish there were a market for it. I've had to rinse my ears out regularly, because what doesn't come out dries and blocks my ear canals."

"You'd make a good hamster," I said.

"Hamster? What do you mean?"

"Your ears seem to behave like hamster ears. Probably for the same reason, too."

"Do they get waxy ears?"

"And dry skins, when they don't get enough of the right nutrients. However, I'd rather go over all of this at once, when you come back to go over your checkup and lab results."

"Lab results?"

"Yes. I don't think you need an unusual amount of lab work done, mostly routine like urinalysis, blood count, and mineral analysis. I also want to make sure you have your blood sugar, triglycerides, cholesterol, and high-density lipids [HDL] tested."

"The cholesterol, triglycerides, and blood sugar tests are for heart attack warning, aren't they? But what's a high-density lipid test?"

"It's a brand-new blood fat test. Researchers have found that it correlates with heart attack potential. The lower it is, the more risk you have."

"I thought high triglycerides or cholesterol were bad, not low."

"You're right. But researchers have found that the 'high-density' fraction is protective."

"So it's a proportion sort of thing, then?"

"Very close to that."

I left the room. Mrs. McMillan got dressed and went to have her tests done.

She returned three weeks later. As she sat down, she said: "Well, am I going to have a heart attack, too?"

"Not today. In fact, I can't tell you for sure whether you'll ever have one or not. But your risk is theoretically higher than I'd like to see. Remember that high-density lipid test?"

She nodded that she did.

"Your blood sugar, triglycerides, and cholesterol were all normal, although the triglycerides and cholesterol were both toward the higher end of normal. The high-density lipid was low, on the edge between moderate- and high-risk groups."

"What do I do about it? I'm trying to eat right, and I do exercise."

"Let's get your skin and ears better."

"My skin and ears? I know I'd like to get my skin problem under control, but I don't care whether I have too much earwax or not. Really, though, I'm more concerned with my heart than my skin or ears. I've lived with them until now."

"I think you can help all three in the same way. You have a much worse dry skin than most people do, but it's probably only because your body chemistry requires more essential fatty acids than most."

"What are essential fatty acids?"

"They're vitaminlike substances, essential to life, found in particularly high concentrations in vegetable oils; safflower, soy, sunflower, sesame, and others. Most of the time people with dry skins can clear up their problem with extra quantities of oils, or oil-bearing seeds or nuts. My usual recommendation is a tablespoonful a day until the skin is better, and then find your own maintenance level. It appears that you, your mother, and daughter have a higher inherited requirement. Remember the hamster I mentioned? In 1952, it was reported that essential fatty acid-deficient hamsters make too much earwax. Like many other fatty acid-deficient animals, they get flaky skin, also [see Christensen in "Further Reading"].

"Your requirement for essential fatty acids probably has a lot to do with your water drinking, too. Membranes, including skin, that lack these nutrients become more permeable, and lose much more water. Like many experimental animals, you're losing a lot through your skin, so you have to drink a lot to replace it.

"Now about your heart. In many people, essential fatty acids help lower the total cholesterol and triglyceride concentrations. In your case, they'll probably raise your HDL level to a safer range.

"Remember you mentioned your mother had high blood pressure? Experimental work in animals shows that essential fatty acids help protect against sodium-induced high blood pressure [see Vergroesen]. However, there's probably another factor here.

"You had a little high blood pressure when you were pregnant, and still have some minor breast swelling before periods. Both of these things occur frequently in women who need more vitamin B_6 than they're getting. I've found that clinically, vitamin B_6 and essential fatty acids are often related.

"Oh, incidentally, about that skin rash around the nose and lips your daughter has, and you've had. Get some skin cream containing vitamin B_6, and have her rub it in. Don't worry if it gets worse for a few days; it frequently does. When it worsens, it'll always reverse and clear up. Almost all cases of 'nasolabial dermatitis' (the technical name for it) clear up with this. Have her take some B_6 and oil by mouth, to help it stay away.

"Now, back to you." I wrote out the following:

1. Vegetable oil: 2 tablespoons daily
2. Vitamin B_6: 100 milligrams, 2 times daily
3. Vitamin E (natural form): 800 units daily

"Why all that vitamin E?"

"That's why I didn't ask you to just take oil the first time you were here. Supplemental oil without extra vitamin E can be biochemically dangerous. The problem is, you can't feel the bad effects, they happen at the cellular level. But vitamin E protects against any possible bad effects."

"OK. What about my vitamin C?"

"For general good health, yes. But not particularly for your dry skin."

"Anything else?"

"You do need a mineral or two. But let's wait a bit. I'd like to see what happens with just what I've written down."

It didn't take long for Mrs. McMillan's symptoms to respond. Within four to five months, she no longer had dry skin. Her excess thirst subsided, and her earwax production settled down to about average. Her HDL-cholesterol rose to a low-risk range.

As advised, she's now cut down the amounts of oil and vitamin B_6 to the quantity needed to keep her particular symptoms controlled.

In her case, she's probably taken most of the biochemical steps needed to prevent a heart attack.

Obviously, her key sign—an extremely dry skin—was worse than most, having genetic as well as dietary factors. But many people with dry skin find that a little more essential fatty acid oil in their diets is a big help.

Why Dry Skin Isn't a Trivial Problem

Essential fatty acid insufficiency may be more common than is known. A key sign, as noted above, is a dry, flaky skin. While dry skin isn't 100 percent due to insufficient fatty acids, the percentage is so high, and the remedy so simple, that I always recommend trying vegetable oil for dry skin first, and only look for other causes if that doesn't work.

Dry, flaky skin very definitely includes dandruff. Most dandruff either disappears or subsides substantially when sufficient fatty acids are provided. If B vitamins and zinc are included, and sugar excluded, even more dandruff can be cleared up.

No one ever died of terminal dandruff, so why should anyone worry about it, or about a little dry skin? Many men feel it's only the women who, for reasons of beauty, should pay any attention to it.

The dandruff or dry skin might not be all that important, but if the skin doesn't have enough essential fatty acids, then usually the heart, liver, brain, and other internal organs don't either. Something much more major than just dry skin could go wrong with one of these organs.

In the case of essential fatty acids, many more of the problems associated with insufficiency are known: these include effects on blood pressure, cholesterol, triglycerides, diabetes, the prostate gland, and a very important group of hormonelike substances known as prostaglandins.

Of course, human biochemistry is highly individual, so not everyone will develop the same pattern of problems from essential fatty acid lack. But the risk is there, as well as the risk of presently unknown problems attributable to lack of this vitamin.

From a preventive point of view, the message is clear: if a nutritional deficiency or insufficiency can be identified with reasonable certainty, even if the symptoms of it seem trivial, it's best to correct the insufficiency before something more serious goes wrong . . . even if we can't be sure what that something might be in any individual case.

Vitamin E should always be taken when extra essential fatty acids are used; otherwise, some of the essential fatty acids could possibly damage cells through a process called lipid peroxidation. Usually, 100 units of vitamin E daily is enough.

Of course, it makes the most sense to get essential fatty acids right in the food. The best sources are the sources of the oils: sunflower, sesame, safflower, and most seeds and nuts. Most of us don't regularly include enough of these in our diets.

FURTHER READING

Cheraskin, Emanuel, and Ringsdorf, W. Marshall, Jr. with Brecher, Arline. *Psychodietetics: Food as the Key to Emotional Health* (New York: Stein & Day, 1974).

Christensen, F., and Dam, H. "A New Symptom of Fat Deficiency in Hamsters: Profuse Secretion of Cerumen." *Acta Physiologica Scandinavica*, vol. 27, 1952, pp. 204–5.

Holman, Ralph T. "Essential Fatty Acids." *Nutrition Reviews*, vol. 16, no. 2, February 1958, pp. 33–35.

Mead, James F., and Fulco, Armand J. *The Unsaturated and Polyunsaturated Fatty Acids in Health and Disease* (Springfield, Ill.: Charles C Thomas, 1976).

Perlenfein, Harold H. "A Survey of Vitamin F." Report #3, February 1942, pp. 21-36, published by the Lee Foundation for Nutritional Research, Milwaukee, Wisconsin.

Vergroesen, Antoine J. "Physiological Effects of Dietary Linoleic Acid." *Nutrition Reviews*, vol. 35, no. 1, January 1977, pp. 1-5.

A teenage girl has severe eczema (also known as atopic dermatitis) on her hands and forearms. Cortisone creams had sometimes helped, but not for long. The nutritional therapy suggested centers around zinc and essential fatty acids, along with vitamin C. In this case, the results were excellent, although great improvement was not noticed until several months had passed. . . . Along with a discussion of the importance of zinc for a healthy skin, and the problems of interpreting various tests designed to measure body zinc levels.

4. A Case of Eczema

"Julie really didn't want to come in today," her mother said. "She's been to so many places about her problem before, and has usually gotten the same kind of treatment, which never works very well. But I persuaded her to try a new approach. I've been reading so much about nutrition and health . . ." she trailed off into silence.

I turned to talk to Julie; she shrank back into her chair. A degree of shyness in younger teenagers isn't unusual, but Julie seemed more shy than most. Her manner was reflected in her clothing: she had on a dress with a skirt to her ankles, and sleeves over her wrists. The neck was high. While this style is certainly popular with many teenagers, it usually disappears on 80-degree days such as we were having.

An explanation wasn't hard to find. What was visible of Julie's hands certainly wasn't pretty. Almost the entire skin surface was red and rough. There were deep cracks in the skin in several places; patches of skin were peeling off here and there.

In contrast, the skin of her neck and face was fairly clear. She had a few pimples—an apparent early teenage acne—but otherwise no sign of the skin condition so obvious on her hands. Her complexion was fair, with blue eyes and long blond hair.

"How long have you had eczema, Julie?"

"As long as I can remember. But it's really bad right now."

"What have you been doing about it?"

"Using some kind of skin junk. But it's not working too well."

"She's using a cortisone skin cream," her mother said. "Sometimes those help, but not usually. That's what I mean— whenever we go to a dermatologist, we usually get some kind of cortisone, and it usually doesn't work. That's why Julie's so discouraged, I guess."

Julie had a very typical—although more severe than most— case of what is variously called atopic dermatitis, atopic eczema, or eczematous dermatitis. Characteristically, it was worse on the areas of skin in front of the elbows, and behind the knees. In these locations, an entire patch of skin from 6 to 8 inches long and from 2 to 4 inches wide was rough, red, cracked, scaly, and, in places, bleeding. The rest of the skin of her forearms varied between nearly normal, and smaller, scattered spots of rough, scaly, red skin. The condition became uniformly bad once it reached her wrists. Her hands were covered with it.

Her legs, except behind her knees, weren't so bad. There were just a few spots scattered further down her calves, but not many.

Julie's fingernails disclosed a telltale clue. As I picked up her hand to look at her nails, her mother said, "I've been reading about those white spots on her nails. They're supposed to be zinc deficiency. I started her taking 10 milligrams of zinc a day two weeks ago, but nothing's happened. We were so hopeful."

Julie's fingernails were indeed characteristic of a problem with zinc metabolism. She had more than 40 white spots scattered about.

"You're on the right track, but 10 milligrams of zinc aren't enough. There may be other factors, too."

While Julie dressed, I asked her mother if she remembered when the problem had started.

"Well, yes, because it came on so abruptly. I nursed Julie

entirely until she was six months old. Within a month or two after I stopped, she suddenly broke out in almost exactly the same places—in front of the elbows, behind the knees. She also got a terrific diaper rash. I took her to the pediatrician and asked if perhaps the cow's milk could be doing it. He said maybe, so we switched to goat's milk. That didn't seem to do much, so we tried a soy formula. She did improve a little after that, but she had some eczema until she was six years old."

"After that?"

"Well, it's been coming on and off ever since. Sometimes she doesn't have any for months, or only a little. Other times it's really bad. But this is the worst I've seen since she was a year old. Of course, she's been going through a growth spurt lately—4 inches in the last 18 months. Can't keep up with her clothing bills! Do you think that could have anything to do with it?"

"That could have a lot to do with it. There's much research that shows zinc to be absolutely essential for proper growth and development. If she's been growing that much, she needed extra quantities of zinc. Some of that same research shows that zinc is especially important for normal sexual maturation. Of course, Julie's right at that age, too."

"Yes, she's developed a lot lately. She's 13, but her periods haven't started yet. Should I be concerned?"

"Not yet. If they don't start in two or three years, then there might be a problem. But don't worry about it now. . . . Another thing you mentioned may be very relevant. Much recent research has confirmed that there is a difference in the availability of zinc to humans from milk of other species, especially cow's milk. While there is zinc in cow's milk, it's bound to that milk's proteins in a different way than in human milk. Some people just can't absorb it properly."

"Is that why the eczema came on when I stopped nursing?"

"Probably, in Julie's case. But it's not necessarily an allergy, it may simply be a problem of bioavailability."

"Should Julie stop drinking milk?"

"For now, yes. Also ice cream and other dairy products. But don't get the idea that milk is the entire culprit in all cases of eczema like Julie's. The real problem appears to be insufficient zinc."

"Do you really think Julie can get rid of this problem?"

"Almost certainly. Julie's type of eczema—starting in front of the elbows, behind the knees—is really not unusual. I've seen lots of similar cases, and nearly every one of them goes away within four to six months with treatment centered around adequate amounts of zinc."

Julie brightened noticeably. "Do you think I'll be better by the time school starts?"

"Well, mostly better. It's May now, and school doesn't start until September. That gives us four months."

"How much zinc should I take?"

"Not so fast. . . . Do you have any problems with too much gas, or constipation?"

Julie looked a little embarrassed. "Well, sometimes, but not always. And it's not really bad."

"Now that you mention it," Julie's mother said, "when she was little I thought maybe she had problems with fatty foods, but I couldn't really tell. I've lost track since she's been bigger."

"There are many things important to good skin health other than zinc. The reason I asked these questions is that some people with skin problems have trouble with digestion and absorption of fat-soluble vitamins A, D, and E, and oils. Even though they eat enough foods with these nutrients, they don't absorb them properly. So I'd like her to use extra in these areas until she's better."

"Can any tests be done?"

"There are only two I'd like you to take for now: a hair test for minerals, and a blood test for digestive enzymes.

"Until you come back, Julie, I'd like you to stop all milk and dairy products, and take the things I'll write down for you":

1. Zinc: 50 milligrams, chelated, 3 tablets daily
2. Vitamin C: 1,000 milligrams, twice daily
3. Cod-liver oil: 1 tablespoon daily
4. Vegetable oil (soy, safflower, sunflower, etc.): 1 tablespoon daily
5. Pancreatic enzymes: 2 tablets with each meal

Julie's mother looked at the list. "You explained all of this except the vitamin C. What's that for? And isn't that an awful lot of zinc?"

"Vitamin C is very important for good healing. Of course, Julie has a lot of skin area to heal. I've found this type of eczema gets better quicker with vitamin C as well as zinc.

"The other items on the list may not even be necessary. In fact, the majority of cases of atopic dermatitis will get better with zinc and vitamin C alone. If you want, you can try this first."

"No, I want to take everything," Julie said. "I want to make sure I get rid of this. None of that stuff will hurt me."

"But . . . isn't that an awful lot of zinc?" Julie's mother was still worried.

"British studies have used as much as 150 milligrams of zinc for months with no toxicity," I replied. "Also, don't forget, we'll cut the amount back as she gets better."

"When should we come back?"

"In six to eight weeks. There's something else I should mention. Don't expect any results for at least two weeks. Studies with radioactive zinc and experimental wound healing have shown it takes that long for substantial amounts of zinc to get built into some of the enzymes involved in the healing of those wounds."

When Julie and her mother returned in midsummer, it was actually 11 weeks later. Once again it was a hot day, but this time, Julie was dressed in shorts and a halter-type top. The change in her condition was very apparent. Her hands were nearly clear; only a few of the deeper fissures remained. The scaling was gone there, as well as in the front of the elbow, and the behind-the-knee areas, where much smaller areas of rough skin remained.

Julie and her mother were of course pleased, as I was.

"How were Julie's tests?" Julie's mother asked.

"The pancreatic enzymes were low, especially lipase, the fat-digesting enzyme."

"I thought so. Julie said she hasn't had any more trouble with gas or constipation since she started on them."

Julie came back again just before the start of school. This

time her skin was completely clear. She had only three white spots left. Even the pimples on her face were gone.

"Will my eczema stay gone this time?" she asked.

"As long as you keep supplying your system with adequate amounts of zinc, it will. Watch your fingernails; you'll probably get a spot or two before your eczema starts to come back."

"Why don't I just keep taking the zinc?"

"If you take nutrients you don't need in excess for too long, some of them can start to cause problems, too. For example, zinc displaces copper. Conceivably, you could develop a copper deficiency in a few years, if you kept taking all that zinc. But that doesn't happen with all nutrients, just some. And generally speaking they're much safer than drugs for the same problems."

I asked Julie to cut her zinc intake to half of what it was, and continue everything else the same. I also advised her it was OK with me if she wanted to try some ice cream every once in a while, but to still stay away from milk. If her skin stayed clear, she could continue to experiment with dairy products.

In the two years since then, Julie's eczema has not returned, and her need for zinc has been reduced. She's continued with 25 milligrams of chelated zinc daily, along with 1,000 milligrams of vitamin C. She doesn't appear to need pancreatic enzymes anymore, and takes cod-liver oil mostly in the winter. She's seen an occasional white fingernail spot, particularly when she's grown a little more; she promptly increased her zinc until it went away.

The type of eczema Julie had is not the only type that responds to zinc-centered therapy. I've seen a variety of skin conditions respond clinically to adequate zinc supplementation. Acne frequently is much improved with zinc.

Why is zinc so effective for a variety of different skin conditions? I certainly don't have all the answers to that, just clinical observation, but perhaps researchers at Johns Hopkins University have a clue. They reported that zinc deficiency suppressed RNA synthesis in the skin but *not* in other organs tested (pancreas, liver, kidney, testes) in their experimental animal, the rat. RNA gives instructions for repairing protein tissues, such as skin, but it can't do this when there is a zinc deficiency (see Hsu and Anthony).

Now obviously, rat results and people results are not always going to be the same. However, considering the human results with use of zinc, this could be a large part of the answer.

The use of zinc in atopic eczema is a nutritional/biochemical treatment I put together from a variety of clues.

In over 40 cases between 1974 and 1979, I saw only one failure. In that case there was partial improvement, but the eczema was so extensive that I'm sure other factors beyond my knowledge were involved.

Particular attention to other associated factors is important, too. Although it didn't turn out to be necessary for Julie, sometimes allergy screening is essential for overall success of zinc treatment. As in Julie's case, if normal absorptive factors such as pancreatic enzymes (or gastric acidity) are low, and not compensated for, zinc won't work very well either. I've observed, but can't presently explain, that zinc absorption seems more related to adequate pancreatic enzymes than to any other factor.

The type of eczema that zinc helps so effectively is given the names *atopic eczema, atopic dermatitis,* and *eczematous dermatitis,* all mentioned in the case report. Since there are no published studies that I know about concerning its treatment by zinc, I'd like to be particularly careful about the description of this skin problem that zinc helps.

One of the hallmarks of the condition is that it appears on the skin in front of the elbows, and behind the knees. While it certainly may appear elsewhere (characteristically on the sides of the fingers, in the "web" spaces, palms of the hands, wrists, forearms, further down the lower legs, and behind the ears), the antecubital and retropopliteal regions are usually the first to appear and last to leave.

In milder cases, the skin reddens and appears and feels rough. As it worsens, scaliness of varying degrees develops as the skin peels off at varying rates. The redness worsens, becoming deeper and brighter. Frequently, in more severe cases, the skin will crack open, and the cracks won't heal. Sometimes bad cases will ooze fluid; occasionally, eczema will become infected, although this is a complication, not an essential part of the problem. Frequently, atopic eczema will come and go. In some it will clear completely between outbreaks; in others, it gets better and worse, but doesn't heal completely. Usually the worse the allergic involvement, the more resistant to healing. Most often, this is a problem of childhood, but it does appear occasionally in adults.

The white spots on the nails identified as a zinc-inadequacy sign by Carl Pfeiffer, Ph.D., M.D., are frequently present, but not always. They are not necessarily a characteristic of atopic eczema. Even when they're absent, zinc-centered treatment helps.

Patience is essential in zinc-centered treatment of atopic eczema. Sometimes no improvement is seen for three to six weeks. Often, the problem is gone by three to four months, but I've seen it take six to eight months in some cases.

In the past year or two, I've emphasized the use of essential fatty acids, along with zinc and vitamin C, in the treatment of atopic eczema. This seems to work just a little faster, and with fewer "worsenings." The essential fatty acids are contained in vegetable oils, such as safflower, sunflower, sesame, and others. Very recently, research work has uncovered the zinc-essential fatty acid connection showing zinc to be crucial to the transformation of some of the nutritionally derived essential fatty acids to their active form.

Whether this is the key to zinc's action in atopic eczema, or the zinc-skin RNA connection, or both, or neither, I'm afraid I can't say. These are all clues, but nothing is definite yet. Whatever the reasons, it certainly works, especially if allergic and absorptive factors aren't neglected.

Just because I've emphasized particularly atopic eczema and zinc doesn't mean zinc can't help other skin conditions. Published research shows that it definitely helps acne. In fact, in any other nonhealing skin condition, I'll usually try zinc as part of the treatment. It's not usually as successful as in atopic eczema, but as long as care is taken not to overdo it, no harm is done.

One other word about zinc. As mentioned in passing in a few of these cases, zinc levels in hair mineral analysis aren't nearly as straightforward as they seem. This is as good a place as any to outline what I've learned about zinc testing by looking at over four thousand hair mineral analyses, and correlating some of them with blood and urine testing, as well as with clinical conditions.

If zinc is reported as low on a hair mineral analysis, it almost always is, and zinc supplementation is indicated. If the zinc is absorbed, the levels will rise on subsequent analysis.

If zinc is reported as normal on a hair mineral analysis, sometimes it is, and sometimes it isn't. Most other mineral test results reported as normal are reliable; zinc is less trustworthy. An experienced nutritional/biochemical practitioner will sometimes suggest zinc supplementation anyway, depending on the clinical state of the patient, especially if the copper level is reported as high while zinc is normal. Follow-up testing usually shows that copper excess has been reduced, while zinc levels stay the same or go up only a little.

When zinc is reported as high on a hair mineral analysis, it usually isn't. That's not a misprint; I really mean isn't. In fact, this situation usually calls for zinc supplementation, and when this is done appropriately, the follow-up analysis shows the zinc level to have gone down, towards normal, not up.

What does appropriately mean? Zinc is a potentially toxic mineral in large excess. So to be safe, when zinc levels on the hair analysis are high, I request a 24-hour urine collection to be done for a zinc test. If this test is reported as high also, I consider that to indicate true zinc excess.

The general rule, however, is that the higher the level on the hair test, the lower the 24-hour urine excretion. On extremely high hair zinc levels, the 24-hour test may be well below the lower limits of normal. On less-high hair zinc levels, the 24-hour test is usually only a little low, or low-normal. When zinc supplementation is taken, follow-up testing (after zinc is stopped) shows hair zinc levels moving towards normal or actually normal. Urine levels usually rise to normal.

In summary, taking zinc supplements when the hair test is high and the 24-hour urine test is low usually causes normalization of both. I don't know why this happens; I've simply observed it over and over again.

I did mention blood testing for zinc also. After having numerous blood tests done for zinc, I came to the tentative conclusion that they usually didn't correlate well with anything, and were a waste of patients' money. So I gave up on those. The urine tests are helpful, though.

Which leads to another minor observation: most studies of hair zinc levels don't seem to take this phenomenon into account. For this reason, they're sometimes less conclusive than they should be.

To return to atopic eczema: if experienced nutritional/biochemical treatment isn't readily available, it's been my observation that 50 milligrams of chelated zinc, 500 to 1,000 milligrams of vitamin C, and up to 1 tablespoon of vegetable oil is safe even for small children with this problem. Of course, vitamin E, 100 units or so, should be used to protect against theoretically possible oxidation of essential fatty acids (see Anderson). These amounts may be too small, or not effective in cases of poor absorption or allergy, but larger amounts should only be used under experienced supervision.

When zinc treatment needs to be prolonged, it's wise to check periodically for zinc-induced copper-deficiency anemia which has been reported as a complication of long-term zinc therapy. Of course, adding copper to the program if necessary will correct this problem. As with any long-term health-care program involving quantities of nutrients larger than present in food or low-dose supplements, it's always advisable to check with a physician knowledgeable in their use.

FURTHER READING

Anderson, T. W. "Nutritional Muscular Dystrophy and Human Myocardial Infarction." *The Lancet*, August 11, 1973, pp. 298–302.

Brenner, R. R. "The Desaturation Step in the Animal Biosynthesis of Polyunsaturated Fatty Acids." *Lipids*, vol. 6, no. 8, 1971, pp. 567-75.

————. "The Oxidative Desaturation of Unsaturated Fatty Acids in Animals." *Molecular and Cellular Biochemistry*, vol. 3, no. 1, 1974, pp. 41-52.

Brewer, George J., and Prasad, Ananda S. *Zinc Metabolism: Current Aspects in Health and Disease* (New York: Alan R. Liss, 1977).

Frankel, Theresa L., and Rivers, J. P. W. "The Nutritional and Metabolic Impact of γ-linolenic Acid (18:3w6) on Cats Deprived of Animal Lipid," *British Journal of Nutrition*, vol. 39, 1978, pp. 227-31.

Hassam, A. G.; Rivers, J. P. W.; and Crawford, M. A. "The Failure of the Cat to Desaturate Linoleic Acid; Its Nutritional Implications." *Nutrition and Metabolism*, vol. 21, 1977, pp. 321-28.

Horrobin, David F. *Personal communication*, September 14, 1978.

Horrobin, David F. et al. "Zinc, Penicillamine and Prostaglandin E_1." *Arthritis and Rheumatism*, vol. 21, 1978, p. 492.

Hsu, Jeng M., and Anthony, William L. "Suppression of Skin RNA Synthesis in Zinc Deficient Rats." Eighth Annual Conference Proceedings, *Trace Substances in Environmental Health*, edited by D. L. Hemphill, 1974, pp. 387-91.

Michaëlsson, Gerd; Juhlin, Lennart; and Vahlquist, Anders. "Effects of Oral Zinc and Vitamin A in Acne." *Archives of Dermatology*, vol. 113, January 1977, pp. 31-36.

————. "Serum Zinc and Retinol-Binding Protein in Acne." *British Journal of Dermatology*, vol. 96, 1977, pp. 283-86.

Miller, Mary Jo. "Zinc Therapy's Success in Acne Reported, but Interest Isn't There." *Skin and Allergy News*, vol. 9, no. 4, April 1978, pp. 158-59.

Pfeiffer, Carl C. *Zinc and Other Micro-Nutrients* (New Canaan, Conn.: Keats Publishing, 1978).

Pories, Walter J., and Strain, William H. "The Functional Role of Zinc in Epidermal Tissues." *Trace Element Metabolism in Animals* (London: E. & S. Livingstone, 1970), pp. 75-77.

Ringsdorf, W. Marshall, Jr., and Cheraskin, Emanuel. "Diet and Dermatosis." *Southern Medical Journal*, vol. 69, no. 6, June 1976, pp. 732–34.

Sandstead, Harold H. et al. "Human Zinc Deficiency, Endocrine Manifestations and Response to Treatment." *The American Journal of Clinical Nutrition*, vol. 20, no. 5, May 1967, pp. 422–42.

Schroeter, Arnold L., and Tucker, Stephen B. "Essential Fatty Acid Deficiency." *Archives of Dermatology*, vol. 114, no. 5, May 1978, pp. 800–801.

Vahlquist, Anders; Michaëlsson, Gerd; and Juhlin, Lennart. "Acne Treatment with Oral Zinc and Vitamin A: Effects on the Serum Levels of Zinc and Retinol-Binding Protein (RBP)." *Acta Dermato-Venereologica*, vol. 58, no. 5, 1978, pp. 437–42.

A 26-year-old man, still suffering from severe acne despite the usual medical treatment, is discovered to have two abnormalities contributing to his problem. One is an allergy to wheat and the other an absorption problem which interferes with mineral nutrition—even blocking most of the potential benefit from zinc supplements he had been taking.

5   A Case of Acne

A thin, slightly pale young man hesitated outside the door to my office.

"You must be Bruce Jensen."

He nodded.

"What can I do for you today?"

"Well, I just thought I'd come in to see if there was anything else I could do for my acne. It's discouraging. . . ."

Mr. Jensen had a moderately severe, although not terribly unusual, case of acne. Luckily, he had only a few scars, but he had several deep cysts scattered on his forehead and cheeks. There were closely packed pimples, whiteheads, and blackheads scattered over the rest of his facial skin.

"What have you tried for it?"

"Practically everything, I think. When I was younger, I took tetracycline regularly. That did slow it down some. I used every acne scrub on the market. The best of them only helped a little. I still use a scrub, though. I figure it can't hurt any."

"You're not using the tetracycline anymore, then?"

"No. I took it from when I was 16 until I was 21, most of the time. It helped, but every time I stopped taking it, the acne got really bad again."

"Why did you stop?"

"I'd been having some minor intestinal problems; when I stopped taking the tetracycline, those cleared up. I also found out I'd been putting an incredible amount of junk into my body. So, by the time I was 23, I'd stopped eating junk food entirely. No more sugar, only whole wheat bread, no soft drinks."

"How old are you now?"

"Twenty-six. That's what's so frustrating. When I was a teenager, everybody said, 'You'll grow out of it. Wait until you're 21.' But here I am. . . ."

"Have you taken any vitamins and minerals?"

"I really got my hopes up when I read about the results some people were getting with zinc. By that time, both my younger brothers had acne, too, so we all tried it. We took 50 milligrams of chelated zinc twice a day. I found out we all had those white spots on our nails that go with zinc deficiency. So I really thought it would work.

"Well, both my brothers got rid of theirs! Mine didn't change much at all. I've still got most of the white spots on my nails."

"Are you still taking zinc?"

"No, it didn't help, so I stopped. I kept eating good food, though, because I want to keep the rest of me healthy."

"Do you have any allergies, as far as you know?"

"No."

"Are there any in your family?"

"My grandfather had asthma. But the dermatologists I talked to said allergies had nothing to do with acne."

"That's a controversial matter. Part of the reason for the debate is that in some persons with acne, allergies play a large part, and in others, they have nothing to do with it. Since your problem is so severe, and long-lasting, I think we at least ought to look at this area."

"If you think it will help."

"I'm also not convinced you should give up on zinc therapy. I know it hasn't worked yet, but there may be a reason for that. I'd like you to start by having two types of tests done. First, an analysis of a hair specimen for minerals; second, a blood test for food allergies."

"I never heard of a blood test for allergies."

"It is relatively new. It's called a radioallergosorbent test (RAST). It determines levels of antibodies for specific allergic substances present in your bloodstream."

"If you have antibodies, you're allergic?"

"Yes."

Mr. Jensen returned three weeks later. "Your allergy test is back," I said, opening his record. "But your mineral test isn't. So let's go over your allergy test."

The test showed an extremely high level of antibodies to wheat, and a moderately high level for corn. There were no significant levels of antibodies for the other foods tested.

"Why were only ten foods tested? I eat more than those."

"Several reasons. As this is still an expensive test, I try to find a way to limit the number to the foods most likely to be a problem. In my experience, these are the most likely. Another doctor might have a different list.

"Also, these are foods that most of us eat frequently. There's little point in testing you for foods you eat infrequently, as they wouldn't be much involved in your problem."

"But I don't have any allergy symptoms!"

"Food allergies can cause many more symptoms than are generally realized. In your case, it's possible that this apparently severe wheat allergy is showing up mostly as acne. However, it's still only theory until proven. You'll have to try, to see if there's really a difference."

"And I switched to whole wheat bread on purpose. It's one of my favorite foods. . . . But I'll try staying off it completely. Corn, too. At least it's an approach I haven't tried."

Six weeks later, he returned. The difference in his acne was apparent. It certainly wasn't gone, but he only had two deep cysts, and about half the number of pimples as before. What remained looked less inflamed.

"I didn't notice any difference for the first two weeks or so," he said, "but then I could see I was getting fewer new pimples and cysts. It has settled down, hasn't it?"

I assured him there was a definite improvement.

"Should I get tested for other allergies, then? It really makes a difference for me. I just wish it wasn't wheat. . . ."

"Before you do that, let's look at this mineral analysis. It might contain a clue to the rest of the answer." I gave him a copy of the test result, and explained how to read it. He studied it for a minute.

"The test shows I'm low in practically all minerals, everything but sodium and zinc; the zinc level is a little high! Looks like I took too much. But what about these spots?"

"Zinc is the most likely mineral of any on this test to show a false elevation when it's really deficient. Calcium and magnesium do that frequently, also. The overall pattern has to be taken into consideration. Actually, this test shows that you're not absorbing minerals in general to the usual degree."

"Could it be because of the wheat allergy?"

"Possibly. However, there's another, more likely, explanation, which may or may not be related to the wheat allergy. There just isn't enough research to fully explain it. It's very possible your stomach isn't secreting sufficient quantities of hydrochloric acid to make full use of the minerals in your diet."

"But I don't have any digestion problems. If I didn't have enough acid in my stomach, wouldn't I notice it?"

"You're right. Most people with insufficient stomach acid have symptoms, but a few don't. It should be checked; otherwise, you could spend months taking minerals with no improvement."

Mr. Jensen shifted uncomfortably. "I don't want to have my stomach pumped," he said.

"I don't blame you. I had that done when I was a medical student. I don't want to repeat the experience. There's another way that's much less uncomfortable."

"What's that?"

"It's a direct test of your stomach's capability to secrete acid." I handed him a small orange plastic capsule, about the size of a large vitamin pill. "This capsule contains a microminiaturized radio transmitter that's sensitive to the pH—acidity or alkalinity—of fluids in which it's immersed. You swallow it, and it radios out from your stomach what the pH is from moment to moment."

Mr. Jensen stared at the capsule. "You're kidding," he finally said.

"Not at all. If an astronaut's heartbeat can be radioed back from the moon, why shouldn't the pH be radioed out of your stomach, with the right technology?"

"Isn't it dangerous?"

"Very, very little. There's not enough electricity to harm anyone. It's plastic, inert, not absorbed, and just passes through your intestines like everything else."

"Who invented this thing?"

"I don't know. It's manufactured by Telefunken in Germany, though, and used in many major medical centers. It's called gastric analysis by radiotelemetry."

Approximately a week later, Mr. Jensen was back for his test. After it had been underway for an hour or so, I went in to check the results.

The recording paper printed by the receiver machine gave a clear answer. It showed that Mr. Jensen's "fasting" (empty stomach) pH was 1.9, well within normal. After he was given a small quantity of test solution, his pH had risen to 4; then his stomach had apparently made enough acid to bring the pH down in a normal length of time. (The higher the number the less acid is present.)

However, when he was given a second quantity of test solution, his pH rose to 6.5, and hadn't come down in over an hour.

"I've been watching the needle indicator," he said. "It won't come back down to the starting point. Isn't it supposed to?"

"You're right. Apparently your stomach can't secrete enough acid to normally acidify the small amount of test solution." I pointed to a copy of another machine recording posted on the wall. "That's a normal test. See how the pH returns to normal much quicker than yours?"

"So my stomach does make acid, just not enough?"

"That's right. The problem is underfunction rather than absent function, called *hypo*chlorhydria rather than *a*chlorhydria.

Actually, partially deficient stomach acid is much more common that totally deficient."

"That's why the zinc didn't help. It wasn't being absorbed."

"Probably. Let's try it and see, though."

When Mr. Jensen's test was done, he came to my consultation office for follow-up. Based on his test, I asked him to start with 3 5-grain betaine hydrochloride or glutamic acid hydrochloride tablets before meals. I recommended he reduce this number only if he experienced heartburn or other discomfort. Also, I wrote up a list of supplemental minerals to make up for his deficiencies, of course beginning with zinc.

"I think the zinc should work better this time," I said. "Most of my patients have good results with it. There's even a report recently in one of the major dermatology journals on the use of zinc for acne (see Michaëlsson).

In the course of the next few months, Mr. Jensen's acne disappeared almost entirely. His color improved; he gained slightly over 10 pounds, reaching a more normal weight.

He also took vitamin B_{12} injections, which he needed due to his malabsorption problem. These helped his energy levels considerably.

Even his self-confidence seemed to improve with the disappearance of his acne. He reported he was "not so shy with the girls anymore."

—————

I should add that acne isn't all the same. Some with acne have definite allergic involvement; some don't. This case of acne also was complicated by nutrient malabsorption; most aren't.

Acne appears to be a preventable disease, in large part a result of the malnutrition of civilization, and not an inevitable accompaniment of adolescence.

In my experience, much acne responds to simple dietary measures, such as:

1. Elimination of all refined sugar, refined flours, artificial flavor, color, and preservatives.
2. Positive dietary additions: as much fresh, raw vegetables

and fruits as possible. Sufficient high-quality protein.
3. Supplements, especially including zinc, essential fatty
acids, vitamins A, B, and C.

FURTHER READING

Nutritional Diseases of Civilization

Schaefer, Otto. "When the Eskimo Comes to Town." *Nutrition Today*, November/December 1971, pp. 8-16.

RAST Test

Berg, Torsten L. O., and Johansson, S. G. O. "Allergy Diagnosis with the Radioallergosorbent Test." *The Journal of Allergy and Clinical Immunology*, vol. 54, no. 4, October 1974, pp. 209-21.

Hoffman, Donald R., and Haddad, Zack, H. "Diagnosis of IgE-Mediated Reactions to Food Antigens by Radioimmunoassay." *The Journal of Allergy and Clinical Immunology*, vol. 54, no. 3, September 1974, pp. 165-73.

Rubin, Lucille D., ed. "The Radioallergosorbent Test: Its Present Place and Likely Future in the Practice of Allergy." *Advances in Asthma and Allergy*, vol. 2, no. 2, Spring 1975, pp. 1-9.

Zinc and Acne

Fitzherbert, J. C. "Zinc Deficiency in Acne Vulgaris." *The Medical Journal of Australia*, vol. 2, no. 20, November 12, 1977, pp. 685-86.

Göransson, Kerstin; Liden, Sture; and Odsell, Lars. "Oral Zinc in Acne Vulgaris: A Clinical and Methodological Study." *Acta Dermato-Venereologica*, vol. 58, no. 5, 1978, pp. 443-48.

Michaëlsson, Gerd; Juhlin, Lennart; and Vahlquist, Anders. "Effects of Oral Zinc and Vitamin A in Acne." *Archives of Dermatology*, vol. 113, January 1977, pp. 31-36.

After many years of psychotherapy and antidepressants, a woman with depression is tested for various biochemical functions. It's determined that, as a result of inadequate stomach acid and pancreatic enzymes, her digestion and absorption of many nutrients is below par. Therapy includes acid and enzyme replacement, as well as vitamin B_{12} injections. . . . This is an example of somatopsychic disease, in which purely physical problems cause mental symptoms . . . with a special word about the B_{12} injection controversy.

A Case of Long-Standing Depression

6

"I'm too young for my life to be over," Mrs. Acton said. "But that's exactly how I feel. Nothing interests me, I have no ambition. I'm depressed a lot. I'm tired all the time. And I can't control my moods; I cry with no reason, or get laughing fits that won't stop. I lose my temper much too quick. I'm tense nearly all the time.

"I know what you might be thinking, but I've already been to see two psychiatrists. In fact, I've been in therapy for 11 years. I've been tranquilized and antidepressed; I'm taking an antidepressant now. But it only helps a little. I don't want to be on drugs forever.

"I would have just given up years ago, but my husband wants me to keep trying. We were so happy for a few years when we were first married. I still love him, so I keep trying. The psychiatrists were his idea. Now he thinks maybe nutrition would help me, so I'm here."

She suddenly looked very sad, and started to cry. "I'm only 36. I don't have anything to look forward to."

I pushed the box of Kleenex closer, and waited for things to subside a little.

"Your husband's right to ask you to try nutritional/biochemical treatment," I said. "Sometimes supposedly mental problems turn out to be a problem with overall body chemistry. Everyone's heard of psychosomatic problems. I wish more were familiar with the concept of somatopsychic illness."

"Somatopsychic? I never heard of that."

"It's just a shorthand way of emphasizing that supposedly 'physical' health problems can cause mental symptoms. But I'm not saying you have that sort of problem for sure, just that it needs to be looked at.

"One way of approaching somatopsychic problems is through other, more physical symptoms. Do you have any symptoms other than mental ones?"

"Not that I know about."

I asked Mrs. Acton a series of questions about symptoms related to various organ systems. All were negative until we came to the digestive tract.

"Well, I do have a little excess gas, and I am constipated quite a bit. But I've been that way for years, and it's never gotten worse. Besides, constipation doesn't cause depression or tension, does it? I've taken laxatives occasionally, which relieved the constipation, but they didn't make me mentally any better."

The rest of the questions I asked Mrs. Acton got only negative responses.

As she was scheduled for a complete examination, I had her go to the examination room. Her physical exam was normal, too. She appeared to be in generally good physical health. Only one very minor abnormality was apparent. She had the beginning of small fatty deposits on the upper eyelids, called xanthelasma. I mentioned them to her.

"Oh, those," she said. "They're supposed to be fat deposits, aren't they? I just started to get them last year. My mother and grandmother had them too, so I never worried about it. Besides, I've had my blood fats checked at a health fair. They were perfectly normal.

"Now, tell me—you are done checking, aren't you? What have you found that might be causing my mood problems? I have a normal checkup, don't I? All the doctors have told me I'm perfectly healthy."

"I don't think your examination is complete until we've done some biochemical testing. After all, most illness starts at the molecular level—unless you get hit by a truck—so chemical testing is very important. I'm the first to admit chemical testing isn't perfect, either, but it's part of a whole checkup.

"However, to answer your question about what I've found so far, not much, but enough. You have those xanthelasma, a little excess gas, and you're constipated."

"Which tests are you thinking about?"

"To start, more or less routine ones. Blood count, urinalysis, and screening types of blood chemistry tests. I usually request mineral analysis of a hair specimen routinely, but for you it's especially important.

"Now, particularly in your case, with what you call mental symptoms, I'd like you to get blood tests for food allergies, and for hypoglycemia. Also, because of your gas and constipation, tests for digestive enzymes, called amylase and lipase, as well as testing your stomach acid production by radiotelemetry. Lastly a blood test for vitamin B_{12}."

Mrs. Acton managed a small smile, the first. "It's a good thing I don't have more symptoms, or you'd be running tests for months. The ones you've mentioned are certainly enough."

Her smile disappeared. "You know, you already asked me about allergy symptoms. I don't have any. Are you sure I need those allergy tests? It seems like you're doing a lot. I don't mean to upset you, but I've read a lot, when I felt like reading, about unnecessary lab tests. They're expensive."

"There are two questions there. First, sometimes the only symptoms of allergy are mental. Second, I know that laboratory testing is expensive. I haven't asked for you to have anything done that I don't think might help. You've had this problem more than ten years. I think an all-out effort is justified if you want to get rid of it."

"All right, I'll get them done. I just wanted to let you know what I was thinking."

"That's fine. I'm doing the same."

"When shall I come back?"

"When your tests are done and returned. If you wish, bring your husband."

Both Mr. and Mrs. Acton returned for reports on her examination and tests. Mrs. Acton was more depressed this time.

"Did you find anything?" Mr. Acton asked. "Is she hypoglycemic?"

"Yes, but her hypoglycemia appears to be definitely secondary to her other problems, so I won't spend much time on it."

"Why not?"

"Because it should go as the other problems are taken care of. Sometimes it's the only biochemical explanation for mental symptoms, but most frequently it's secondary to other problems. It looks that way in Mrs. Acton's case."

"So what did you find with all those tests?"

"That Mrs. Acton's stomach is making some acid, but it's an abnormally low amount. That's called hypochlorhydria. Her pancreas isn't producing enough digestive enzymes. Consequently, she isn't digesting and absorbing her nutrients properly. Her mineral analysis shows this clearly. She has abnormally low levels of calcium, magnesium, iron, copper, manganese, zinc, chromium, selenium, and lithium."

"Why doesn't she have more physical symptoms?"

"She will, if this isn't corrected. Right now, she's young enough, apparently, to tolerate this kind of malnutrition physically, and show only excess gas and constipation as physical symptoms."

"But she's been eating fairly well, and I've been giving her vitamins."

"I know, she told me. But that doesn't help enough if digestion and absorption are poor."

"How about her other tests?"

"They're normal."

Mrs. Acton spoke for the first time. "Even those allergy tests?"

"Yes."

"I thought so. I'm just not allergic."

"Remember our discussion? I know what you might be thinking. But the money wasn't wasted. Sometimes symptoms like yours have been almost entirely caused by food allergy."

"Now what do we do?" Mr. Acton asked.

"I'd like you to do this in two steps. First, I'd like her to take some corrective action to help digestion, and a series of vitamin B$_{12}$ injections. After we see how much this does, I'd like her to add on the specific nutritional supplements needed."

"Why not everything at once?"

"I usually do like to start a comprehensive program all at once. But in Mrs. Acton's case, I want to find out what vitamin B$_{12}$ will do by itself."

"Didn't you do a vitamin B$_{12}$ blood test?" Mrs. Acton asked.

"Yes, and it was normal, but on the low side," I replied.

"So why should I need any? And why can't I swallow it?"

"I've learned that any time a person has digestion and absorption problems, a series of vitamin B$_{12}$ injections should be tried, and frequently will produce good results. This is nothing new. It's mentioned in textbooks. Second, it usually works better when injected than when swallowed, as its absorption is very tricky."

"But my blood test is normal."

"That's another thing any nutritionally oriented doctor learns quickly. A normal blood test does not always reflect normal tissue levels. For example, people with severe osteoporosis almost always have normal blood calcium levels.

"However, you have another indication that your individual metabolism might need more vitamin B$_{12}$ than most. You remember your xanthelasma?"

"Those fat things on my eyelids? I wondered why you were so interested in those."

"Very often, those go away with vitamin B$_{12}$ injections [see

Merck Service Bulletin]. So I guessed that either your absorption was poor, or you just needed more."

"So you did guess all this from my gas, constipation, and those fat deposits."

"Yes, now let's see how it all works."

To improve her digestion and absorption, I asked Mrs. Acton to take 3 betaine hydrochloride tablets, 5 grains each, before meals. I cautioned her to stop them immediately if she had any adverse symptoms. I asked her not to take any form of aspirin, or any anti-inflammatory medicines while taking the acid, because of increased danger of ulcers. Also, I advised her to use 1 or 2 1,300 milligrams pancreatin tablets. The number should be estimated by how many it took to relieve her excess gas, and relieve constipation, along with the acid.

However, most important for her mental symptoms, I asked her to take an injection of vitamin B_{12}, 100 micrograms, twice weekly to start. Since vitamin B_{12} and folic acid are "metabolic partners," I also asked her to use 1 milligram folic acid twice daily.

Her response was striking. Both Actons reported that the effect of each B_{12} injection was obvious within 24 hours after taking it. (They also reported it "wore off" after just 2 to 3 days. She quickly learned when she needed another one.)

Mrs. Acton's mental attitude was entirely different with the B_{12}. She reported she had "energy and ambition." She could control her emotions "for the first time in years." Her depression lifted, and tension dissipated. Her anger fits (which her husband said were worse than she had told me) became a thing of the past. She reported she was interested in life again and that it felt like a second honeymoon.

Of course, vitamin B_{12} injected twice weekly (she learned to give her own shots) was definitely more than usual. I assured her there were no known side effects, and that as her food started to digest and assimilate better, she could start to taper the injections down to a less-frequent maintenance level. But considering how low her overall nutrient levels were, it would take months of good diet, and numerous supplements, which I listed for her, before her nutrient levels would be generally normal. In the meantime, vitamin B_{12} injections were a harmless enough way to control her somatopsychic illness.

———————

Let me be the first to admit that vitamin B_{12} therapy, by injection, is very controversial. The orthodox medical viewpoint holds that vitamin B_{12} therapy should only be employed in cases of proven pernicious anemia with achlorhydria.

The preventive point of view is that pernicious anemia is an "end-stage" of vitamin B_{12} deficiency, which can take years to develop. While it's developing, many bodily malfunctions may occur which vitamin B_{12} can prevent totally.

Most physicians who employ nutritional/biochemical means have learned to try injectable vitamin B_{12} in any case of suspected nutrient malabsorption. Sometimes, nothing much happens; occasionally, the results are spectacular, as in Mrs. Acton's case. Usually, the results are somewhere in between.

Most nutritionally oriented physicians have also learned that, as with many other nutrients, normal blood levels of B_{12} are frequently meaningless as guidelines to therapy.

Of course, if vitamin B_{12} were dangerous, more caution would be in order. But to the present, no toxic overdose has ever been reported.

Frequently, it's asked why B_{12} is so much more successful by injection than by tablets. The answer lies in the "absorptive mechanism" for vitamin B_{12}. It's so involved that there are numerous "breakdown points" possible, many more than for any other nutrient.

I also suspect that, as with many other B vitamins that function as parts of coenzymes, many more people than generally realized have a subclinical cellular enzyme deficiency compensable by extra vitamin B_{12}.

Particularly when mental, emotional, or "nervous system"

disease is involved, vitamin B_{12} is always worth trying. If treatment is continued, it should be accompanied by folic acid, at least 5 milligrams daily, and frequently more.

FURTHER READING

Merck & Co., Inc., *Vitamin B_{12}: Merck Service Bulletin* (Rahway, N.J.: Merck, 1958).

Somogyi, J. C., and Tashev, T., eds. *Early Signs of Nutritional Deficiencies* (New York: S. Karger, 1976).

Depression is usually not the kind of problem that is resolved with a single element solution; in these three cases, it is. The three are put together to emphasize the importance of biochemistry and nutrition in mental illness, which is one of the most promising areas of current research. In a case of premenstrual depression, the answer turns out to be vitamin B_6. . . . A case of depression with insomnia is alleviated with the amino acid tryptophan. . . . A case of depression in a man who had a terrible temper was improved with the help of niacinamide.

Three More Cases of Depression 7

Although it's just beginning to surface in most "everyday" medical care, there's an increasing amount of biochemical research being reported from university medical centers that should radically change the focus of medicine over the next generation. The more such work is done, the more researchers are examining the functions and therapeutic uses of vitamins, minerals, amino acids, fats, carbohydrates, proteins, and hormones in the treatment of disease.

Of course, that is really nothing new at all. Some physicians have made use of all these elements in their practices for years. Pioneers in natural care go back several generations in our country, and further overseas. University researchers have reported useful vitamin and mineral work for many decades. What is new is the increasing professional and public focus on more natural means of health care.

Some of the most exciting research is in the area of mental health. Researchers have developed biochemical tests to predict manic-depressive illness in persons who have not yet had the manic part of their illnesses. Other researchers have found that diet definitely has an effect on the levels of hormones and neurotransmitters in the brain. Even a professor of psychiatry at Harvard Medical School has stated that schizophrenia is a biochemical illness (*Clinical Psychiatry News,* January 1976). The psychiatrist of the future will need to be as knowledgeable in biochemistry and biology as he or she is in psychology.

Instead of one case, in this chapter I'd like to briefly describe three cases with a common psychological symptom: depression. Each had a fairly simple, single element solution for the depression involved, but as I'll point out at the end, a single element cure is usually not the ultimate answer.

Menstrual Depression

Gail Peters scarcely sat down in the consultation room when she burst into tears and sobs. She was an attractive young woman apparently in her mid-twenties, but her red, bloodshot eyes over dark, puffy half-circles certainly detracted from her appearance. They betrayed much recent crying and loss of sleep.

When she regained her composure, she apologized. "I'm sorry," she said, "I promised myself I wouldn't do that, but I couldn't help it. That's part of the problem; I get so depressed over nothing. I'm so cranky and irritable even I can't stand it."

"How long has this been going on?"

"Years. But it's been lots worse the past two years. I'm afraid if it doesn't stop, we're headed for a divorce."

"Why's that?"

"My husband, John, doesn't have much patience with my moodiness anymore. He used to tolerate it better, but now he calls me the Wicked Witch of the West, and leaves the house. Every month I hardly see him for a week or ten days. He goes to work early, stays late, and sometimes comes home at all hours."

"Every month?"

"Yes. It gets worse before my menstrual periods, much worse. I cry at the least thing; when I'm not crying, I'm screaming or yelling. Sometimes I don't realize I'm doing it until halfway through. Then I can't stop."

"And after your period?"

"It's better for a while. John stays home more. But the closer my period gets, the closer it is to 'witch time'—that's what John calls it." She started to cry again.

"Are you taking birth-control pills?"

"Not anymore. I thought that might be causing it, so I stopped. For a few months I was a little better, but it's worse again. That's another thing; since I'm off the Pill, and I don't want an IUD, birth control is a problem. That hasn't helped our marriage any, either."

"Do you eat sugar or white bread?"

"Yes, lots of both. I know I shouldn't, but that's what I'm doing here, to find out if changing my diet will change my depression and moodiness."

"You're right. It definitely will help. So will some vitamins, for now."

I wrote her a note as follows:

1. Vitamin B_6 (pyridoxine): 100 milligrams, 3 times daily
2. B complex tablet (with at least 50 milligrams of pyridoxine): 3 times daily

"Isn't that a lot of B_6?"

"Yes, but it won't hurt. If you want the Wicked Witch of the West to go away, and John to stay home, you'd better use it."

After general advice about a good diet, I asked Mrs. Peters to return after three menstrual periods had gone by. Of course, she was to come in sooner if there was no improvement, but I really didn't expect to see her before then. We'll see the outcome later.

Depression and Insomnia

Mrs. Eleanor Trumbull had been in for one or two visits before she mentioned her most serious health problem. She'd mentioned only minor problems before, discussed diet a little, and left. I had a vague suspicion there was something else on her mind, but had a feeling it would be best not to push.

As she came in this time, she seemed more determined. "I'll come right to the point this time, Doctor," she said. "I've been depressed for years. Sometimes it gets so bad I can't get anything done around the house for days."

"Is there any pattern to it?"

"No, that's the problem. Nothing particular seems to cause it. My children are grown. My husband and I have been married for 35 years and get along well. We've tried to analyze it, but it doesn't help. I've even been to two psychiatrists, but neither one could help me. One gave me an antidepressant drug, but it made me feel nervous and 'high,' so I wouldn't take it after that."

"Do you get nervous or anxious?"

"Not especially. Mostly just 'down'; don't want to go anywhere, do anything. Sometimes it's not so bad; when I was younger, it even went away for months at a time. But the last few years it's been steady."

"Have you noticed any other symptoms that seem to go along with it?"

"Just one. The more depressed I get, the worse my insomnia gets. Sometimes I feel if I could just get a good night's sleep, it would all go away."

"How long have you had insomnia?"

"About as long as I've been depressed. But it varies, too."

Reaching for my note pad, I said, "I think there may be a solution for both your problems. I'd like you to get some trypto-phan, and use 1 gram (1,000 milligrams), 3 times daily. Make sure one dose is right before bedtime."

"Is that a drug?"

"It's an amino acid; one of the building blocks of protein."

"Do I get it at the drugstore?"

"No, at the health food store."

"Are there side effects?"

"If you take more than you need, you might feel drunk or fuzzy in the head. But this wears off; then don't take as much."

"How do you know I need it?"

"Because of your depression and insomnia. When those two symptoms coexist, tryptophan is usually the remedy."

"I'll try it, as long as it isn't another drug. When should I come back if it doesn't work?"

"Two or three weeks, either way. But I'm pretty sure it will work. What I want you to come back for is to talk about reducing the dosage."

'A Depressed Volcano'

During my entire first interview with William Nesbitt, he never smiled or laughed. His overall mood could best be described as grim. He was a muscular, somewhat overweight truck driver; for our entire talk he sat straight upright, arms crossed.

"I feel so down and out sometimes I feel like just driving my car right off the road," he said. "Life's no fun anymore—hasn't been for years. Nothing I do helps. My wife wants me to see a psychiatrist, but I don't need a headshrinker."

"Why did you decide to come here?"

"I finally figured there must be something physical the matter. Also, my temper."

"What makes you think it's physical?"

"Last few months, driving, I've started to have practically blackout spells. Had to pull off the road several times or I would have keeled right over."

"Anything else happen?"

"Yea, after a couple of those spells, I got real nervous and shaky. Heart was pounding. But there wasn't any pain, so I didn't figure it was a heart attack."

"Are you still having spells?"

"My wife reads a lot on health. I couldn't get an appointment right away, so she figured out I was having spells when I hadn't eaten for several hours. She told me to eat something when I felt a spell coming on. I used to drive all day without eating. Now, if I eat something, it helps. She says it's hypoglycemia."

"What about your temper?"

"Well, I always had a quick temper. But it's really bad now.

I notice my wife and kids always stay away from me when I'm home. I figured it was because I was so depressed, and I guess that's part of it. But my wife says that the least little thing she or the kids say makes me fly off the handle." Mr. Simpson looked especially grim. "She says I'm like a volcano—a depressed volcano, always down but always ready to erupt."

He shook his head. "Do you figure there's any connection between being depressed and those spells? I'll go see a psychiatrist if you say so, but . . . (he looked almost hopeful) . . . couldn't it be physical? Maybe hypoglycemia?"

"I'm almost positive you're right. I've heard this type of problem often; it is usually hypoglycemia. You'll need a glucose tolerance test. In the meantime, to help both your depression and your temper, get niacinamide at the health food store. Start with 500 milligrams of the time-release kind twice a day, and work up to 2,000 milligrams twice a day, slowly. If you have any nausea, cut back. And don't take any for two days before your test. Take an equal amount of vitamin C."

"My wife told me I might need that test. But she said it takes six hours. I won't be able to come back for that for nearly a month because of my work. Isn't there anything else I can do?"

"From the sound of things, you should read a book on hypoglycemia, and start changing your diet. But don't worry about being depressed and your temper. I'm sure the niacinamide will help with that. If it doesn't, let me know."

————————⬩————————

Obviously, each of the three problems described above could not be called simple depression. Mrs. Peters had the all-too-common premenstrual syndrome caused by an imbalance between estrogenic hormones and B vitamins, particularly B_6. Mrs. Trumbull had what could be best described as a "relative" tryptophan deficiency. Mr. Nesbitt had an apparent case of hypoglycemia: low blood sugar.

But in each case, depression was the symptom most bothersome to the person involved, so attacking that problem came first.

Even though the treatment was only symptom relief, at least it was nontoxic symptom treatment. Equally important, it worked in these cases, as it does in almost all cases like them.

Each patient noted a marked lessening of depression at his or her return. Mrs. Peters's "witch" was indeed gone; Mrs. Trumbull was no longer "down," and was sleeping "like a log." Mr. Nesbitt smiled when he told me he wasn't thinking of driving off the road anymore, and that his sense of humor was back.

At subsequent consultations with all of these patients, I tried to help them put their psychological problems into a perspective of overall health improvement and maintenance. Mrs. Peters has been able to reduce her dosage of vitamin B_6 to "none some months and a few pills others" by getting rid of all sugar and white flour, and adopting a natural food diet.

I might add that I've worked with at least 600 women with various premenstrual symptoms over the last eight years; in every case, the premenstrual problem was eliminated or nearly so with sufficient amounts of pyridoxine.

Like most B vitamins, pyridoxine is nontoxic even in high doses. Some women have exceeded Mrs. Peters's dose; but 99 percent don't need to. The only reaction I've ever known was in a child who took 3,000 milligrams one day, and got a rash. This rash promptly disappeared after the pyridoxine was stopped.

One of the few general rules in nutritional/biochemical medicine is, "If it's premenstrual, try B_6!"

Mrs. Trumbull, by concentrating on eating foods high in tryptophan (which her body apparently requires to a greater degree than most), has been able to slowly reduce her supplemental dosage to between ½ and 1 tablet daily.

Tryptophan is not as "foolproof" a therapy for depression as pyridoxine is for premenstrual symptoms. I've certainly seen cases where it didn't work at all. In depression and insomnia together, however, it is usually quite effective. I always keep tryptophan in mind for use in depression.

Even if it isn't 100 percent effective for depression, studies have shown it works almost as well as commonly prescribed antidepressant drugs. And of course, any synthetic drug is likely to have many more side effects than a substance naturally present in the body. Given these studies, and my own observation, I no longer use antidepressant drugs. The side effects from tryptophan are much less, mostly involving drowsiness. I've found tryptophan, other vitamins and minerals, proper diet, and psychotherapy when necessary are much more effective than drugs for depression.

Mr. Nesbitt, working hard at getting rid of his hypoglycemia, was able to drastically reduce his niacinamide supplements. After working with a psychologist on changing some of his emotional response habit patterns, he was able to stop it entirely, without returning to his former depressed "volcanic" state.

Vitamin B_3, by which I mean both niacin and its close cousin, niacinamide, seems particularly helpful for mental symptoms associated with hypoglycemia. Not only depression, as in Mr. Nesbitt's case, but also anxiety and nervousness are much improved by B_3. Fits of anger, fairly common in teenagers and men with hypoglycemia are also better controlled.

Niacin and niacinamide are both forms of vitamin B_3, but do have some differences. The most obvious difference is that niacin in sufficient quantities will dilate smaller blood vessels. Many unaware vitamin takers have accidentally discovered this when they've suddenly become very hot, and noted that their skins were bright red and intensely itchy after taking a dose of niacin. Fortunately, this effect isn't harmful, and usually passes in 30 to 60 minutes. Niacinamide won't do that.

Niacin also will lower serum cholesterol; niacinamide's effect on cholesterol varies from none to small. Niacin will raise the blood sugar, sometimes a helpful effect in hypoglycemia. Niacinamide seems to do this to a smaller degree.

I usually recommend niacinamide in doses of 500 milligrams, from 1 to 4 times daily in these conditions, of course, as long as there's no nausea.

Since niacinamide doesn't produce uncomfortable flushing, it's frequently used when higher doses of vitamin B_3 are required. However, many patients have told me they prefer niacin because the flush reaction "isn't that bad," usually passes after a few weeks, and it "feels better" than niacinamide. This seems particularly so in alcoholism. I have no explanation for that.

Vitamin B_3 is one of only 2 B vitamins (the other is B_1, thiamine) with potentially harmful side effects in very high doses (megadoses). Excess vitamin B_3 usually affects the liver first. The earliest, and ordinarily key symptom of excess B_3 is a persistent nausea. Vomiting doesn't usually follow; the nausea could best be described as "low-grade." However, liver function tests taken at this time frequently show elevated levels of several liver enzymes.

If niacin or niacinamide is reduced in dosage or discontinued, this effect as well as the nausea disappears. There appears to be no permanent liver damage.

The only bad cases of B_3 side effects I've seen have been when the warning symptom of nausea was ignored.

For each of these people, fairly high doses of natural antidepressives were very helpful at the beginning of their progress toward better emotional and physical health.

Each was also fortunate in being able to discontinue or nearly discontinue the supplement involved; some persons with similar problems don't seem to be able to do so.

A valid question might be asked: Why not leave off the unnaturally high doses of even natural substances, and let the ultimate correction come more slowly through proper dietary changes? I personally have no objection to this approach for those who'd rather take it, and try to help my patients in that manner when they prefer.

Most, however, would agree with Mrs. Peters, who didn't want to be depressed one day longer than she had to. As long as the quicker, higher supplement route appears safe, I'll go along with those who prefer it.

Lastly, there are those who, because of inherited or biochemical damage, need higher levels of certain nutrients than can ever be gotten entirely from foodstuffs. Especially in the area of mental health, this at present appears to be a sizable number of persons. For someone unfortunate enough to be in this group, whether called "schizophrenic," or whatever, extra doses of the necessary nutrients will probably be a lifelong need.

None of our three depressed patients was in the schizophrenic group. All had what could be and has been called neurotic depression. But as we can see from their response to vitamin and dietary treatment, some neurotic depression has a biochemical basis.

As emphasized in the cases above, and throughout this book, single element therapy is absolutely no substitute for overall dietary improvement, getting rid of toxic junk foods, and building in maximum possible good nutrition.

In fact, some critics of nutritional therapy claim that high-dose vitamin treatment is pharmacological rather than nutritional, and therefore no different than drug treatment. Since drug treatment, according to these critics, is "proven," and vitamins and minerals aren't, drug therapy is preferable.

Considering drug side effects, I disagree.

As illustrated in these cases, when overall nutritional correction takes place, high-dose vitamins can often be cut back or eliminated.

Mrs. Peters, Mrs. Trumbull, and Mr. Nesbitt all illustrate further the "somatopsychic" principle: in each case, a nutritional/biochemical derangement affecting the entire system, producing particularly mental symptoms, was corrected by very physical means: nutrient therapy.

FURTHER READING

Anonymous. "Schizophrenia Is 'Without Doubt' Biologic Disorder." *Clinical Psychiatry News*, vol. 4, no. 1, January 1976, pp. 1, 31.

Jensen, K. et al. "Tryptophan/Imipramine in Depression." *The Lancet*, November 8, 1975, p. 920.

Kline, N. S., and Shah, B. K. "Comparable Therapeutic Efficacy of Tryptophan and Imipramine: Average Therapeutic Ratings Versus 'True' Equivalence. An Important Difference."

Current Therapeutic Research, vol. 15, no. 7, July 1973, pp. 484–87.

    Pauling, Linus, and Hawkins, David, eds. *Orthomolecular Psychiatry* (San Francisco: W. H. Freeman, 1973).

    Rao, Bapuji, and Broadhurst, A. D. "Tryptophan and Depression." *British Medical Journal,* February 21, 1976, p. 460.

An 8-year-old boy has many bouts of flu, earache, colds, bronchitis, and other infections, causing him to lose many days from school. Examination reveals that the boy's immunity seems to be low, along with low vitamin levels. A new diet approach has no noticeable effect for several weeks, as the body's cells need considerable time to build new resistance. After some months, his infections cease and his swollen tonsils shrink. . . . With a note on allergy and recurring infection.

8   A Case of Recurrent Infection

I first met Bobby MacDonald two days before Christmas of 1974. He was the last patient on a not-very-busy afternoon. As he came in with his mother, part of the reason for our "slow day" was again apparent: like many others, they were carrying sacks of recent purchases, boxes, wrappings, and ribbons in various stages of organization.

"Excuse me," Mrs. MacDonald said, as she looked around for a place to set her things. "We've just been shopping, and I thought we'd do a little wrapping while waiting. Can I put my things here?"

Scarcely pausing for an answer, she put her packages on the filing cabinet, motioned her son to sit down, and sat down herself.

As soon as all seemed settled, I asked what I could do for them.

"It's Bobby. He has just a little earache, on the right side this time, I think. But he's had so many of them, we've learned to come in early. Isn't that right, Bobby?"

Bobby appeared resigned to it all. However, he nodded his head in agreement.

I asked Bobby when his ear had begun to hurt.

"I don't know," he replied. Looking at his mother, he ventured tentatively: "Yesterday?"

"He got a cold a week ago," Mrs. MacDonald said. "I started giving him his decongestant right away, but I guess it didn't help."

"Did you give him any vitamin C?"

"No. The pediatrician I've taken Bobby to said it wouldn't do any good. But that's why we're here. Bobby just gets one infection after another. This year, so far, he's missed 17 days of school. Last year he missed 33 days and almost got held back. The year before, he missed 27 days. There's got to be some better way of keeping him healthy!"

"What type of problems has he had?"

"Nothing really unusual. That's the problem. He's had lots of colds, the flu, earaches, tonsillitis, bronchitis, and even pneumonia once, but he didn't have to go to the hospital. You name it, he's had it! But he's been checked for anemia, white blood cells, and. . ." She paused to think. "I believe it was an immunity test. All that was normal."

"Was that called electrophoresis?"

"That's it! Expensive, too," Mrs. MacDonald replied.

"Well, let's go check your ear, Bobby," I said. We all got up and went into the examination room.

As Bobby climbed onto the examination table, I asked what grade he was in.

"Third," he said.

"How old are you?"

"Eight."

"Do you have any brothers or sisters?"

"Yes."

"He has three," Mrs. MacDonald said. "Two brothers, one sister."

"Do they get sick as often?"

"Not as much as Bobby. But they do get their share. Five or

six colds a year and we all get the flu every winter."

As Mrs. MacDonald suspected, Bobby was starting to get another ear infection. Other than this, he appeared to have a typical viral cold, with very slightly red throat, runny nose, and swollen glands.

"I'm glad we decided to come in," Mrs. MacDonald declared. "Now what? Do you use vitamin C, or antibiotics, or what?"

I explained that at this stage, an antibiotic would be necessary. But if vitamin C had been started early enough, the ear infection might have been prevented.

"What antibiotic?" Mrs. MacDonald asked. "Ampicillin?"

"Yes," I replied. "He's had it before?"

"Of course. It usually works. We're just adding up for our taxes, and my husband says this year Bobby's had 9 bottles of ampicillin, 2 bottles of erythromycin, and 13 bottles of decongestant!"

"I'd like you to use the decongestant, too, this time," I said. "Also, lots of vitamin C."

"How much is lots?"

"As much as he can take without getting gas or diarrhea. If that happens, then he's gone past the 'intestinal tolerance' level, and his body can't use quite all of it, so cut the dose down a little. He could possibly take as much as 6 to 10 grams a day, or more."

Mrs. MacDonald paused for a minute. "That's 6,000 to 10,000 milligrams. Is it safe?"

I advised that over a short period of time, a week or two, it was entirely safe, and would be of definite value.

"What about preventing all this in the first place?"

"I'd like you to bring Bobby back after a week to see if his ear is better. We can discuss that then," I answered.

"That's fine," said Mrs. MacDonald. "I guess we've got to get rid of this problem first, anyway."

I also made sure to ask Mrs. MacDonald to give Bobby *Lactobacillus acidophilus* while he was taking his antibiotic, and for two days after, to keep the intestinal bacteria as normal as possible during antibiotic treatment.

When they returned a week later, we went right to the examination room to check Bobby again.

His ear was much better; in fact, practically normal. His nose was still a little runny. The glands in his neck were still swollen, though. I mentioned this to Mrs. MacDonald.

"That's not unusual, is it?" she asked. "Bobby has swollen glands most of the time, even when he's well. I asked our doctor before; he got a white blood cell count, and said not to worry about it. Our oldest son has that a lot, too."

I explained that while not unusual, chronically swollen lymph glands weren't normal, either. In children with recurrent infections, they're often present.

Bobby's tonsils were also large; they practically touched in the middle of his throat. They weren't red or inflamed though; it wasn't an acute infection.

"His tonsils have been that way for years," Mrs. MacDonald informed me. "I was told they should be taken out, but I'd rather not have that done. Is there anything else to do?"

"Yes, I'll get to that in a little bit. First, let's talk about a basic diet strategy to prevent so many infections."

"No vitamins?"

"Of course, vitamins. But they won't help nearly as much if the food he eats every day isn't the right sort."

So I wrote out for Mrs. MacDonald, as I usually do, a note containing recommendations. This is what the note said:

1. Absolutely no sugar. Honey is OK, but no refined sugar on or in anything.
2. No white flour. All bread and cereal products must be whole-grain.
3. Avoid all refined foods. Bobby should have whole, natural foods, as fresh as possible.

"Why no sugar?" Mrs. MacDonald asked.

"There are so many reasons for not eating sugar, it would take hours to list them. Why it's important for recurrent infections is that experiments have shown that refined sugar, sucrose, depresses the immune system. That, of course, impairs the ability to fight infections [see Cheraskin]."

Going on to recommendations 2 and 3, I reminded Mrs. MacDonald that refined flour, even when enriched, has much less of many of its original vitamins and minerals. As many of these vitamins, particularly the B group, are crucial to fighting infections, Bobby was probably somewhat deficient in them. The same reasons applied for refined, synthetic, or other processed foods. Much of their original nourishment is gone. These foods are optimum for no one, but they should particularly be avoided by someone like Bobby, who's not in the best health.

"I want to check you for a few other things, too, Bobby. Could you take off your shirt and shoes and socks?"

It didn't take long to check, but the examination showed definite clinical signs of deficiencies in vitamins A and D, and zinc, plus inadequate function of the thymus gland.

Mrs. MacDonald had heard of zinc, and vitamins A and D, but said she'd never heard of a thymus gland.

"The thymus gland is located underneath the sternum, or breastbone. It's very important to the control of many factors of immunity to infections," I explained.

"Isn't that a very rare problem?" Mrs. MacDonald asked.

"No," I replied. "I find the same signs of thymus gland malfunction in the majority of children with repeated infections. I've asked many mothers to give their children dietary treatment for it, and it usually works well."

"How can I tell?" she asked.

"Usually, enlarged tonsils return to normal, and swollen glands reduce to normal size."

"Is it safe?"

"Have you ever eaten sweetbreads?" I asked.

Mrs. MacDonald made a face. "Yes," she said. "My mother used to serve those."

"Well," I said, "sometimes the foods called by that name varied, but most frequently they included pancreas, thymus, and other internal organs of an animal."

"You mean I have to feed that to Bobby?"

"Yes and no." I could see Bobby making a face this time. "There are food tablets of compressed thymus glands."

As time was growing short, I made another list for Mrs. Mac-Donald. It read as follows:
1. Vitamin C: 500 milligrams with each meal (more if he gets sick)
2. B complex: 10 to 20 milligrams of each B vitamin in each; one with each meal
3. Combination, natural source, vitamins A and D: 10,000 IU of A and 400 IU of D, 3 a day
4. Zinc: 25 milligrams, chelated, one a day
5. Thymus tablets: 1, 3 times a day.

Mrs. MacDonald took the second list. "How long will he need all this?"

"We'll have to wait to see how he does."

"When should we come back?"

"Two months. But remember, there's very little point in giving him all the vitamins unless you change the way he eats, too."

"I know," Mrs. MacDonald said. "I've been thinking of changing the whole family, and now I will."

Three weeks later, Bobby and his mother were back. Mrs. MacDonald looked discouraged.

"He's got another cold," she said, "and he's been taking all his vitamins. It was such a struggle to change the whole family. Now what?"

"I didn't eat any sugar, either!" Bobby said.

I checked Bobby, and cound find no sign of complications of his viral cold. I told Mrs. MacDonald so, and she relaxed a little.

"He doesn't need an antibiotic, then?"

"No, just his vitamin C."

"Can I give him the decongestant?"

"If it makes him more comfortable."

"Aspirin?"

"Only if his fever is very high. Don't be discouraged that he's gotten this cold. It's only been three weeks since Bobby started his nutritional program. It takes longer than that to rebuild and repair body cells. At least, he hasn't any complications this time."

February 14, Valentine's Day. Bobby's mother was pleased. "He hasn't had a cold since the last time we were here."

"Good," I said. "Has he had any problems with his diet or vitamins?"

"What kind of problems?"

"Upset stomach, rash, diarrhea; any sort of reaction."

"Not that I've noticed. She looked at Bobby. "He hasn't told me of any."

I asked Bobby. "Have you noticed any problems with your vitamins, Bobby?"

"No," he said.

"I've noticed one thing," Mrs. MacDonald observed. "Bobby hasn't been as tired as he was before. He's started doing more things. And his mood seems better and more stable."

"Good."

"Do I continue giving him the other vitamins?"

"Yes. I'd like you to come back in—let's see—April, unless Bobby has any other problems before then."

Our visit was brief in April. I asked how Bobby had been doing.

"He hasn't missed any school since January," Mrs. MacDonald replied. "He hasn't had one cold, and neither has anyone else in the family. I figured those vitamins wouldn't hurt anybody, so we all take them."

She paused. "Are there any changes I should make in Bobby's supplements?"

"Since he's had as little as possible of B vitamin-depleted foods since January, please eliminate one B vitamin tablet. And with summer coming soon, you can probably eliminate one vitamin A and D capsule."

I checked Bobby briefly.

"Yes, that should be OK now. But please continue the thymus in his diet. He still has signs of need for it."

"Fine," Mrs. MacDonald said. "When should I bring him back?"

"September, before school."

When I checked Bobby again in September, he no longer had clinical signs of problems with vitamins A or D, or zinc, or his thymus.

"How do his tonsils look now?" Mrs. MacDonald inquired.

"Perfectly normal for his age."

"Not big anymore?"

"No."

His tonsils, which in January nearly touched each other, now were reduced in size to normal. He had no detectably swollen lymph glands.

"What about the B complex vitamins and vitamin C?" she asked.

"I'd like him to continue the vitamin C. If you add brewer's yeast in some of the things he eats, you can discontinue the B vitamins. You can also discontinue the thymus."

A year later Bobby was back for a preschool checkup. It was a pleasant surprise to see Bobby and his mother again.

Bobby had grown, of course. He was going to be in fifth grade, and was transferring to a different school.

"Bobby's doing fine," Mrs. MacDonald reported. "He had a few sniffles once or twice, but I increased his vitamins C and A and they went away. He didn't miss a day of school all year."

"Yeah, just me and Jeff didn't miss any," Bobby said.

"We're really pleased. You know Bobby's father is an engineer at Boeing, and he didn't believe in nutrition when I first brought Bobby in. But now that he's seen how Bobby's doing, he's started reading my nutrition magazines and books. He's been down to the health food store himself, and says he's been feeling better, too. We all do."

Not every child with frequent, recurrent infections does as well as Bobby did, with a prompt reduction of his infection rate to practically zero. But many do, and for those whose infections don't clear as well and as promptly, other tests and treatments are necessary, and are usually successful in achieving an appreciable reduction in the occurrence of infections.

———— ◆ ————

Bobby MacDonald was a "textbook example" of what happens to so many children on a basic junk food diet: not seriously ill, but chronically developing minor infections, and never fully healthy. Although he could have passed a physical examination as "perfectly normal" between each infectious episode, a deeper look at his body chemistry would have shown subclinical malnutrition, with cellular level inadequacies in various vitamins and minerals.

It might be argued that a refined, sugared diet can be proven to meet minimum daily requirements (now called Recommended Dietary Allowances). As you might suspect, it's my observation that minimum daily requirements produce minimum daily health. Is that good enough for you, or your children?

Bobby had an excellent outcome, based simply on changing from basic junk food to a basic natural diet, and adding in the most important (for his problems) of the missing vitamins and minerals. As noted above, many children do well with this approach, but not all.

For most of the remainder of children with recurrent infections, who only improve to a degree with Bobby MacDonald's program, the answer lies in one word: allergy.

Whenever recurrent infection persists, I'll usually recommend screening for allergy. I've found the radioallergosorbent (RAST) test to be the most useful, quite accurate, and in children particularly, the most humane method of testing for food allergy. Since this testing technique is still relatively expensive, the entire diet isn't tested at first. Instead, the child's blood is tested for several foods which traditionally have been found to be highly allergenic. Each individual practitioner will have a different basic list; mine includes wheat, milk, eggs, corn, citrus, tomato, legumes, and beef.

If this test turns up entirely negative, with no sign of allergy to these foods, it's usually not worthwhile to pursue allergy testing further.

However, in most children with recurrent infections who don't respond well to basic natural foods with vitamins and minerals, the test is usually positive for one or more of these foods. Despite the expense, further testing of frequently eaten foods not on the above list is very worthwhile.

At least in our local medical community, the RAST test is at present controversial. Many physicians won't use it, or deny that it works; some insurance carriers balk at paying for it. But hundreds of persons I have worked with have shown considerable improvements with its use.

A few other notes about Bobby's program: Chelated zinc, like any chelated mineral, is simply complexed with amino acids, much as it occurs in nature. Since high doses of minerals are usually not directly obtainable from natural sources, chelation mimics nature as closely as possible. The usual natural sources of vitamins A and D are fish-liver oils. Except in cases of allergy, these are usually best.

FURTHER READING

Axelrod, A. E. "Nutrition in Relation to Acquired Immunity." *Modern Nutrition in Health and Disease,* by Robert S. Goodhart and Maurice E. Shils (Philadelphia: Lea & Febiger, 1973), pp. 493–505.

Cheraskin, Emanuel. "Sucrose, Neutrophilic Phagocytosis and Resistance to Disease." *Dental Survey,* vol. 52, no. 12, December 1976, pp. 46–48.

Golden, Michael H. N.; Jackson, Alan A.; and Golden, Barbara E. "Effect of Zinc on Thymus of Recently Malnourished Children." *The Lancet,* November 19, 1977, pp. 1057–59.

Nalder B. N. et al. "Sensitivity of the Immunological Response to the Nutritional Status of Rats." *Journal of Nutrition,* vol. 102, 1972, pp. 535–42.

Pauling, Linus. *Vitamin C and the Common Cold* (San Francisco: W. H. Freeman, 1970).

Pekarek, Robert S.; Hoagland, Anna M.; and Powanda, Michael C. "Humoral and Cellular Immune Responses in Zinc Deficient Rats." *Nutrition Reports International,* vol. 16, no. 3, September 1977, pp. 267–76.

Most people don't imagine that teenagers suffer from digestive problems, but increasingly, we are seeing in them the same problems usually associated with adults. In this case, although Jennifer was eating well and taking vitamins, her diet was lacking in one critical component—fiber, or roughage. She had to endure much pain before the cause was found, but in a way, she was lucky. Many adults with her condition will eventually require surgery.

9

A Case of Cramps from a Low-Residue Diet

Jennifer Walters was 14 years old. Her mother had brought her in for a checkup. As she explained, Jennifer had a very persistent symptom that "just wouldn't go away." She'd been checked several times at clinics in California, where they'd lived until recently, and "everything turned out OK." But her symptoms continued, so her mother decided to try once again "to see if maybe a nutritional approach might help."

Jennifer was fairly cheerful and answered questions readily. I asked her to describe her symptoms.

"It's these cramps," she said. "I get them all the time. Sometimes they don't hurt too bad, but sometimes it hurts so much I have to go to bed. Twice I had to go to the hospital."

"Where do you hurt? Is it menstrual cramps?"

"No, my period just started last year, and I've had these since I was . . ." she looked at her mother, ". . . about 9 or 10 years old, I think."

"That's right," Mrs. Walters said. "In fact, Jennifer had mild cramps when she was 7 or 8, too. But she didn't have them very often, and there was only a little pain, so we didn't pay much attention."

"Can you show me where the pains are when you have them?"

"Well, they aren't in just one place. They happen in different places at different times."

"Is there any one area that's worse than others?"

"Not really."

"Please trace with your finger the general area on your abdomen where it hurts."

Jennifer outlined most of her lower abdomen, and most of the upper area as well, with the exception of the uppermost region between her ribs, over her stomach.

"That covers nearly everywhere, doesn't it?"

"The doctors said it was intestinal spasms," Mrs. Walters observed. "They tried different antispasm medicines, but some of them made her sleepy. Finally we settled on these." She rummaged through her purse, and pulled out a bottle to show me. "They usually work if Jennifer takes them in time, and they don't make her drowsy."

"Do they stop the pain, Jennifer?"

"Mostly. But sometimes they just cut it down some."

"I know you've had your abdomen checked lots of times, but you haven't been here before, so I'd like to check you now."

Jennifer and her mother went into the examination room. I checked her entire abdomen; it appeared to be completely normal. So as not to overlook anything, I checked her chest and spine also; these too appeared normal.

"That's what all the doctors say," Mrs. Walters said. "It's so frustrating."

"Don't give up yet. Frequently a normal physical examination gives just as important information as an abnormal one. If nothing else, it tells us a few things that aren't wrong."

I turned to Jennifer. "I know you've been asked a lot of questions before, but we have to go through them again to try to figure this out."

"That's OK," she replied.

"Do you get nauseated?"

"No."

"Ever any steady pain?"

"No."

"Any bleeding with bowel movements, or black ones?"

"No."

"Diarrhea or constipation?"

"No diarrhea. But I usually only go every two or three days. . . . Mom says that's constipation, but one doctor said that's OK."

"I know. A professor at my medical school told us that, too. But it really isn't healthy function. Let's continue . . . do you get fevers when you hurt?"

"No."

"Urine ever turn brown?"

"No. Why would it do that?"

"There's a rare disease that causes intestinal cramps that also causes the urine to turn reddish brown."

"Is that called porphyria?" Mrs. Walters asked. "Jennifer was checked for that; it's a urine test, isn't it?"

"Yes. While we're on that subject, what other tests has Jennifer had? X-rays?" I asked.

"Oh, yes. She had an upper GI [gastrointestinal test] twice— once when she was 10, and again last year. She had a barium enema last year. All those were negative. She's had several blood tests. I even insisted on a glucose tolerance test because her grandmother has diabetes, and I thought maybe Jennifer had low blood sugar. But it was perfectly normal, too."

"Are there any allergies in your family?"

"Not that I know about. We've thought about that, but these cramps happen when she's eaten all sorts of different foods."

"Usually, I'd expect some diarrhea, too, if it was caused by food allergy," I said. "Are there any illnesses in the family?"

"On her father's side, nothing major. But her grandparents, my parents, have had lots of problems. Her grandfather's had two heart attacks, and is getting emphysema. Her grandmother has diabetes, high blood pressure, and has had a terrible time with diverticulitis. She's had surgery twice already. I hope Jennifer isn't going in that direction. . . ." She looked worried. "But her x-rays were normal."

"I'm sure you know that's very unusual until later in life. But perhaps that's a valid concern for the future. Now that we've talked about all these other things, we need to go over Jennifer's food intake."

"She doesn't eat any junk," her mother said. "She's very good about that, even though a lot of her junior high classmates aren't. We've raised her on good foods."

"Good. But I need the exact details, anyway. Jennifer, what do you usually eat for breakfast?"

"Eggs and milk or juice. Sometimes grapefruit."

"Anything else?"

"No. Oh, Mom makes me take my vitamins."

"Which ones?"

"B, C, and E, I think."

"Lunch?"

"Whatever they have at school. Usually it's hamburgers or hot dogs, or spaghetti or macaroni. That kind of junk. I never get anything from the machines except apples. Never any sugar stuff."

"All white bread and white flour?"

"Yes, but I know that's not good for you, so lots of times I don't eat the hamburger buns and rolls."

"I've been thinking of having her take her lunch, but both her father and I work."

"She's old enough to make her own, isn't she? If this is what I suspect it is, that would definitely be a good idea."

"I suppose she is old enough. But what is her problem? You haven't done any tests yet, or anything."

"She's had all the tests I can think of already. Besides, I just have a suspicion so far . . . it hasn't been proven. Let's finish with her diet history first, though. Jennifer, do you eat at home after school?"

"Sure. Usually a banana or an orange. Sometimes some crackers with peanut butter."

"How about dinner?"

"Lots of different things. Usually meat—chicken, roast, fish. I always have milk."

"Vegetables?"

"Oh, yes. Corn or peas or beans. Sometimes potatoes."

"Salads?"

"Yes, sometimes."

"What kind?"

"Lettuce and tomatoes."

"Do you eat any bread?"

"Not very often."

"How about granola?"

"No."

"I don't get granola because they all seem to have sugar in them," Mrs. Walters observed.

"How about carrots, celery, turnips, spinach, cabbage, beet greens. . . ."

Jennifer made a face. Her mother said, "Every once in a while Jennifer will have a carrot. But she's never liked most vegetables since she was a little girl. I actually have a hard time getting her to eat a raw vegetable salad. I've told her that not eating vegetables would give her constipation. But do you think it would give her these terrific cramps, too? Don't you think it might be something more serious? I thought maybe she had a serious vitamin or mineral deficiency."

"It's certainly possible to develop vitamin and mineral deficiencies eating the way Jennifer does. A vitamin K deficiency is one of the first that comes to mind. It's found mostly in deep green, leafy vegetables. Some children who eat this way will even get nosebleeds because of not enough vitamin K.

"But in Jennifer's case, it's probably just the lack of bulk and fiber in her diet, over several years, that's led to increasingly severe spasms. Her intestines are unusually reactive; but her problem isn't unusual at all, just more severe. In the past few years, I've checked many children and teenagers with recurrent intestinal spasms. Very frequently, a lack of dietary bulk and fiber is the source of the problem."

"You don't think you need any further tests?"

"Not really. I'd like Jennifer to decide which of the raw, bulky, fibrous vegetables she can stand, and eat at least two or three a day. Also, give her 2 tablespoons of unprocessed bran a day. Last, you can find granolas made with honey, and no sugar, at the health food store. Try that for breakfast for a while."

"If it's as simple as that, why weren't we told before?"

"Remember, I said this was only a theory until it's proven. I think it's a pretty good theory. But we won't know for sure until Jennifer tries it. If it doesn't work, we'll know shortly."

Mrs. Walters and Jennifer gathered their things and left. As they went down the hall, I could overhear Jennifer saying, "Yuk, spinach. . . ."

I had asked Mrs. Walters to bring Jennifer back in a month. When they returned I asked Jennifer about her spasms.

"I haven't had any since I started all that raw vegetable stuff," she answered. "I can't stand it. The granola with honey is OK though."

"This is the first entire month she's had without spasms in several years," Mrs. Walters said.

"I can't understand how raw vegetables stop cramps," Jennifer observed.

"It's because your intestines need a certain amount of bulk and fiber to work properly. When they weren't getting it, they had to work harder—contract more—to push everything through. The pressure inside them was higher. In some people, that adds up to cramps and spasms.

"I want to mention just one other thing to you. You know about your grandmother's intestinal problem with diverticulitis, and the surgery she's had to have?"

"Sort of."

"Apparently, you've inherited the same 'insides' she has. If you continue to eat lots of raw vegetables, granola, and other bulky fibrous foods, you can probably avoid that kind of problem completely. If not, you have a good chance of getting the same thing when you're older."

"Oh." Jennifer thought for a minute. "OK. But do I have to keep taking that bran stuff?"

"Probably not, if the rest of your diet has enough bulk and fiber. Try stopping it; only restart if the spasms start to return a little. I wanted you to use it just to make sure."

"I have just one question," Mrs. Walters said. "Why didn't any of those other doctors tell us this? I get so mad when I think of all the pain Jennifer's had!"

"Please try to understand something, and not be too mad. If you needed major surgery, you wouldn't consult a dermatologist, would you? Or me, for that matter. If your problem is nutritional or biochemical, you're most likely to get help from doctors who specialize in nutritional biochemistry."

Despite the severity of her cramps, and the pain she'd been through, Jennifer was fortunate that her inadequate diet gave her symptoms at an early age, when it could be corrected with no permanent damage to her.

Millions of Americans aren't so lucky. The type of diet followed by Jennifer, technically called "low residue," appears to be capable of leading to worse problems than simply cramps. There's a good deal of evidence to show that a low-residue, or low-roughage diet, devoid of natural fiber and highly refined (and for good measure laced with sugar and chemicals), can ultimately lead in many persons to much more serious diseases, including diverticulitis, colon cancer, and heart attacks in certain people.

So changing Jennifer's diet at age 14 may well have prevented these and other problems later in life. Many teenagers aren't so lucky.

Hardly anyone in the last four to five years has been able to avoid the barrage of publicity surrounding the topic of dietary fiber. Articles have been published in many popular magazines; even major medical journals have published articles on the subject (although usually with words of caution about accepting the idea too readily). So I won't go into a long, detailed explanation here, but will try to summarize it briefly, particularly as related to Jennifer's problem.

Over tens of thousands of human generations, our intestines have become adapted to relatively large quantities of bulk and roughage. With proper amounts of bulk, it is relatively easy for the intestinal muscles to propel the contents through. If sufficient bulk is not supplied, the intestinal muscles have to work much harder squeezing and contracting. In Jennifer's case, this excess squeezing and contracting led to severe pain. Jennifer's case was more severe than most, but not really all that unusual. Children are frequently brought in for relatively vague abdominal pains that are caused by nothing more than inadequate roughage.

Years of such abnormal squeezing and contracting can lead to herniations of the muscle wall of the colon. That is all that diverticulosis is. These little hernias on the colon wall are very susceptible to infection with abnormal colon bacteria. Infection of diverticula, called diverticulitis, is often very painful and occasionally requires surgical treatment.

Just as bad, if not worse, it takes two to three times as long for a low-roughage diet to be moved through the colon. During this unnaturally long time, certain colon bacteria (also present in unnaturally large numbers because of the low-roughage diet) have the opportunity to break down normal bile acids (produced by the liver as part of the digestive process) into cancer-causing substances. On top of this, some of the chemical additives to our diets can be carcinogenic (cancer-causing). Between the internally produced and externally added carcinogens, and their extra time in the colon, societies on refined low-roughage diets have the highest rate of colon cancer in the world.

Incidentally, there is an old, but excellent medical test, revived by nutritional/biochemical practitioners, that detects the presence of substances in the urine caused by abnormal bacteria in the colon, the types associated with the formation of carcinogens. While this is not a test for cancer, if positive, it may indicate a higher degree of potential for cancer. Taking steps to correct a positive test, such as adding fiber and *Lactobacillus acidophilus* bacteria to the diet, should theoretically reduce the production of carcinogens, and thus the potential for cancer.

This test, called Obermayer's test, or indican test, can be performed rather simply with a routine urinalysis. (Remember this is not a test for cancer, but a preventive type of test.)

What about heart attacks? At first glance, it seems a little unlikely that more roughage in the colon will lead to less problems for the heart. But researchers have found that high-residue diets, depending on their composition, can lower cholesterol or triglycerides. Certainly this doesn't prevent all heart attacks; but from the epidemiologic evidence, as well as the experimental evidence, it appears it will help prevent a substantial number. There is also evidence that straining at stool can lead to sudden heart attacks in susceptible people; preventing this straining is certainly worthwhile.

If all this weren't enough, it seems likely that a collection of other problems, including appendicitis, gallstones, constipation, hemorrhoids, varicose veins, phlebitis, and obesity are all related in varying degrees to low-roughage diets.

So, you can see that Jennifer's cramps were just the tip of the iceberg of the problems she could have had later in life, if her intestines hadn't complained, loudly and painfully. As I mentioned at the beginning, Jennifer was lucky.

In the next chapter, we'll look at one result of a low-residue diet in an adult. At the conclusion of that chapter, there is a long list of further reading on the subject of food fiber and health.

FURTHER READING

Usually, I like to list as many references as might be helpful. However, an excellent compilation of the best references has already been done by David Reuben, M.D., in the bibliography of his book, *The Save Your Life Diet* (New York: Random House, 1975).

I recommend his summary highly for both general reading and specialized reference.

A woman is taking tranquilizers for intestinal cramping and related symptoms for which no physical cause can be found. An investigation of her diet reveals a lack of fiber to be the underlying problem. She also has sensitivities to certain foods which cause pain. A diet prescription is offered, along with an explanation of why colon problems are so common in certain countries, rare in others.

A Case of Colitis 10

One typically rainy day in October, Mrs. Debbie Davis visited our office in Kent. She was a short, pleasant woman; although overweight, that was not the problem she had come to consult about.

She told me that she had had colitis for approximately five years. This had been a variable problem, not particularly responding to treatments, but coming and going "on its own" until settling down during the previous year.

Unfortunately, she had been involved in an auto accident in April. Following this, her colitis once again began to act up, but this time worse than ever before. Her symptoms for most of this year had included:

• Intestinal cramping, from mild to severe. This sometimes came "on its own" but often seemed set off by foods, particularly high carbohydrate ones.

• Alternating constipation and diarrhea.

• Intermittent mucus discharge.

• Frequent blood in mucus and with bowel movements.

These symptoms were much the same as she'd had before. It

seemed, though, that the stress of the accident had made them all much worse than previously.

As the year progressed, Mrs. Davis had found more and more aspects of her life impaired by what originally had seemed "strictly a physical problem." In addition to the above, she said, she was chronically tired, and had very little energy. She was starting to get headaches. Perhaps worst of all, for three months she'd been having spells of depression, a problem she'd not had before.

Mrs. Davis was 28 years old. She'd never been highly social, but for the past six months had hardly gone out at all. If she attended a party, her symptoms were frequently set off, forcing her to return home. Although her husband was sympathetic to her pain, he was showing signs of increasing impatience with her inability to live a relatively normal life. As Mrs. Davis said: "I really can't blame him, either! After all, I'm only 28 and shouldn't be sick like this."

She also was beginning to blame herself. One doctor had told her that "colitis patients are just nervous," and had given her Valium, a much-prescribed tranquilizer. Predictably, that hadn't worked.

In the months since her accident, she had sought help from a number of doctors. As we went through the list of tests she'd had done, all of which had turned out negative, it became increasingly clear that she had none of the usually diagnosed bowel problems.

X-rays of both the upper and lower gastrointestinal tracts had been done, and later repeated. The "upper GI" was negative for stomach or duodenal ulcer. She said her small intestine on the same "upper GI" was also normal, eliminating an inflammatory bowel disorder (of unknown cause), called regional enteritis.

She said her "lower GI" was also normal. Although this procedure, as well as sigmoidoscopy (looking into the colon with a long, lighted tube), had been done to look for ulcerative colitis, neither this nor any sign of cancer had been found. The only positive finding, accounting for her bleeding, had been a "redhot" case of internal hemorrhoids. ("I'd certainly agree with that description!" Mrs. Davis said.)

Also, numerous stool examinations had been done. No abnormal bacteria (medically referred to as "pathogens") had been found. There was no evidence of parasites. Analysis of composition showed no sign of malabsorption (which can have a variety of causes, including cereal-grain sensitivity or celiac disease).

She'd also tried a milk- and dairy product-free diet for eight days, to see if lactose intolerance (inability to handle milk sugar, caused by deficiency of an intestinal enzyme, lactase) was her problem. "I had to stop that before the two weeks I was supposed to do," she said, "because I was getting *worse* and cottage cheese was all I could tolerate."

Despite the normality found, her symptoms continued. So, she'd been treated with a long and depressing list of medications. In addition to the tranquilizer, she'd been given two or three different antibiotics "just in case of a germ that hadn't been found," several types of antispasmodics, and painkillers. None of these had come near to solving the problem. But the antispasmodics and painkillers did help her tolerate the symptoms. At that time, she was taking regularly one medication of each type.

As Mrs. Davis said: "I'm not one to give up, so I started checking into this on my own. I read books and articles and decided vitamins might help." Several weeks before, she'd started herself on a full range of vitamins. Her present intake included a multiple vitamin, calcium, iron, vitamins C and E, lecithin and alfalfa tablets, as well as a protein powder.

She reported that this had helped for a few days. But then her symptoms had returned "as bad as ever." For the week or two prior to her appointment, she'd been able to eat only cottage cheese, and hadn't been able to get her vitamins down.

I asked her what her usual diet would be if she were not having a problem with colitis. She listed for me the following:

Breakfast: bacon, eggs, toasted white bread, and decaffeinated coffee

Lunch: usually nothing

Dinner: meat, potatoes, noodles (made of white flour) or rice, and one of several vegetables, including corn, peas, or beans

Snacks: much fruit, ice cream, and quite a bit of white bread

She also ate many refined carbohydrate snack foods. This

diet pattern was a major clue to the solution of her problem. Another part of the puzzle was her observation that "I never had any of this problem before I was 23." Although celiac disease, lactose intolerance, ulcerative colitis, and many other bowel diseases can start in adults (as well as children), I thought this observation was worth pursuing. So I asked what type of food she had eaten as she was growing up.

She thought for a minute. "Well," she started, "my mother always had whole wheat bread." As she went over the rest of her answer, it was obvious she had replaced a relatively fiber-rich, unrefined diet with highly refined, processed, and sugared fare. As she said later, "I just thought my mother was old-fashioned. All my friends ate the same as me, and it didn't seem to hurt them."

At this point Mrs. Davis' problem seemed apparent. I didn't ask her to have any further tests performed. Her examination showed only abdominal tenderness over the area of the colon; all else appeared relatively normal.

I explained that her problem was not unusual, just more severe than most, and was caused by a refined carbohydrate diet with practically no roughage, needed by the intestines for proper function. Her problem was further aggravated by the antibiotics she'd taken, which would wipe out normal intestinal bacteria, needed for proper bowel function.

To help with her problem, I recommended several things:
1. A bowl of sugarless bran cereal every day (to add roughage) or, even better, two rounded tablespoons of unprocessed bran flakes taken with cereal or yogurt.
2. Replacement of all white bread and cereal products with whole-grain products (also to provide proper roughage).
3. A dose of *Lactobacillus acidophilus* each day, either liquid or capsule, to replace the normal bacteria previously eliminated by antibiotics.
4. Avoid all sugar. This is because sugar is a gastrointestinal irritant, and with her problem, would only make things worse.

5. Tablets made of whole animal intestinal substance, cold processed. Even though her previous tests had detected no definite intestinal damage, it was impossible to tell if there was any "microscopic" or molecular-level damage. If there had been any, the whole intestinal substance should provide all the components necessary for any needed cellular repair to her own intestine.

Mrs. Davis agreed to try these suggestions. However, she wanted to know "what to do about my depression, headaches, and tiredness." I said I thought these were probably caused by poor nutrition, due to her bowel problem, and further aggravated by the stress of her auto accident. Many studies have shown that stress—emotional, physical, surgical, etc.—causes nutrient losses much higher than usual. As these nutrients are frequently not replaced, whatever condition may have existed before often gets worse. And new stress-related symptoms may appear.

It was my opinion that the headaches, depression, and tiredness were in her case stress-related, and should clear (although perhaps slowly) with the program recommended. If not, there were nutritional treatment programs specifically for these problems that could be tried.

I asked her to check back in six to eight weeks, or, of course, sooner if things weren't going well.

When Mrs. Davis returned in December, she appeared much happier and less nervous than before. She'd been sticking closely to the recommended program, with good results. Her cramping had nearly disappeared; she'd had but two mild attacks in the past month; her alternating diarrhea and constipation were gone. She no longer had any mucus discharge; she'd had no bleeding for six weeks.

Although her tiredness was still something of a problem, it had lessened. Her headaches were much less severe; she was no longer suffering depression. She'd been able to resume normal activities, and was able to go out when she wanted.

She confessed, however, that once, "just to see," she'd tried several pieces of candy. Shortly afterward, she had an upset stomach and cramps once more. She decided not to try it again. She wanted to know if she'd always have to stay with the program recommended.

I advised her she could discontinue the tablets of intestinal substance, but that unless she wanted the colitis to return, the rest of the program recommended would be lifelong. Also, it was good for her health in general, anyway!

I haven't seen Mrs. Davis for several months now. Her husband was in recently, and told me she was doing well. The colitis seemed to be gone. "And you know what?" he said. "She's even losing some weight!"

Mrs. Davis' problem was truly not unusual. As noted by a major medical textbook, colitis (also called "irritable colon," "mucous colitis," "spastic colon," or "nervous colon") is considered to account for more than 50 percent of all gastrointestinal illness. This same textbook states the cause to be unknown and puts heavy emphasis on emotional causes, and treatment for supposed psychiatric disturbance. It has been my experience that this is only rarely the case.

Basing treatment on restoration of proper bowel function with proper nutrition and replacement of normal bacteria when necessary, I have observed the vast majority of cases cured with nothing else required.

Restoration of proper nutrition (with particular emphasis on roughage) might seem only the logical thing to do. However, logic in this case has been supported by a series of brilliant and painstaking investigations by British physicians, led by Denis Burkitt, John Cleave, and Neil Painter.

In summary, they have shown that many common diseases including colitis, appendicitis, diverticulitis, and even colon cancer are actually not common at all, but rare in certain areas of the world where diets are high in the natural fiber found in unprocessed, unrefined foods. These diseases are apparently only common in Westernized, industrialized areas where much of the diet is highly refined. Making the situation even worse is the addition of truly enormous quantities of refined sugar, which serves only to aggravate an already poor dietary situation. "Topping off" low-residue, high-sugar diets in many Western countries is an antibiotic-related abnormal bacterial content of the bowel.

Frequently, as in Mrs. Davis' case, it requires correction of all three of these "problems of civilization" to achieve good intestinal health once more. Unfortunately, while our minds may be adapted to civilization, our bodies, including our intestines, are still in their natural, "primitive" state. If we insist on ignoring this fact, in one way or another, our bodies will let us know.

If we follow the lead given by Drs. Burkitt, Cleave, Painter, and others working on aspects of this problem, perhaps we can make these illnesses—colitis, appendicitis, diverticulitis, and bowel cancer—a rarity on our "space age" part of the planet as well.

FURTHER READING

Balasegaram, M., and Burkitt, Denis P. "Stool Characteristics and Western Diseases." *The Lancet,* January 17, 1976, p. 152.

Burkitt, Denis P. "Relationships Between Diseases and Their Etiological Significance." *The American Journal of Clinical Nutrition,* vol. 30, February 1977, pp. 262-67.

———. "Diet and Diseases of Affluence." *Qualitas Plantarum—Plant Foods for Human Nutrition,* vol. 27, no. 3-4, 1977, pp. 227-38.

———. "The Link Between Low-Fiber Diets and Disease." *Human Nature,* December 1978, pp. 34-41.

Burkitt, Denis P., and Painter, Neil. "Dietary Fiber and Disease." *Journal of the American Medical Association,* vol. 229, no. 8, August 19, 1974, pp. 1068-74.

Burkitt, Denis P., and Trowell, H. C., eds. *Refined Carbohydrate Foods and Disease: Some Implications of Dietary Fibre* (New York: Academic Press, 1975).

Burkitt, Denis P., and Tunstall, Maria. "Common Geography as a Clue to Causation." *Tropical and Geographical Medicine,* vol. 27, 1975, pp. 117-24.

Cleave, T. L. "The Neglect of Natural Principles in Current Medical Practice." *Journal of the Royal Naval Medical Service,* vol. 42, no. 2, Spring 1956, pp. 55-83.

————. "Bran and Diverticular Disease." *British Medical Journal*, May 13, 1972, pp. 408-9.

————. *The Saccharine Disease* (New Canaan, Conn.: Keats Publishing, 1975).

Manning, A. P.; Heaton, K. W.; and Harvey, R. F. "Wheat Fibre and Irritable Bowel Syndrome." *The Lancet*, August 27, 1977, pp. 417-18.

Painter, Neil S. "Dietary Fiber—a Simple Way to Deal with Diverticulosis." *Modern Medicine*, vol. 42, no. 21, October 14, 1974, pp. 28-32.

————. "Bran and the Irritable Bowel." *The Lancet*, March 6, 1976, p. 540.

————. *Journal of the Royal Society of Medicine*, vol. 71, no. 4, April 1978, pp. 305-6.

Painter, Neil S., and Burkitt, Denis P. "Diverticular Disease of the Colon: A Deficiency Disease of Western Civilization." *British Medical Journal*, May 22, 1971, pp. 450-54.

Painter, Neil S.; Almeida, Anthony Z.; and Colebourne, Kenneth W. "Unprocessed Bran in Treatment of Diverticular Disease of the Colon." *British Medical Journal*, April 15, 1972, pp. 137-40.

Reuben, David. *The Save Your Life Diet* (New York: Random House, 1975).

Trowell, Hugh. "The Development of the Concept of Dietary Fiber in Human Nutrition." *The American Journal of Clinical Nutrition*, vol. 31, October 1978, pp. S3-S11.

The patients, who eat a generally good diet, both go to work early in the morning. Both are plagued by fatigue, especially in the afternoon. An examination of their eating pattern quickly pinpoints the problem, and shows that *when* you eat can be just as important as *what* you eat.

A Case of Afternoon Fatigue

11

Jim and Susan Oldham came in for their appointments together. Like many couples, they liked to sit in on each other's visits and as they'd explained to the receptionist, "We seem to have the same problem, so we'll just go together."

Jim was tall and muscular; he appeared to be at least six foot-six and quiet. Susan was no more than five-foot-one, bouncy and talkative. She immediately took the lead in the discussion.

"We don't really have any bad symptoms or anything," she said. "Neither one of us is really sick. We're wondering if it's all psychological or something, because sometimes there isn't any problem. But we thought we'd come in and talk to you about it first."

"You haven't said what the problem is yet."

"Oh, yes. Well, it's this tiredness. What's so strange is we both have it pretty much the same, and started feeling bad about the same time. We thought it must be something catching like a virus or something, but we both had mononucleosis already, so it can't be that. You can't get mononucleosis twice, can you? I had diseases twice. . . ."

"Hold on. You said tiredness, but I need more details. Are you tired all the time? Sometimes? Has this been a problem for a few weeks, a few months?"

"We didn't feel this way when we got married. That was 18 months ago, when Jim got out of the Navy. He enlisted just after high school. We both went to the same high school but we didn't want to get married then. So he joined the Navy and I went to business college. I got out 3½ years ago. . . ."

"I think we'd better get more specific about the tiredness. When did you personally notice you were getting more tired?"

"About the same time Jim did. At first we didn't talk to each other about it, but then I found out he'd been having the same trouble. . . ."

"I mean, how many months ago?"

"Oh. Well, I noticed it seemed to start just after our first anniversary, so it must have been about six months ago. I think that's right, isn't it, Jim?"

"Yeah."

"Have you been tired every day since then?"

"No, it's not every day except lately it seems to be nearly every day. At first, it was worse during the week and not on weekends, so we thought we were just working too hard. But we have to, because we're trying to save some money toward when we have a baby, and we had to buy a new car and pay for the apartment. . . ."

"So now you're tired every day?"

"Nearly every day, except vacation. That's why we thought maybe it was psychological, maybe we didn't like work or something. I'll have to admit I don't have the most exciting job."

"Are you tired all day?"

"No, it's not nearly so bad in the morning, except lately I've been noticing a little in the morning. Maybe it's because we stay up late many nights."

"So what time of day do you start to get tired?"

"It's really bad at three or four o'clock in the afternoon. Some days I can hardly get my work done. I make more typing errors, and forget things, because I just want to take a nap. My girl friend says maybe I've got that hypoglycemia thing like her girl friend had. She always went to sleep in the afternoon, too."

"So you get tired at about three o'clock every day?"

"Well, except that sometimes I get a little tired at 11:00 or 11:30 A.M. But it's not nearly as bad and I don't really notice it after lunch. Isn't that strange?"

I thought perhaps I had an idea of what the problem might be, so I turned to Jim, as I thought we might get to the bottom of the matter sooner that way.

"Susan says you've had the same problem with tiredness?"

"Yes."

"Every day?"

"Yes."

"Worse in the afternoon?"

"Yes."

"You're tense when you get home?"

"Yes, but it's just my job. The boss is a real . . . , and I'm working really hard to get ahead and out of that department anyway."

"You've had no other symptoms except this tiredness? No headaches, no other pains, no fever, nothing else?"

"Not that I know of."

"Are you tired after dinner?"

"Come to think of it, not so bad. But it's really bad at the warehouse afternoons. Gets so I don't want to lift another thing."

"Do you do anything to feel better?"

Jim looked a little guilty. "I didn't tell Susan, because she was raised right, not to eat any junk or anything. But I sneak a Coke every once in a while. It really seems to help."

I thought perhaps a few more questions would help to clarify the problem, but I had to ask Susan.

"You lived at home until you were married?"

"Yes. I didn't really want to move out because I wanted to save my money. Of course I paid rent as soon as I went to work."

"Your mother did the cooking?"

"Yes. My mother's been a real health food type since we were little. She read everything Adelle Davis ever wrote, and raised us kids according to what she said. That's why I didn't think I had that hypoglycemia, because I never eat any sugar. Jim and I don't have any sugar or junk food at home, eat only good food, only fresh stuff, nothing canned except soup every once in a while. . . ."

I've heard this pattern so often that I thought it was time to get to what probably were the key questions.

"But what do you eat for breakfast?"

"Oh, some juice or coffee."

"Nothing else?"

"I just don't have time. My company starts early, not as early as Jim's job, but I have to be to work at 7:30 A.M., and I stay up too late at night to get up much before I have to leave. Besides, I've been too tired lately."

"Lunch?"

"Oh, just a salad. I've been trying to keep my weight down. My father always said that's a good way to turn your husband off if you get too big and fat. . . ."

I turned to Jim.

"What do you eat for breakfast?"

"Since I got this job, I haven't been eating breakfast. I get there at 6:00 A.M., and I don't want to wake Susan. So, I have some coffee out of a machine or something. I don't put any sugar in it, though."

"And lunch?"

"Mostly I miss lunch because I'm working so hard to get done. That boss won't hire enough people to get the job done. Besides, if I work hard, I can probably get out of there in a few months or so."

I looked at both of them. "There's your answer," I said. "There's no need to do any lab tests, or worry about psychological problems. All you both need to do is eat some protein for breakfast, and a little more for lunch. The whole problem should clear up in a few weeks."

"But we eat enough protein," Susan said. "I know about protein; we both get home early enough that we have an early dinner, and I make sure there's enough protein in it. Later in the evening I always make a protein snack. We both get more protein than the Recommended Dietary Allowance. I know Jim's big, but I make sure he gets enough protein for his size."

"Sometimes I think that what's needed in nutrition is not more doctors, but more wise grandmothers. My grandmother always used to tell me to eat a good breakfast if I wanted to feel good. However, since you're here, let me tell you about the Iowa Breakfast Studies. Have you ever heard of those?"

"No," Susan replied. "What's that?"

"Over 20 years ago, several scientists supported by several cereal companies spent lots of time, money, and effort proving what most grandmothers could have told us: if you don't eat breakfast, you won't do as well as you could do at school or work. They showed that if their test subjects ate 1 ounce of protein in the morning, that their performances at specific tasks were better than those who ate no protein, or less than 1 ounce. One of the measurements they made was of blood sugar. Those who ate protein had higher blood sugar levels for longer than those who didn't. Those persons' blood sugar levels went sufficiently low that it began to affect their performance at various tasks.

"Neither group had either hypoglycemia or diabetes. All blood sugar readings were within normal. But the lower normal levels brought on by not eating enough protein weren't enough to sustain optimum performance.

"So, like you, these test subjects weren't sick. They just weren't performing up to par because of what they ate, or, in this case, didn't eat.

"I hear about this kind of problem very frequently. I know if you skip protein at breakfast, and have none at lunch either, you're bound to get more tired the longer you do it. You'll probably feel very briefly better after a salad for lunch, and of course you'll get a lift from a caffeine-sugar soft drink. But with that, your blood sugar will go even lower later, and you'll get cranky.

"If you're in a hurry, you needn't take much time to eat, especially if it's just an ounce or two of protein. Eat a hard-boiled egg on the way to work. Or a piece of cheese, or a big glass of milk. Even protein tablets will do. Have cottage cheese in your salad at lunch. Remember, *when* you eat can be as important sometimes as *what* you eat."

"Are you sure that's all it is?" Susan asked. "I thought it was really bad."

"Let me just quote my grandmother once more. 'Eat the right food at the right time, and you'll do better.' If you don't, come back and tell me I was wrong!"

The next time I saw either of the Oldhams was when Susan came in for her Pap smear, several months later. When I asked her what had happened, she told me (in several hundred words or more) that both the Iowa Breakfast Studies and my grandmother had been completely correct.

FURTHER READING

Arnold, Samuel J. et al. "Asking Your Patient About Breakfast." *Medical Tribune,* vol. 17, no. 15, April 21, 1976, p. 7.

A Complete Summary of the Iowa Breakfast Studies, reprinted January 1976 by the Cereal Institute, 1111 Plaza Drive, Schaumburg, IL. 60195.

After surviving a heart attack, a man seeks some nutritional alternative to a cholesterol-lowering drug his cardiologist suggests. He is put on a whole new dietary program calculated not only to lower cholesterol, but to normalize many other risk factors associated with heart disease. After six months, his cholesterol has been reduced from 396 to 220, and triglycerides from 685 to 110. He's also lost 20 pounds. His chances of having another heart attack are probably much reduced.

A Case of Heart Disease

12

Orville Henderson didn't look well. His complexion was pasty and just a little gray. There was slight puffiness beneath his eyes, and an obvious case of dandruff showed on his suit jacket. He seemed a little nervous and tense, even though slumped in his chair.

"I just got out of the hospital," he said. "Heart attack; I almost didn't make it. Never thought it would happen to me; I suppose you hear that a lot. But it's not in my family, and, to tell you the truth, I hadn't seen a doctor since I was discharged from the Army in 1946. My wife kept after me, but I never had the time. Too busy building the business. I sell insurance.

"I never really gave it much thought until I got a terrific chest and arm pain and landed in the coronary care unit. I've had more time to think now; I want to prevent this from ever happening again. I'll do whatever's necessary."

"Have you talked to the doctor you had in the hospital about this?"

"Yes. And he's supposed to be one of the best cardiologists.

He wants me to start on an exercise program soon. I'll go along with that. But he wants to give me a drug to get my cholesterol and triglycerides down, as well as a low-fat diet. I'm not so sure about that; my wife won't hear of it. She says it's not necessary to use drugs to get cholesterol down, that diet, vitamins, and minerals will do it. So that's why I'm here. Will that work, really?"

"It will; and in a much more healthy way."

"What do you mean—more healthy?"

"Taking drugs to lower cholesterol is like clamping a lid on a pot that's boiling over. That's not really a good solution; a better way is to turn the stove down. That's what diet and supplying needed nutrients does."

"That makes sense," Mr. Henderson said. He handed me a slip of paper, a copy of his laboratory results. "I had these done last week at the cardiologist's. I thought it would save time if I brought them along."

"Thank you." I read over the slip. It showed a cholesterol of 396 milligrams percent (normal is 150 to 250, although some say as high as 300 is normal), and triglycerides 685 milligrams percent (normal is 35 to 160). "I'll agree with one thing: these blood fats do need to be reduced."

"I don't understand one thing. What does 'Type IV' mean?"

"That's part of a classification system of blood fat abnormalities worked out by Dr. Donald Fredrickson a few years ago. They're categorized in Types I through V according to the types, amounts, and proportions of different blood fats. Each type is associated sometimes with other metabolic problems."

"What about Type IV?"

"That may be the most common. It's usually related more to diet and lack of exercise; sometimes people with Type IV problems have abnormal blood sugar tests, high uric acid levels, or low thyroid function. Speaking of that, if you haven't had these tests done, you should."

"I don't think I have."

I made a note to schedule Mr. Henderson for these tests. "Also, while we're talking about tests, there's another one I'd like you to get done. That's a mineral analysis using a hair specimen."

"You had my wife take one of those last year, didn't you?"

"Yes, it was very revealing, too."

"I know. She's been taking these vitamin and mineral pills ever since. She is feeling better, though."

"Good. That should take care of tests for now. Let's talk about diet."

"We've already started on that. I've cut out all the eggs, butter, cheese, and fatty meats. My wife says I'll have to cut out all the sugar, too, but I haven't yet. What's that got to do with getting the cholesterol down?"

"It's got a lot more to do with cutting down triglycerides. But before we talk about that, why are you cutting out all the eggs and so on? Did your cardiologist ask you to do that?"

"No, he just told me to go on a low-fat diet. But from everything I've read I thought that was necessary. . . ." He looked confused.

"Only a few patients of the hundreds I've treated for high cholesterol have had to severely limit dietary intake. Usually, it's a problem of correcting the metabolism rather than diet."

Mr. Henderson thought a minute. "Adjusting the stove again, huh?" he said.

"Yes, in a way. Now, I want you to diversify your meat intake more; much more fish and poultry, and less beef and pork. Don't eliminate eggs and cheese, though; you can use a little butter. I'll only ask you to stop them if your cholesterol doesn't revert to normal. Eggs are an excellent source of protein."

Mr. Henderson still looked puzzled. "What about unsaturated fats? Aren't they important?"

"Yes, they are. I don't mean to de-emphasize those. Please make sure to include at least 1 or 2 tablespoons of pressed vegetable oil in your diet each day. You can use it as salad dressing, or mixed with other foods. Also, for snack foods, use sunflower and sesame seeds, or other oil-bearing seeds or nuts."

"My wife says these are healthy, too, but won't it increase my calorie count?"

"Some. However, with your level of triglycerides, what's more important is the carbohydrate count. I want you to make sure to limit your carbohydrates for the present to 60 to 90 grams daily. If you're not familiar with that, you can get a carbohydrate counter.

"To reduce your levels of triglycerides it's important not only to reduce carbohydrate, but to control what types of carbohydrate you consume. Refined sugar of any type or quantity has to go. Many studies have shown that it directly increases the triglyceride count."

"I knew you'd say that. My wife's been after me about it for years. But in my kind of business all this health food stuff is difficult to do. I eat out a lot, and restaurants and clients don't understand. If you're different, it's not always good for business." He paused. "I guess I'd better, now."

"If you're going to have the best chance of preventing recurrence, yes. Also cut out refined flour, and any other types of refined food. As much of your food as possible should be uncooked, whole, and natural. When it is cooked, cook it as little as possible. The problem with food refining is that it removes most of the essential vitamins and minerals. There isn't always that much to begin with after chemical farming on nutrient-depleted soil.

"I also want you to cut out all the alcohol for now. You may be able to use some again later on, but for now, none. It raises triglycerides."

Mr. Henderson looked glum. "If heart attacks weren't fatal, I don't know if I'd do all this," he observed. "How long before I can have a drink?"

"Six months at least. While on the subject of drinks—you know caffeine is out, too, don't you?"

"I guessed as much."

"There are two food items I'd like you to add to your diet, onions and garlic."

"What for? In my business, that could be a problem. But I always have liked those a lot. . . ."

"Studies have shown that they help hold down cholesterol levels. Remember, those are part of an overall program. You don't have to eat any set number of onions a day, or take garlic twice daily, just make sure to include them whenever you can.

"Now, about supplements. . . ."

Mr. Henderson interrupted. "Wait a minute. I want to make sure I have this food thing straight first. Let's see: less beef and pork, more fish and fowl, but I can have eggs, cheese, and some butter. I should use at least one tablespoon of oil daily and eat seeds and nuts for snacks. No processed snack foods or other processed foods, no sugar, no white flour. As much raw food as I can. No booze for at least six months, and no coffee. And onions and garlic added when I can. Is that it?"

"Exactly."

Mr. Henderson shook his head. "I'm going to be a regular health food nut."

While Mr. Henderson was going over his foods, I wrote out a list of supplements, as follows:

1. Vitamin C: 2 grams (2,000 milligrams), 3 times daily
2. Lecithin: 19-grain capsules; 5, twice daily, or 1 tablespoon of granules twice daily
3. Niacin: 250 milligrams capsule (time-release), 1, twice daily
4. Dolomite tablets: 3, twice daily
5. Vitamin E: 800 units daily
6. B complex vitamins: a "50" formula; 1, 3 times a day.

I gave it to Mr. Henderson. "This may not be everything; it depends on what your tests show."

Mr. Henderson read it over. "Could you please explain what each of these is supposed to do?"

"As much as I can in the time we have left. Vitamin C is to help keep plaque out of arteries. Also, it helps activate an enzyme called lipoprotein lipase that helps bring triglyceride levels down as well.

"Many years ago, Dr. Lester Morrison of Loma Linda University School of Medicine demonstrated the cholesterol-lowering effects of lecithin. Others have found the same thing.

"Niacin has even found its way into nonnutritional medical practice as a cholesterol-lowering agent, although it's simply a form of vitamin B_3. Most important, it has been reported as effective in reducing the recurrence rate of heart attacks.

"Dolomite is made up of calcium and magnesium, both of which help lower cholesterol levels. The vitamin E is to help with healing, and the B vitamins are there because you've been eating refined foods for so long."

Mr. Henderson thought for a moment. "You mean if I stop eating refined foods, I might not need the B vitamins after a while?"

"That's right. Not only that, you might not need most of these supplements at all, and others at pretty much of a reduced rate."

At that, he brightened just a little. "I'm glad to hear it. No offense, but it's always seemed to me that all this vitamin popping is overdone."

Even though it was time for the next appointment, I didn't want to let that particular remark pass by. "What business did you say you were in, Mr. Henderson?"

"Insurance. Why?"

"How many of your clients are sufficiently insured?"

"Not as many as I'd like. That's not your point at all, is it?"

"No. If nothing else, 'vitamin popping' is relatively cheap health insurance. And this doesn't even take into account demineralized soils, foods robbed of nutrients by processing, transportation, storage, cooking. . . . Not to mention the effects of air and water pollution."

"Yeah, I guess so. When should I come back?"

"Have your cholesterol and triglycerides rechecked in six weeks. We'll go over those and your other tests then."

Mr. Henderson looked considerably healthier on his return. Most noticeably, he'd lost weight. The puffiness under his eyes was gone. He even seemed less tense.

"I've lost 12 pounds," he announced. "I'm even getting to like these health foods my wife's stuffing me with. Between that and the exercise, I feel better than I have in years. My cardiologist says he's never seen such a fast improvement. He's even let me return to work already. How are my tests?"

"Slow down a second. I'll look them up. Let's see . . . your cholesterol is 310, and your triglycerides, 322. Not normal yet, but definitely improved."

"Good. What about my other tests?"

"Your thyroid function test was normal, but on the low side. Your glucose tolerance test, though, was about as close to being diabetic as you can get without actually having diabetes."

Mr. Henderson looked uncomfortable. "What do I have to do about that?"

"Nothing you're not doing already."

"Oh, good. I thought I'd have more things to take."

"I'm afraid you do, but not for that. Let's look at your mineral analysis."

"Oh, yeah . . . I'm really interested in how that came out."

Mr. Henderson's mineral analysis showed several problems. Magnesium, chromium, selenium, and manganese were all too low; zinc levels were higher than usual.

Mr. Henderson studied the report for a minute. "I guess I should take all those minerals that are too low," he said. "But what do I do to get that zinc level down?"

"Take zinc supplements."

"What?"

"Hair mineral analyses are trickier than they look. Nearly always if the zinc levels are high on this test, taking zinc will bring them down to normal."

"That doesn't make sense."

"I know. But I've watched it work in practice hundreds of times. In fact, the highest hair zinc levels I've seen have had low urine and blood concentrations."

"OK, if you say so. What do I get?"

"Get chelated zinc, 50 milligrams, and use twice daily."

"And the other things?"

"Remember, you're already taking a source of magnesium; the dolomite. For manganese, I'd like you to use a 20-milligram chelated supplement twice daily."

"That's another two pills. . . . And there are two left to go."

"Yes, but they're very important. Both low selenium and low chromium have been suspected of contributing to a higher rate of heart attacks. For that matter, so has low magnesium."

"Looks like I had them all going against me, doesn't it?"

"Fortunately, it's not too late to correct it."

"I know. . . . Well, what about the other two?"

"Luckily, you get off with only one here. Yeast products are very high in both selenium and chromium. I'd like you to use two tablespoons of brewer's yeast a day."

"All right. Anything else?"

"No. Just stick to it all, and repeat your cholesterol and triglyceride tests in two months."

Two months later, Mr. Henderson's cholesterol was found to be 250, and his triglycerides, 140. As he'd continued on his diet and exercise, he'd dropped another 8 pounds, to 170. We had just a brief visit, as I didn't want him to make any changes yet. I asked him to return in another three months.

At that visit Mr. Henderson came in looking positively elated. "I couldn't wait," he said. "I already found out from the nurse about my tests. The cholesterol's 220, and the triglycerides, 110. How about that? I'm down to 160 pounds now—not bad for five-foot-nine, especially at my age. Now, I've been good, and watched my diet, taken all my vitamins. When can I cut down some?"

"How are you feeling?"

"Fantastic. Better than in years. My skin's better. Even my dandruff's gone. I had that since college."

"Even if you do cut down on the vitamins, you shouldn't go off your diet. Sugar and refined foods are still out."

"I understand that. But I can have more carbohydrates, and a drink every once in a while, can't I?"

"Yes. Just watch your weight, and keep exercising. If it starts to go back up, you'll have to tighten up again."

"That's fair enough. I even like my diet now, and it's not really a problem, even on business. I usually have fish and salad and skip the white rolls and desserts. We have fruit at home instead. But what I really want to know is, what about those pills?"

"Why don't you cut them all by half. Then we'll get your tests done again in a while, to see if everything's still OK."

"That's for sure. I plan to get my blood tests and mineral tests done regularly. Anything I can do to prevent another recurrence."

It's been 3½ years since Mr. Henderson's heart attack. He's stayed with his diet, and keeps up fairly well with exercise. His vitamin and mineral list has been pared down gradually, while following his tests, to vitamins C and E, 2 lecithin capsules, with brewer's yeast for B vitamins, and kelp as a natural source of minerals. His tests have remained normal. Of course, three years really isn't a long time, and I can't say absolutely he'll never have more heart problems. But I think he's done everything he can to prevent further heart attacks. As Mr. Henderson himself has come around to saying, "Taking just a few vitamins, in addition to a good diet and enough exercise, is cheap enough insurance."

Preventing Heart Attacks

Heart attacks from coronary atherosclerosis may be one of the most easily preventable epidemic diseases of modern civilization, particularly in younger age groups from 40 to 70.

Coronary atherosclerosis refers to the blockage and narrowing (sclerosis) of the blood vessels to the heart (coronary arteries). The blockage consists of largely fatty deposits (atheroma) containing large quantities of cholesterol and triglycerides. Most of us are familiar with the term *cholesterol*. Triglycerides are simply another form of fat, the same as "stored fat" in the all-too-familiar locations, but circulating in the blood. Unlike cholesterol, triglycerides are made in the body principally from carbohydrates eaten.

The accumulation of much biochemical research shows that complex carbohydrates, found mostly in unrefined foods such as grains, potatoes, and fruits, cause many less triglyceride problems than simple carbohydrates, which are nothing more than sugar in one form or another.

Unfortunately, some medical nutritional authorities continue to insist that the connection between diet and coronary atherosclerosis is not fully proven, and are willing only to admit that "too much saturated fat" is probably a problem. This position is justified by the fact that no one has so far been able to work out a "one-step-at-a-time, straight-line connection" from diet to blocked blood vessels, including each of the biochemical steps along the way. According to the orthodox point of view, no proof can be established until this is done.

In fact, this type of "A to B to C" proof may never be accomplished, because it probably doesn't exist. Coronary atherosclerosis appears to be another example of a disease with many causes, many modifying influences, and many interrelated and cross-linked pathways of metabolism. Many nutrients, literally from A to zinc, have been found to be involved with varying degrees of importance in atheroma formation. Lack of exercise is certainly important; a few scattered bits of evidence indicate that factors besides diet and exercise may be involved.

Many insights into health and disease, particularly widespread disease, have been gained through another branch of science called epidemiology. Epidemiology is the study of health and disease patterns in large groups of people, comparing population groups, sometimes on a worldwide scale. A study of epidemiologic data, combined with a nutritional/biochemical point of view, makes it very clear that refined foods, deficient in various vitamins and minerals, eaten to excess, combined with very little exercise, are almost invariably associated with high rates of coronary atherosclerosis and heart attack.

Conversely, population groups living on whole, natural, unrefined foods, and getting more exercise, have low rates of heart disease. Ironically, epidemiologic studies have also shown that the one "bogeyman" of many nutrition authorities, high-animal-fat diets, may not be necessarily causative of coronary atherosclerosis. Two population groups, the Masai tribe of Africa, and Greenland Eskimos, both living on almost exclusively animal diets, have a much lower incidence of heart disease than Western populations. Their diets are unlike "civilized" high-animal-fat diets in that they are whole, natural, unrefined, and generally unprocessed.

The epidemiologic evidence is fairly clear in associating highly refined, highly processed, sugar- and additive-laden food with a high level of heart attacks. The weight of evidence from biochemical research is finally starting to catch up with epidemiology on this point.

Unfortunately, medicine is not practiced by epidemiologists or nutritionally oriented biochemists. So the myth of "we don't know what causes heart attacks" is likely to persist in the medical community for years yet.

FURTHER READING

Chromium
Boyle, Edwin; Mondschein, Benjamin; and Dash, Harriman H. "Chromium Depletion in the Pathogenesis of Diabetes and Atherosclerosis." *Southern Medical Journal*, vol. 70, no. 12, December 1977, pp. 1449-53.

Newman, Howard et al. "Serum Chromium and Angiographically Determined Coronary Artery Disease." *Clinical Chemistry*, vol. 24, no. 4, April 1978, pp. 541-44.

Schroeder, Henry A. "Frontiers in Trace Element Research." Presented at the international symposium *Trace Elements and Brain Function*, October 1973, Princeton, N.J.

Epidemiologic Studies
Burkitt, Denis P. "Some Diseases Characteristic of Modern Western Civilization." *British Medical Journal*, February 3, 1973, pp. 274-78.

Cohen, A. M.; Bavly, Sarah; and Poznanski, Rachel. "Change of Diet of Yemenite Jews in Relation to Diabetes and Ischaemic Heart-Disease." *The Lancet*, December 23, 1961, pp. 1399-1401.

Ho, Kang-Jey et al. "Alaskan Arctic Eskimo: Responses to a Customary High Fat Diet." *The American Journal of Clinical Nutrition*, vol. 25, August 1972, pp. 737-45.

Mann, George V. et al. "Atherosclerosis in the Masia." *American Journal of Epidemiology*, vol. 95, no. 1, 1972, pp. 26-37.

———. "Cardiovascular Disease in the Masai." *Journal of Atherosclerosis Research*, vol. 4, 1964, pp. 289-312.

Prior, Ian A. M. "The Price of Civilization." *Nutrition Today*, July/August, 1971, pp. 2-11.

Schaefer, Otto. "When the Eskimo Comes to Town." *Nutrition Today*, November/December, 1971, pp. 8–16.

Folic Acid

Oster, Kurt A. "Evaluation of Serum Cholesterol Reduction and Xanthine Oxidase Inhibition in the Treatment of Atherosclerosis." *Recent Advances in Studies on Cardiac Structure and Metabolism*, vol. 3. (Baltimore: University Park Press, 1973).

Garlic and Onion

Bordia, Arun K. "Effect of Garlic on Human Platelet Aggregation in Vitro." *Atherosclerosis*, vol. 30, no. 4, August 1978, pp. 355–60.

Bordia, Arun K. et al. "Effect of Essential Oil of Garlic on Serum Fibrinolytic Activity in Patients with Coronary Artery Disease." *Atherosclerosis*, vol. 28, 1977, pp. 155–59.

———. "Effect of Essential Oil of Onion and Garlic on Experimental Atherosclerosis in Rabbits." *Atherosclerosis*, vol. 26, no. 3, 1977, pp. 379 86.

Jain, R. C. "Onion and Garlic in Experimental Atherosclerosis." *The Lancet*, May 31, 1975, p. 1240.

———. "Effect of Garlic on Serum Lipids, Coagulability and Fibrinolytic Activity of Blood." *The American Journal of Clinical Nutrition*, vol. 30, no. 9, September 1977, pp. 1380–81.

Jain, R. C., and Konar, D. B. "Garlic Oil in Experimental Atherosclerosis." *The Lancet*, April 24, 1976, p. 918.

———. "Effect of Garlic Oil in Experimental Cholesterol Atherosclerosis." *Atherosclerosis*, vol. 29, 1978, pp. 125–29.

Sainani, G. S.; Desai, D. B.; and More, K. N. "Onion, Garlic and Atherosclerosis." *The Lancet*, September 11, 1976, pp. 575–76.

Sharma, K. K. et al. "Effect of Raw and Boiled Garlic on Blood Cholesterol in Butter Fat Lipaemia." *The Indian Journal of Nutrition and Dietetics*, vol. 13, no. 1, 1976, pp. 7–10.

Lecithin and Cholesterol

Adlersberg, David, and Sobotka, Harry. "Effect of Prolonged

Lecithin Feeding on Hypercholesterolemia." *Journal of Mt. Sinai Hospital*, vol. 9, 1943, pp. 955-56.

Krumdieck, Carlos, and Butterworth, C. E. "Ascorbate-Cholesterol-Lecithin Interactions: Factors of Potential Importance in the Pathogenesis of Atherosclerosis." *The American Journal of Clinical Nutrition*, vol. 27, August 1974, pp. 866-76.

Morrison, Lester M. "Serum Cholesterol Reduction with Lecithin." *Geriatrics*, vol. 13, January 1958, pp. 12-19.

Magnesium and Atherosclerosis

Anderson, T. W. et al. "Ischemic Heart Disease, Water Hardness and Myocardial Magnesium." *Canadian Medical Association Journal*, vol. 113, August 9, 1975, pp. 199-203.

Heggtveit, H. A. "Magnesium and Myocardium: The Influence of Magnesium Deficiency and Magnesium Loss Secondary to Ischemia and to Drugs." Second International Symposium on Magnesium, University of Montreal, Quebec, Canada, 1976.

Malkiel-Shapiro, B. "Further Observations on Parenteral Magnesium Sulphate Therapy in Coronary Heart Disease: A Clinical Appraisal." *South African Medical Journal*, December 20, 1958, pp. 1211-15.

Parsons, R. S.; Butler, T.; and Sellars, E. P. "The Treatment of Coronary Artery Disease with Parenteral Magnesium Sulphate." *Medical Proceedings*, November 14, 1959, pp. 487-98.

Seelig, Mildred S., and Haddy, Francis J. "Magnesium and the Arteries: I. Effects of Magnesium Deficiency on Arteries, and on the Retention of Sodium, Potassium, and Calcium. II. Physiologic Effects of Electrolyte Abnormalities on Arterial Resistance Dietary Magnesium Deficiency." Second International Symposium on Magnesium, University of Montreal, Quebec, Canada, 1976.

Niacin and Coronary Artery Disease

Anonymous. "Clofibrate and Niacin in Coronary Heart Disease." *Journal of the American Medical Association*, vol. 231, no. 4, January 27, 1975, pp. 360-81.

Eisen, Milton Earle. "Effect of Vitamin A, Niacin and Riboflavin on Vascular Lesions." *American Journal of Surgery*, vol. 95, March 1958, pp. 438–44.

Schlierf, G., and Hess, G. "Inhibition of Carbohydrate-Induced Hypertriglyceridemia by Nicotinic Acid." *Artery*, vol. 3, no. 2, April 1977, pp. 174–79.

Refined Sugar and Heart Disease

Ahrens, Richard A. "Sucrose, Hypertension, and Heart Disease: An Historical Perspective." *The American Journal of Clinical Nutrition*, vol. 27, April 1974, pp. 403–22.

Reiser, Sheldon. "Effect of Dietary Fiber on Parameters of Glucose Tolerance in Humans." Presented at the 176th ACS National Meeting, Florida, 1978.

Roberts, A. M. "Effects of a Sucrose-Free Diet on the Serum-Lipid Levels of Men in Antarctica." *The Lancet*, June 2, 1973, pp. 1201–4.

Selenium and Heart Disease

Shamberger, Raymond J. "Selenium in Health and Disease." Symposium on Selenium-Tellurium in the Environment, University of Notre Dame, Indiana, May 1976, pp. 253–67.

———. "Selenium and Heart Disease." *Executive Health*, March 1979.

Shamberger, Raymond J. et al. "Selenium and Other Trace Metal Intakes and Heart Disease in 25 Countries." Twelfth Annual Conference on Trace Substances in Environmental Health, Columbia, Missouri, 1978.

Vitamin C and Atherosclerosis

Ginter, Emil. "Cholesterol: Vitamin C Controls Its Transformation to Bile Acids." *Science*, February 16, 1973, pp. 702–4.

Sokoloff, Boris et al. "Aging, Atherosclerosis and Ascorbic Acid Metabolism." *Journal of the American Geriatrics Society*, vol. 14, no. 12, December 1966, pp. 1239–60.

Spittle, Constance R. "Atherosclerosis and Vitamin C." *The Lancet*, December 11, 1971, pp. 1280–81.

Turley, S. D.; West, C. E.; and Horton, B. J. "The Role of

Ascorbic Acid in the Regulation of Cholesterol Metabolism and in the Pathogenesis of Atherosclerosis." *Atherosclerosis,* vol. 24, 1976, pp. 1–18.

Verlangieri, Anthony J., and Bakos, Etel et al. "Influence of L-Ascorbic Acid on Aortic Mucopolysaccharides in Cholesterol-Induced Rabbit Atherosclerosis." *Federation Proceedings,* vol. 35, no. 3, March 1, 1976, p. 661.

Willis, G. C. "The Reversibility of Atherosclerosis." *Canadian Medical Association Journal,* vol. 77, July 15, 1957, pp. 106–9.

Willis, G. C.; Light, A. W.; and Gow, W. S. "Serial Arteriography in Atherosclerosis." *Canadian Medical Association Journal,* vol. 71, December 1954, pp. 562–68.

A woman with high blood pressure (164/114) and early diabetes is asked to go on a fairly "radical" diet: completely vegetarian, emphasizing raw foods. Exercise and vitamins are also prescribed. Eighteen months later, her blood pressure is down to 130/72, her blood sugar normal, and her weight lower as well.

13   A Case of Diabetes and High Blood Pressure

Stella Anders was in for a follow-up report and discussion of her physical exam, which she'd had done two to three weeks previously. She'd said when she came in that she had no specific problems she knew about, just "a feeling that I'd better get a checkup." Unfortunately, I had to let her know that her vague uneasy feeling had been correct: her examination and laboratory tests had turned up several problems.

"First, let's go over the things we discussed during your examination," I said. "Remember I mentioned your blood pressure was too high?"

"Yes, I think I told you it had been borderline for years even though I've been on a low-salt diet."

"It's more than borderline now. Your reading, which we rechecked, was 164/114. Any persistently elevated blood pressure over 140/90 is a potentially serious problem. Studies have shown a higher risk for strokes and heart attacks, and also for kidney problems."

"What do I do about it?"

"Before you do anything about it, we need to do two further things. We need to fit it into your overall health picture at present; second, further tests are needed to assess any signs of damage. Some of your blood and urine tests were for kidney function, since your blood pressure was high. Your blood tests were normal, but your urinalysis showed a trace of sugar."

"Sugar? Does that mean diabetes?"

"I'm afraid so. Remember what you told me about your family medical history?"

Mrs. Anders looked visibly more worried. During the medical history I'd taken at her last visit, she'd told me her grandmother had died of kidney failure, following a stroke and several heart attacks. She'd had diabetes and high blood pressure for several years. Mrs. Anders' mother, still alive after several strokes, was confined to a wheelchair.

"There's a chance of reversing this, isn't there?"

"I think so. It'll require a lot of work, though."

"That's just what I'll have to do. I don't want to spend my last years in a wheelchair."

"Let's go through the rest of your tests. Your triglyceride test was 220 (normal is 35 to 160). That often goes with diabetes, too.

"Your hair mineral analysis showed some problems. The chromium level was so low that the lab could scarcely find it. That's probably got a lot to do with your blood sugar problem. However, your test also shows a need for zinc, potassium, and manganese. It's a fairly typical pattern for diabetes.

"Lastly, let's go back over some other physical findings. You're five-foot-five and 152 pounds. . . ."

Mrs. Anders looked embarrassed. "I've been meaning to do something about my weight for years. I just haven't had proper motivation. I don't have any excuse now."

"Remember I said I'd like to get a little further information? Your urine sugar and your family history almost certainly add up to diabetes for you, but I want you to get a glucose tolerance test to see how bad it is. Your blood tests for kidney function were OK; I'd like to avoid kidney x-rays unless your blood pressure doesn't come down. Diabetes and hypertension are so frequently associated that we can be fairly sure you don't have a primary kidney problem causing hypertension. However, I would like you to get a stress electrocardiogram done in view of both the hypertension and diabetes. . . . Finally, I'd like you to get food allergy testing done."

"Skin tests?"

"No, those aren't very accurate for food allergies. They're fine for inhalants, pollens, dust, and so forth, but not nearly as good as blood testing for food allergies."

"Blood tests?"

"Yes, based on a radioactive assay for antibodies to specific foods."

"OK." She rose to go. "Should I get all those things scheduled right away?"

"As soon as you can. Please make an appointment for two to three weeks from now, when all the results should be back."

On Mrs. Anders' return, we went over her follow-up tests.

"Your treadmill electrocardiogram was normal, no sign of coronary artery disease. Unfortunately, your glucose tolerance test was worse than I suspected. The fasting level was 104; but from there it went to 336 and 312 at the first and second hours."

"What's normal?"

"Usually 160 and 140."

"Does that mean I need insulin?"

"No."

"How about those pills to lower blood sugar?"

"There's a lot of controversy about them. Some doctors think they cause more people to die of cardiovascular disease. Other doctors deny it."

"What do you think?"

"I ignore the whole thing, because synthetic drugs are totally unnecessary to control blood sugar. Proper diet, vitamins, and minerals will almost always do the job. In the few cases where it doesn't, particularly in juvenile-type diabetes, I recommend insulin. But your case will probably be similar to most maturity onset types, and not require it."

"That's good. What about my other test?"

I looked through her record for the allergy test results. "This will probably be a surprise to you. The antibody testing showed high levels of antibodies to corn and wheat. Those are probably the two most common food allergies."

"But I thought you had to have symptoms like hives, or sinus problems, or asthma to be allergic."

"Not at all. Some of the most unusual symptoms can be associated with food allergies. In some people, blood sugar problems can be partly a result of allergies."

"Well, I certainly seem to have enough causes for my diabetes. Not enough chromium or other minerals, overweight, maybe food allergies. . . . Now what about my high blood pressure?"

"Some of the same factors may be involved. Overweight certainly contributes. And Dr. Arthur Coca found years ago that some persons with hypertension had chronic undetected allergies. . . . So no corn or wheat by-products or derivatives, either. But before we discuss diet any further, I want to go over something else."

"What?"

"Exercise."

"For an old lady like me?"

"You're only 61. In some areas of the world, that's barely middle-aged. If you want the best chance of staying out of the wheelchair you mentioned, exercise is a key. Many studies have shown exercise to be important to reducing high blood pressure. You probably know that. You might not be aware that exercise also can improve carbohydrate tolerance."

"What kind of exercise?"

"Any sort of vigorous exercise; running, swimming, riding a bicycle. The important part is making up your mind to actually do it. Pick out an exercise you enjoy, so you'll be more likely to stick with it. A little common sense is necessary, too. If you haven't exercised in a long time, start with only a few minutes a day, and gradually increase. I'd like you to work toward from 45 minutes to one hour daily of vigorous exercise. It's not dangerous. Your treadmill test showed you can take it."

"Do I really need that much, though? It's hard to find the time."

"Then you should *make* the time."

"I know you're right. I'll work on it."

"Let's think about diet. With the diabetic problem, it'll of course be necessary to eliminate all refined sugars, refined carbohydrates, and processed foods. Following this, there are two basic approaches; the high-protein, controlled-carbohydrate type, or the raw-food, high complex-carbohydrate type of diet." [These diets are explained in some detail in chapter 17, "A Case of Palpitations."]

"What do you recommend?"

"Sometimes it comes down to a matter of individual lifestyle. But in your case, there's another consideration; your blood pressure. High-protein diets aren't usually helpful in blood pressure control. In fact, if you're really serious about getting your health problems under control as rapidly as possible, I'd recommend a fairly radical change from the type of diet you told me about."

"Radical change? What's that?"

"I'd suggest you consider the total elimination of all animal products from your diet. Fresh, raw vegetables and fruits should make up approximately 60 percent of your total food intake. For protein, you'd need to rely on unroasted nuts, seeds, and proper combinations of vegetable products."

"This, and all that exercise? Why don't you recommend climbing Mount Rainier to the top? Twice a week! Do you know how much of a change all this will be?"

"Yes, I do. Remember, I didn't tell you to do it, just to consider it. You're responsible for your own health, ultimately. I'm here only to make informed recommendations. The choice is up to you."

"I know. But why such a large change?"

"Because you have more than just a little high blood pressure, as well as diabetes. This is probably the best way to attack both. Many studies have shown that vegetarians have much lower blood pressures, as well as a much lower rate of heart attacks, strokes, certain types of cancer, and other health problems."

Mrs. Anders was back in two weeks. "Well, I went home and talked to Herbert. We decided there's no point growing older together without keeping our health as long as we can.

Herbert really surprised me. He decided to go on this program with me. He's had a borderline high blood pressure for a few years, too. He's decided to take up the exercise, too."

I was happy to hear that. If both Anders were adopting the program, they'd be more likely to stay with it.

"You told me you were taking vitamins B, C, and E. . . . I think I'd better give you a list. However, if you stick to the diet strictly, and have 60 percent raw foods, you won't need these as long as otherwise."

Mrs. Anders' list of supplements included her own vitamins, B, C, and E. In addition, her physical examination had shown a need for extra vitamin B_6. So I asked her to add on 50 milligrams, 3 times a day. For the chromium shown lacking on her mineral analysis, I asked her to use 2 tablespoons of brewer's yeast daily. I also asked her to obtain supplemental sources of zinc, potassium, and manganese, all shown lacking on her mineral test.

I suggested taking 2 tablespoons of vegetable oil daily, containing unsaturated fatty acids. Safflower, sunflower, soy, sesame, flaxseed; any of these or other vegetable oils would do. Much recent research indicates that unsaturated (or "essential") fatty acids can decrease both serum cholesterol and triglyceride levels, help reduce elevated blood pressure, and normalize many abnormal biochemical factors in diabetes (see Vergroesen).

"I'd like you to come in every 60 days or so for a blood pressure reading and an after-eating blood sugar test. If all goes well, we can stretch the intervals out later."

Mrs. Anders stuck to her diet and exercise plan rigidly. By the end of 18 months, her blood pressure was 130/72, "lower than in years." Her weight had come down to 128; her overall muscle tone and appearance were much better. Her two-hours-after-eating blood test for sugar returned to 120, perfectly normal.

At 18 months' time, she insisted on another glucose tolerance test. I pointed out that the refined sugar involved in the test wasn't good for her metabolism. She hadn't had any for a year and a half and it would likely make her feel ill.

Mrs. Anders replied that she knew all that, but for her own

satisfaction, she wanted an exact comparison. "It'll make me feel it's all been worth it," she said. "Besides," she said with a smile, "you're the one who told me I had to make my own health decisions. As long as it won't kill me or hurt me badly, I want it done."

I had to admit she had several good reasons for doing it. We were both pleased when this test, too, came out entirely normal.

⎯⎯⎯⬥⎯⎯⎯

Vegetarian diets are in fact healthier for most people. Many studies have confirmed the finding that there is much less hypertension, heart disease, stroke, gallbladder disease, and other disease including cancer in vegetarian populations.

So why don't I emphatically recommend vegetarianism for all of my patients if it's so much healthier?

As noted before, medicine is as much of an art as a science. What seems scientifically obvious isn't always easy to put into practice. Further, nutritional/biochemical medicine is as much a matter of culture change as it is applied science. For most people, radical change in any aspect of life is naturally resisted; small, stepwise changes are much more acceptable, particularly in such a personal matter as daily diet. Outside interference, even with the best intention, is likely to be resented, consciously or subconsciously.

For example, take Mr. Orville Henderson in chapter 12, "A Case of Heart Disease." The chances are great that if anyone had tried to alter his diet before he had his heart attack, even with clear proof of benefit, he wouldn't have done it. Ask Mrs. Henderson! In going over a recovery program with him following his heart attack, it became obvious that the changes I suggested were about as "radical" as he was willing to accept. Would vegetarianism have been better for him? Of course . . . but how helpful would it have been if he'd decided not to come back, because it was just "too much"?

On the other hand, Mrs. Anders's problems could be solved much more effectively by a vegetarian program than in any other way. In her case, whether she was ready for such a change or not, the only responsible approach was to present this alternative first. Fortunately for her, she accepted this idea. Unfortunately, more than half the people for whom vegetarianism is the best alternative solution for their health problems choose a different alternative, at least in my recent experience.

Are there dangers in a vegetarian diet? (Interestingly, I hear this question most from parents of teenagers who've suddenly decided to swear off meat.) The usual problems are three: vitamin B_{12}, iron, and protein. None of these problems is insurmountable.

Vitamin B_{12} is found almost exclusively in foods of animal origin. Lacto-ovo vegetarians, who eat eggs and dairy products have no problem. Of course there are vitamin B_{12} tablets, which should probably be used by all pregnant strict vegetarians.

It's sometimes difficult to obtain enough iron on a vegetarian diet; I've found a disproportionate number of anemic vegetarians. However, an awareness of this problem is usually enough to encourage the eating of spinach and other iron-containing foods.

The protein problem is not nearly as bad as imagined by most people who are used to eating meat. The solution lies in successful matching of foods with complementary protein patterns, such as corn and beans, or cereal grains and milk. This complementary amino acid matching creates more complete proteins, which are more useful to the human body.

Complementary protein matching is extremely well explained in the paperback *Diet for a Small Planet* by Frances Moore Lappé. High-complex carbohydrate and raw-food diets are becoming increasingly popular at university centers for diabetes control. While most of these programs aren't 100 percent vegetarian, they come close, and frequently represent an effective compromise between the average diet and vegetarianism.

For those who haven't encountered the term *complex carbohydrate*, this is just another way of saying unprocessed, unrefined vegetables, grains, and fruits, such as whole brown rice, other whole grains, unprocessed potatoes, and the whole range of vegetables and unjuiced fruits (juicing usually removes fiber and bulk).

So why can't university scientists just say "unprocessed, unrefined vegetables, cereal grains, and fruits" instead of the involved-sounding "high-complex carbohydrate diet"? I suspect the real, deep down reason is that they'd sound too much like us "health food nuts" . . . and we couldn't have that, could we? The term *simple carbohydrates* refers chiefly to sweeteners such as sucrose, corn syrup, or honey. Technically, refined carbohydrates such as white flour and corn grits are complex carbohydrates, but are not that much better than simple carbohydrates.

In case you're wondering, I do in fact recommend—gently—that vegetarianism is the healthiest dietary pattern for most people (there does seem to be a small minority who "can't get along," principally energy-wise, without some meat or fish) but I certainly don't insist on it, or get upset or bothered with people who choose to remain meat eaters. After all, as has been mentioned before, there's more to life than health, or trying to stay healthy, and we all are entitled to eat our way through life in any way we see fit.

FURTHER READING

Allergies and High Blood Pressure
Coca, Arthur F. *The Pulse Test: The Secret of Building Your Health* (New York: Lyle Stuart, 1967).

Carbohydrates and Blood Fat
Macdonald, I. "The Effects of Dietary Carbohydrates on High Density Lipoprotein Levels in Serum." *Nutrition Reports International*, vol. 17, no. 6, June 1978, pp. 663-68.

Singh, Inder. "Low-Fat Diet and Therapeutic Doses of Insulin in Diabetes Mellitus." *The Lancet*, February 26, 1955, pp. 422-25.

Carbohydrates and Diabetes
Himsworth, H. P. "High Carbohydrate Diets and Insulin Efficiency." *The British Medical Journal*, July 14, 1934, pp. 57-60.

Kiehm, Tae G.; Anderson, James W.; and Ward, Kyleen.

"Beneficial Effects of a High Carbohydrate, High Fiber Diet on Hyperglycemic Diabetic Men." *The American Journal of Clinical Nutrition*, vol. 29, no. 8, August 1976, pp. 895-99.

Trowell, H. C. "Dietary-Fiber Hypothesis of the Etiology of Diabetes Mellitus." *Diabetes*, vol. 24, no. 8, August 1975, pp. 762-65.

Chromium

Boyle, Edwin; Mondschein, Benjamin; and Dash, Harriman H. "Chromium Depletion in the Pathogenesis of Diabetes and Atherosclerosis." *Southern Medical Journal*, vol. 70, no. 12, December 1977, pp. 1449-53.

Pal, B., and Mukherjee, S. "Chromium in Nutrition." *Journal of Applied Nutrition*, vol. 30, no. 1 & 2, 1978, pp. 14-27.

Tuman, Robert W.; Bilbo, James T.; and Doisy, Richard J. "Comparison and Effects of Natural and Synthetic Glucose Tolerance Factor in Normal and Genetically Diabetic Mice." *Diabetes*, vol. 27, no. 1, January 1978, pp. 49-56.

Wise, A. "Chromium Supplementation and Diabetes." *Journal of the American Medical Association*, vol. 240, no. 19, November 3, 1978, pp. 2045-46.

Essential Fatty Acids

Vergroesen, Antoine J. "Physiological Effects of Dietary Linoleic Acid." *Nutrition Reviews*, vol. 35, no. 1, January 1977, pp. 1-5.

Raw Foods and Diabetes

Douglass, John M. "Raw Diet and Insulin Requirements." *Annals of Internal Medicine*, vol. 82, 1975, pp. 61-63.

Douglass, John, and Rasgon, Irving. "Diet and Diabetes." *The Lancet*, vol. 2, no. 7,998, December 11, 1976, pp. 1306-07.

Vegetarianism

Anholm, Anne C. "The Relationship of a Vegetarian Diet to Blood Pressure." *Preventive Medicine*, vol. 7, no. 1, March 1978, p. 35.

Anonymous. "Vegetarian Diet and Vitamin B_{12} Deficiency."

Nutrition Reviews, vol. 36, no. 8, August 1978, pp. 243-44.

Burslem, John et al. "Plasma Apoprotein and Lipoprotein Lipid Levels in Vegetarians." *Metabolism,* vol. 27, no. 6, June 1978, pp. 711-19.

Chang, Mei Ling W., and Johnson, Margaret A. "Effect of Dietary Vegetable and Type of Carbohydrate on Lipid Metabolism in Rats." *Nutrition Reports International,* vol. 18, no. 3, September 1978, pp. 337-44.

Ellis, F. R., and Sanders, T. A. B. "Angina and Vegan Diet." *American Heart Journal,* vol. 93, no. 6, June 1977, pp. 803-5.

Ellis, F. R.; West, E. D.; and Sanders, T. A. B. "The Health of Vegans Compared with Omnivores: Assessment by Health Questionnaire." *Plant Foods for Man,* vol. 2, 1976, pp. 43-52.

Frader, Joel; Reibman, Bonnie; and Turkewitz, David. "Vitamin B_{12} Deficiency and Strict Vegetarians." *New England Journal of Medicine,* vol. 299, no. 23, December 7, 1978, p. 1319.

Lappé, Frances Moore. *Diet for a Small Planet* (New York: Ballantine Books, 1975).

Phillips, Roland L. et al. "Coronary Heart Disease Mortality Among Seventh-Day Adventists with Differing Dietary Habits: A Preliminary Report." *The American Journal of Clinical Nutrition,* vol. 31, no. 10, October 1978, pp. S191-S198.

Sanders, T. A. B., and Ellis, F. R. "Serum Cholesterol and Triglycerides Concentrations in Vegans." *Proceedings of the Nutrition Society,* vol. 36, no. 1, May 1977, p. 43A.

Scharffenberg, J. A. "Diet, Serum Cholesterol, and Heart Disease." Paper presented at the American Association for the Advancement of Science Meeting, February 15, 1977, in Washington, D.C.

The patient has two distinct problems. The first is bursitis. For this condition, shots of B_{12} and several supplements are recommended. The second condition involves a fibrous ridge of tissue on the hand, which proves to respond well to very high doses of vitamin E.

A Case of Bursitis and Dupuytren's Contracture

14

It was obvious from the way Mr. Karpovitch walked that he was in pain. He held his right arm close to his side, and moved his shoulder very stiffly.

Before I could say anything, he informed me what the problem was.

"It's just my old bursitis acting up again," he said. "I couldn't get it to go away with heat packs and aspirin, so I came in for a phenylbutazone prescription. That always takes it away in three or four days."

Mr. Karpovitch had been in before, but not about bursitis, or for an overall history and physical exam. So his bursitis was a surprise to me.

"You've had it before, then?"

"Yes, so many times I've really lost track. Lots of times I get rid of it by taking a day or two off work, resting, and taking lots of aspirin and vitamin C. I usually put on hot packs, too. Sometimes it won't go away with that, so I need a prescription. That's happened six or seven times now. But it goes away after that."

"Since you haven't been in before for your bursitis, do you mind if I have a look at it? There may be something else to do for it, with fewer potential side effects."

"Side effects? What do you mean?"

"The drug you mentioned is a very powerful anti-inflammatory drug. Like all other drugs of its type, it can cause upset stomach, gastrointestinal bleeding, even ulcers. It also can cause blood cell problems; the list of side effects is a long one."

"Is that why they always told me to take it with milk or food?"

"Yes. That helps prevent some of the stomach problems."

"I didn't know it was so serious."

"Potentially, yes. If you know about the problems and guard against them, in actual practice, the complication rate seems low. I've prescribed this type of drug in the past when nothing else worked. After all, even if it is a potentially toxic drug, if nothing else would get you better, then I would use it with proper precautions."

Mr. Karpovitch could move his right arm forward until it was nearly level with his shoulder. He could also move it to the rear. Each time he was stopped by pain. The most painful motion was to the side; he couldn't get his arm even close to shoulder level. Just the effort brought a grimace of pain.

"I had to shave with my left hand this morning," he said. Three small Band-Aids attested to this unusual effort.

"I'm sorry, but I'm going to have to poke at your shoulder to find the painful area."

"I figured as much. One doctor did that so he could put a shot of cortisone into it. Is that what you're going to do?" he asked.

"Not that either."

The most painful spot in his shoulder was right at and below the "point." Other areas were a little tender, but most seemed to radiate from the extremely sore central location. It appeared to be a typical subdeltoid or subacromial bursitis.

"Have you ever had an x-ray of your shoulder?"

"Ten years ago. Didn't show anything. Bursitis doesn't show up on x-rays, does it?"

"Not usually. When it gets calcified, you can see the calcium, though. With the number of episodes you've had, you might have calcifications by now."

"Do you want me to get an x-ray?"

"I think so. But you can start treatment before then."

"That's good. Can I get my shirt back on?"

"Just a minute. Let me see your hands." I thought I'd seen something in the palms of both hands.

He held them out. "Turn your hands over, please."

When Mr. Karpovitch turned his hands palms up, another problem was perfectly apparent. Each palm had a distinctive ridge of fibrous tissue extending from the base of the fourth finger back into the palm of the hand, following the line of the tendon. The one on the right was much worse than the left. It was about $2\frac{1}{2}$ inches long, and $\frac{3}{4}$ inch wide at the midpoint. The thickening was very dense, and his fourth finger was beginning to be pulled downward toward his palm. On the left a similar ridge was just getting started. In medical terms, such dense ridges of tissue are called Dupuytren's contractures.

"How long have you had those? You've never mentioned them."

"I didn't think there was anything you could do. My father had them, too, and finally had to go get them operated on. I was just waiting for mine to get bad enough. The one on the right's been there for about six years. It's gotten much worse in the past year or two; about the same time the other one was getting started. Do they have something to do with bursitis?"

"No direct connection that I know about. But there is a natural treatment that usually dissolves them, and helps bursitis a little bit, too. Why don't you put your shirt back on, come back to my office, and we'll go over treatment for both problems."

When Mr. Karpovitch was seated again, I said, "Let's go over your bursitis first, as that's more acute. Do you think you can learn to give yourself injections?"

"I knew there was a catch. Injections of what? Why can't I come in here to get them?"

"Injections of vitamin B_{12}. You could come in here to get them, but it would be much less expensive for you, and more convenient to give them to yourself. You see, you need 1,000 micrograms—one cubic centimeter—a day for 10 to 14 days. Then you start to taper off slowly."

"That's a lot of shots! Why can't I take vitamin B_{12} pills?"

"They just don't work as well as injections. Vitamin B_{12} is a difficult vitamin to absorb sometimes."

"How fast does it work?"

"Not quite as fast as the phenylbutazone usually does. Pain relief ordinarily starts between the first and second days; pain is usually gone in five to ten days. However, the vitamin B_{12} is more sure. Once the pain is gone, it stays gone, and doesn't recur as soon as treatment stops. That happens sometimes with anti-inflammatory drugs."

I wrote Mr. Karpovitch a prescription for enough vitamin B_{12} to last two weeks, and asked him to see the nurse for instruction in self-injection before he left.

"There are two other things I'd like you to take for the bursitis. One is vitamin C, as you already mentioned. That's for its general anti-inflammatory properties. I'd like you to use 2 grams, 4 times a day. Cut back only if it gives you gas.

"Also, I'd like you to get some dolomite tablets. I've found that most people with bursitis need either calcium or magnesium, or both. Dolomite is an excellent, inexpensive source. Please use 3 tablets, 2 times a day."

"You want me to take calcium even though I might have calcifications?"

"Yes, more often than not, it's needed. To find out for sure, I'd like you to get a mineral analysis done, using a piece of hair."

"I've heard of those. Wanted to get one done before now, but this is as good a time as any. Is that everything? How about vitamin E?"

"For bursitis in the acute phase, 800 to 1,200 units daily is a good idea. Sometimes even more help comes from higher doses. But I was coming to vitamin E, as that's also the treatment for your Dupuytren's contractures."

"It is? But I've been using 200 units a day for nearly six months, and nothing's happened."

"That's not nearly enough. I've never seen Dupuytren's contractures go away with anything less than 3,000 units daily. To be on the safe side, I usually recommend 2,000 units, twice daily. This type of treatment takes persistence. Usually results don't even begin to show for four to six months. I know of one case that took nearly a year to begin to get results. Once it starts to work, though, the contractures are usually gone in a year or two. Very advanced ones sometimes don't clear completely."

"How do I know when it starts to work?"

"The fibrous tissue becomes much softer, more pliable. Once it does, start to work it as much as you can. This will help, too."

"That's good news. I wasn't looking forward to an operation." He paused. "Let's see if I've got all this: the main treatment for my bursitis is vitamin B_{12} shots every day. The vitamin C and dolomite help it out. The vitamin E, 2,000 units, twice a day— that's a lot—is for the contractures, and will help the bursitis, too. Is that all?"

"Yes. Remember I want you to get your shoulder x-rayed, and a mineral analysis."

"I'll do those both today. When should I come back?"

"In a week. But call back sooner if your shoulder doesn't begin to improve."

The first thing Mr. Karpovitch did on his return was to swing his right arm in all directions. "Look at that," he said. "That B_{12} worked faster than you said. The pain started to go away in the middle of the night after I left here and was completely gone in five days. Why didn't you say it could work that fast? Can I stop taking those shots now?"

"I didn't say it would work that fast because it usually is a little slower. But I'm happy it went faster for you. Don't stop the shots yet; in fact, I'd like you to continue for several months. Of course, not every day. You see, your x-ray showed calcification in the area of the bursa."

"But why do I have to continue these injections if the pain's gone?"

"Because I'd like you to get the calcification gone, too."

"You mean it goes away?"

"Very frequently. But it takes months to a year or two. Meanwhile, I want you to take daily injections for another week. Then taper to 3 a week, 2 a week, 1 a week, and maintain at 1 every two weeks for at least six months.

"You can reduce the vitamin C to 2 or 3 grams daily now that your bursitis pain is gone. I'll need to look at your mineral analysis before changing the dolomite, though. It hasn't returned from the laboratory yet; it probably will take another week. Call in and ask the nurse, please."

"Fine. Sure am glad that bursitis pain is gone. You know, I've heard of heat and aspirin treatment, cortisone injections, short-wave treatments, phenylbutazone and other drugs, but I never heard of vitamin B_{12} treatment. Is that something new?"

As is all too frequent with vitamin treatment, I had to explain that it wasn't new, just neglected. "No, it's not new. As far as I know, it was originally described by I. S. Klemes, M.D., in 1953 and later in 1957 in *Industrial Medicine and Surgery*. His reports cover nearly 60 cases, and it worked in all but 3. I've only seen it fail once, myself."

"That's good enough for me. When should I come back?"

"Six months. Don't forget to call about the dolomite dose."

When Mr. Karpovitch's mineral analysis arrived, it showed extremely low levels of calcium and magnesium. Since this is so frequently associated with insufficient vitamin D intake, I asked the nurse to have him add 2,000 units of natural vitamin D daily, and continue the dolomite dose the same.

In six months his x-ray showed a beginning resorption of the calcium in his shoulder. I asked him to continue treatment, and to get x-rays every 6 months. At the third interval, 18 months, the calcium was completely gone. Of course, he'd had no recurrence of symptoms. At this point, I asked him to cut back to mainte-nance of 1 cubic centimeter of vitamin B_{12} every 60 days, and 2 dolomite tablets daily, as his mineral analysis was much improved. Vitamin D was cut back to 800 units daily.

Five months after starting vitamin E treatment, Mr. Karpovitch phoned in to say that his Dupuytren's contractures had definitely softened. He of course continued his vitamin E, and at the time of this writing, after three years' treatment, his left hand has been completely clear for over a year. The right palm contracture is down to $1\frac{1}{4}$ by $\frac{1}{4}$ inch and is entirely flexible.

As stated above, I know of no direct connection between bursitis and Dupuytren's contracture. That they both occurred coincidentally in this patient is somewhat unusual.

Most bursitis doesn't become calcified. The cases that do, like Mr. Karpovitch's, tend to be chronic, and more severe than others. Beyond these observations, there is no explanation of why calcification happens. The consensus of nutritional/biochemical opinion is that it isn't caused by excess calcium; in fact, frequently calcium deficiency is found, as in this case. Magnesium deficiency is also suspected of being a factor. It's my opinion (but I have no proof) that changes in the body's natural electrical field, localized in the shoulder, are also involved.

The relationship of vitamin B_{12} to calcification, or rather to clearing it up, is a mystery. The observed results are clinical; the biochemistry is unknown.

I should add that most of my patients with uncalcified bursitis are helped by injected vitamin B_{12}, on the same schedule as in this case. Several of them "ward off" the bursitis with their own individual maintenance schedule.

Aside from Dr. Klemes's report, I've seen no other reference to treatment of bursitis with vitamin B_{12}.

After this case report appeared originally in print, observant readers wrote in to say I'd not mentioned the possible effect of vitamin E on hypertension. That was a valid criticism, so I should say a little more about it. No less an authority than Wilfred Shute, M.D., one of the developers of vitamin E therapy, has pointed out that in a few persons with uncontrolled hypertension, as little as 200 to 400 units can elevate the blood pressure. It should be reemphasized that this happens in a very small number of all those with hypertension or a tendency toward it, not everyone with hypertension.

Even so, persons with this problem and especially their physicians should be aware of the possibility. This and many other details of vitamin E treatment can be found in Dr. Shute's recent book listed below.

It's been noted by an astute clinician that more than 90 percent of persons with Dupuytren's contracture have abnormal glucose tolerance tests (see Leake). I've found this to be so; however, Mr. Karpovitch, when tested later on, turned out to be one of the minority without that abnormality.

FURTHER READING

Dupuytren's Contracture
Gibson, H. R. B. "Dupuytren's Contracture." *British Medical Journal*, vol. 2, August 23, 1952, p. 446.

Leake, Chauncey D. "New Sign for Incipient Diabetes." *Geriatrics*, vol. 23, October 1968, p. 92.

Ross, James A. "Dupuytren's Contracture," *British Medical Journal*, July 26, 1952, p. 232.

Shute, Evan. "Scar Tissue and Collagenosis." *The Heart and Vitamin E* (New Canaan, Conn.: Keats Publishing, 1977), p. 125.

Vitamin B$_{12}$
Klemes, I. S. "Vitamin B$_{12}$ in Acute Subdeltoid Bursitis." *Industrial Medicine and Surgery*, June 1957, pp. 290–92.

Vitamin E
Shute, Wilfrid E. *Dr. Wilfrid E. Shute's Complete Updated Vitamin E Book* (New Canaan, Conn.: Keats Publishing, 1975).
———. *Health Preserver: Defining the Versatility of Vitamin E* (Emmaus, Pa.: Rodale Press, 1977).

A woman has been on prolonged medication for repeated infection and irritation of the bladder and urethra. At the same time, she has chronic diarrhea, which she'd been told was not related to her other problem. Tests having ruled out anything more serious than a urethra which may be too small, the patient goes on a fast to see if symptoms subside. Subsequent blood tests pinpoint a number of foods which are causing her bladder irritation. The bowel problem, a result of antibiotics, disappears with *Lactobacillus acidophilus* treatment.

A Case of Chronic Bladder Irritation and Bowel Upset

15

"Basically, I have only two problem areas," Mrs. Arends said. "My bowels and my bladder. If one isn't acting up, the other is. It's been going on for years like that, so I really don't have much hope for a permanent cure, but I thought maybe you could tell me some better way to control it than these. I hate to be taking drugs all the time."

She put three prescription bottles on my desk. One was for an antidiarrheal medication; the second, a painkiller for the urinary tract; the third, an antibacterial frequently used for urinary tract infections.

"How long have you been taking these prescriptions?"

"Fifteen years or so—of course, not these same exact medications. I haven't been taking this one (she indicated the antidiarrheal) as long as the others, since I didn't start having bowel trouble until two or three years after the bladder trouble started."

"Why don't we start at the beginning: what kind of bladder problem have you been having? When did this start?"

"Just after I got married; I was 23. I'm 38 now. I got a terrific bladder infection. The doctor said that was very common for just getting married. He even called it 'honeymoon cystitis,' or something like that. He gave me a prescription for a sulfa drug. The infection went away, and everything was fine, I thought.

"That first year I had 5 bladder infections. Actually, I've had so many over the years that I lost track after counting 20 or so. I've been through every antibiotic in the book.

"Not only that, but after two or three years, I started getting what the urologist calls a bladder and urethral irritation. It's hardly left me ever since. Most of the time, when I urinate, it hurts. I have to go eight or ten times a day; lots of times when I do, there's nothing there. Sometimes I burn a little, sometimes a lot. Every once in a while it's pain-free, but only for a few days. Then it's back again. Lately, the burning has been all the time."

"The burning doesn't come from infections?"

"Oh, no, that's a different kind of burning. It took me a little while to learn that. When I was younger, I used to rush to the doctor every time I had pain. My husband threatened to buy a house near the doctor's office so I could just go over there to the bathroom. But with this kind of burning, the urine tests always came out negative. No pus cells, no bacteria. So after a while, I learned which kind of burning was infection, and which was just, well, burning.

"That's why I take this," she said, indicating the painkiller. "I try to take it as little as possible, but when the pain gets bad, or I just get tired of it, I do use it. I was worried I'd get addicted, but the doctor said no, it was just for urinary tract pain, and not addicting."

"You can always tell when you have an infection, then?"

"Oh, yes. I've almost quit going in for tests. I was right every time for three or four years. Even one time when the laboratory said I didn't, I made them check again, and they'd made a mistake. So, finally, my doctor said it was just a waste of my time and money to keep coming in, I should just phone in when I needed a prescription."

"You saw a urologist and had tests?"

"Oh, of course. I've had my kidneys x-rayed twice. My urologist has looked up into my bladder with that little tube lots of times. The only thing he ever found the matter was that my bladder looked irritated. I could have told him that without even looking!

"Right now, I'm getting dilated every few weeks. That does seem to help a little. The urologist says my urethra's too small."

I made a few notes. "Now, what about the bowel problem?"

"I don't really know if it's a problem or not. Sometimes I think it's just nerves, because I *am* tense about this bladder thing. But until I got this prescription (she indicated the antidiarrheal) it really made traveling or just leaving home for a few hours difficult. Mostly, I get sort of a diarrhea; not really, but very loose. Some days I have to go six or seven times: that always seems to happen during trips. Other days I don't go at all, although that's much less often."

"Is there any bleeding, pain, or any other symptom?"

"No, just the diarrhea and occasional constipation. I've had upper and lower x-rays and even been checked with that awful long tube. I'll never do that again! But it was all normal. So when it gets bad, I just take the medicine. But I try to keep that to a minimum, too."

"When did you say you started having bowel problems?"

"When I was 25 or 26; two or three years after I started having bladder trouble. I've always thought there must be some connection, but the doctors said there wasn't. Do you think there might be?"

"Possibly. Let me ask you a few more questions. Have you had a vaginal discharge or infection?"

"Oh, yes, I've had a little yeast infection for years. But it really doesn't bother me much. A gynecologist I saw once said some women just have them chronically, that if the symptoms weren't too bad just to ignore it. Of course, he pointed out that with all the antibiotics I have to take for my bladder it's not too much of a surprise. So I really don't pay any attention to it anymore. It's just there along with the bladder and bowel problems. . . . It seems like nothing down south there works quite right."

"How's your health otherwise?"

"Good, I think. Well, I'm tired a lot and get a headache now and then, but I don't really think those are health problems."

"Does anyone in your family have allergies?"

"My son has a little hay fever. Let me think . . . my father had asthma as a child, but that went away, and he hasn't been bothered for years. What's that got to do with me, though? I've never had any allergy problems."

"Maybe, or maybe you don't know you do. One of the first things to check when a person keeps getting infections is allergy."

"I've never heard of an allergic bladder."

"It certainly happens. Any organ in the body can react in an allergic way. Some people even have brain and nervous system allergy. But that's getting away from your problem. Since you've had all the other usual tests, why don't we check that?"

"I'm willing to try anything if you think it might help. How do we check?"

"There are several different ways . . . skin tests, blood tests, pulse testing. . . . But before you do any of that, I'd like you to think about trying a very basic sort of self-test for food allergies: fasting."

"I've done that before. It didn't seem to change anything."

"How long did you fast?"

"A day or two."

"That's not nearly long enough. I think you have food allergies; bladder allergy is usually to food. So, to tell if food is bothering you or not, the simplest and cheapest way is to not eat. Unfortunately, it usually takes four to six days to make a reliable decision. The first day or two, symptoms frequently get worse; but if your symptoms clear up and leave on the last days of the fast, it's usually a very clear indication of food allergy. Actually, this applies to any food-allergy-caused symptoms, not just bladder problems."

"I can see how that might tell about foods in general, but how does it tell which foods are the problem?"

"It doesn't. But frequently if you come off the fast carefully, one food at a time, with plenty of time between each food, you can find out which ones cause symptoms. Remember, though, there are other ways of testing for allergies. Fasting, especially for four to six days, isn't easy. It really shouldn't be done at all by some people."

"I think I'd like to try: I could stand to lose some weight anyway. But . . . couldn't it take a long time, just weeks to figure out which foods are problems by only eating one at a time? If something does cause symptoms, don't you have to wait until the symptoms go away before trying anything else? Otherwise, you'd get confused. What if the symptoms don't go away for two or three days? I could spend from now until Christmas just checking foods for allergic symptoms!"

"Those are some of the drawbacks to that system, although it usually isn't that bad. I've seen some people do it very successfully. Another option is to combine methods. Since extensive food-allergy testing is relatively expensive, why not see if you have food allergies at all by fasting, and then if your symptoms do clear after three to five days, and stay gone until you start to eat again, then get the standard testing done. That way, you could be more sure the money spent would be worth it."

Mrs. Arends thought for a minute. "That makes sense. . . . I just have water, right?"

"Distilled water. Some people are bothered by chlorine, fluoride, or other things in the water."

"I think I'll do it. Then what kind of testing do we do if it works?"

"I prefer to do blood testing, the radioallergosorbent test, RAST for short. It's the simplest and I've found it quite reliable."

"Good. Let's do it." Mrs. Arends got up to go; then she sat down again. "I almost forgot. What about this bowel problem? Do you think that's allergy too?"

"It could be, but more likely it's caused by the same thing that's caused your yeast infection . . . antibiotic therapy. Has anyone ever advised you to take *Lactobacillus acidophilus* when you take antibiotics?"

"No, what's that?"

Lactobacillus acidophilus bacteria are among those used to make home yogurt, buttermilk, and other sour milk products. They're also vital to restoring your internal body ecology to normal. When you take antibiotics, they kill the germs you don't want . . . in your case the infectious ones in your bladder. But they also kill many perfectly normal, in fact indispensable, bacteria that live in all of our intestines. These friendly bacteria help digest food for us, produce essential vitamins, and help keep bowel function normal. If they're not replaced, symptoms such as yours occur frequently, particularly with repeated courses of antibiotics.

"But whether you have symptoms or not, anytime you take any antibiotics for any reason they should always be followed by an *acidophilus* 'chaser.' *Acidophilus* won't interfere with the antibiotics, and will help keep your internal body ecology normal."

I advised Mrs. Arends to take a tablespoon of *Lactobacillus acidophilus* suspension, or 3 or 4 capsules, twice daily for at least two to three weeks in view of the length of time she'd had her problem.

I also gave her a printed outline of a "yogurt/*Lactobacillus acidophilus*" treatment for her yeast infection, described in chapter 43, "Surviving Drug Therapy."

She looked skeptical. "I can believe my bladder problem might be allergy," she said. "But are you sure the rest is as obvious as that? Why didn't someone tell me before? That's an awfully simple answer."

"Elementary, my dear Watson. . . . What I mean is, it all depends on your perspective. From the point of view of body ecology, it seems obvious. . . . However, nothing's proven until it's tried. I may be wrong, but it can't hurt. Try it and see."

Mrs. Arends did; her bowel symptoms and chronic yeast problem cleared up after two to three weeks.

More important, she found that on the third, fourth, and fifth days of her fast the burning when she urinated completely disappeared. Her urination decreased to three to four times daily. Her tiredness disappeared (a frequent result when intake of allergenic food is stopped).

Subsequent food-allergy testing disclosed she was allergic to milk, eggs, tomatoes, peppers, oranges, and bananas. As long as she didn't eat these foods, her symptoms disappeared. She has had no further bladder infections.

A woman in the last weeks of pregnancy has begun to retain large amounts of water. Her blood pressure is also rising, and tests show there is protein in her urine. While her regular obstetrician monitors her progress, she is told to eat more protein and take magnesium and vitamin B_6 among other things. The threatened state of toxemia is averted; she sheds the water she's retained, and has a healthy delivery. . . . With a special note on why toxemia of pregnancy has not yet been eradicated.

16 A Case of Preeclampsia (Early Toxemia of Pregnancy)

Preeclampsia is a name given to the first stages of a problem which is also called toxemia of pregnancy. The symptoms of preeclampsia are unusual weight gain, rising blood pressure, and protein found in the urine, all associated with edema (water retention). Early detection of preeclampsia is one of the main tasks of routine prenatal care. That is why any prenatal visit to the doctor involves being weighed and having a urine specimen and blood pressure reading taken.

As might be guessed from the name *preeclampsia*, it is only the first stage of the problem. If untreated, it can proceed to eclampsia. In this stage, symptoms worsen, and the pregnant mother goes into convulsions and/or coma. Although in recent years the mortality rate for both mothers and babies from eclampsia has dropped, it has not yet been eliminated. Since much of the evidence showing how to prevent toxemia dates back to the 1930s, it appears to me that the conquest of this health problem is long past due.

On an unusually hot day for the Seattle area, with the temperature in the nineties, Barbara Morton appeared at the office. She hadn't been in for over a year, and had come in on a semi-emergency basis for a problem with her pregnancy. I'd not even known she was pregnant. When she first called I'd advised that she check back with her regular obstetrician, who would be more familiar with her recent medical history than I. However, her mother, also a patient of mine, called in to say that the obstetrician had advised there was nothing further he could do at present. Barbara's mother, Mrs. Johnson, was quite sure that nutrition had something to do with her daughter's problem. So we made the appointment.

Barbara and her mother came in together. Although Barbara was 23, married for two years, and had been away from home since age 17, she and her mother were close. In fact, Mrs. Johnson's degree of worry was much greater than her daughter's.

"I'm sorry to have been so pushy about this," Mrs. Johnson said, "but I don't think Barbara realizes how much of a problem she has, or how bad it can get. I keep telling her I lost my first baby this way, and nearly died myself. She doesn't realize how quickly things can go bad."

"It's not that I'm not worried, Mom," Barbara replied. "It's just that with, well, more modern treatment methods. . . ."

"Treatment methods aren't any better than they were when I lost my baby," declared Mrs. Johnson. "At least, most places. I know; I've been keeping track."

"Before we do anything about treatment, let's have a look at the problem," I said, trying to fit a word in.

Mrs. Johnson looked surprised. "Isn't it obvious what the problem is? Look at her ankles; like regular balloons. And her hands are so puffy you can't see the tendons, and under her eyes. . . . It looks exactly like that toxemia I had way back then!"

"Let's get some background first," I replied. "Barbara, when is the baby due?"

"September eighth."

"Are you sure of that?"

"Yes, as much as I can be. I got pregnant the first month after I stopped my birth-control pills. I know that's not good, but. . . ." She stopped.

"Is this your first pregnancy?"

"Of course it is!" her mother answered. "I raised all my girls right."

"Mother! I'm sure the doctor isn't interested."

"I just wanted him to know."

"Let's get back to Barbara's problem. Let's see . . . that means you have about six weeks left."

"Yes, thank goodness."

"When did this swelling start?"

"A little bit, two weeks ago. I noticed my ankles were a little puffy. But it really got bad this week. I've gained 8½ pounds in the past seven days. My obstetrician really got upset about that, but he was worried before then, too."

"Why?"

"Well, my usual blood pressure the first few months was about 110/60. But three or four weeks ago, he said it was starting to go up. It's been going up slowly ever since. I had it checked two days ago; it was 140/96. Is that really bad high blood pressure?"

"It's not really very high for a single blood pressure reading. But when you're at this stage of pregnancy, and your usual blood pressure is 110/60, then it's much too high."

"See, I told you!" Mrs. Johnson said.

"Do you remember any problems with your urinalysis?" I asked.

"This week, the doctor said there were some traces of protein in my urine." Barbara suddenly looked more worried. "He said if my blood pressure and fluid got a lot worse, he might have to give me diuretics. He says he doesn't usually like to do that; there's more evidence diuretics aren't good. But sometimes there's nothing else to do to stop it from getting worse."

"Nothing else to do! That's nonsense!" Mrs. Johnson declared. "I've been reading about some doctors—a Dr. Tom Brewer especially—who say that preventing toxemia is just a matter of proper nutrition. Tell Dr. Wright what you eat, Barbara!"

"Mother. . . ."

"It is important, Barbara. As long as we're talking about it anyway, why don't you, please?" I said.

Barbara looked a little defensive. "I've been following all the good nutrition rules you told me about. So has David. We've decided we're going to have good nutrition in our family from the start. We don't eat any sugar or white bread. Since I quit work when I got pregnant, I buy hardly any canned or packaged things anymore. Everything is fresh or frozen, and I make my own bread."

"Can you tell me specifically the type of things you eat every day?"

"For breakfast, I have whole wheat toast and tea, herb tea. At lunch, I have a sandwich with whole wheat bread, usually sprouts and bacon and tomato, or a little peanut butter. For dinner, some nights we have raw or steamed vegetables, and fresh fruit. Other nights, fish or chicken and rice and vegetables. We're trying to stay away from beef and heavy, red-type meat. They seem to be bad for the health. . . ."

"Barbara, your diet has been quite good at avoiding all the foods you shouldn't eat. But it sounds like you are short on protein. What about eggs, cheese, nuts, seeds?"

"I stopped eating eggs because they made me sick to my stomach when I first got pregnant. I haven't tried them since. I never have been much of a cheese eater. Is protein very important?"

"Extremely so, for prevention of toxemia problems. As far back as 1935, a lack of sufficient protein in the diet was linked to an increased incidence of toxemia by Dr. Maurice Strauss of Harvard University. This observation has been repeated over and over since then. Women with toxemia of any degree sometimes have lower serum albumin levels. And this type of protein in the bloodstream is necessary to keep fluid from leaking into the tissues, where it's called edema. The less serum albumin, the greater the tendency to edema."

"Why does that make my blood pressure go up?"

"That's not been worked out, step by step. But increased protein isn't the only answer."

"So I don't just go home and eat more protein?"

"Not at this point. With an extra 8½ pounds of fluid this week, and your blood pressure going up, we'd better do some other things, too. First, let's check your weight, blood pressure, and urine once more."

The results weren't encouraging. Barbara's weight was 158 (she was five-foot-two). Her blood pressure was 142/100. Her urine showed traces of protein.

I asked Barbara if she was taking any vitamins for her pregnancy.

"Well, my prenatal multiple vitamin with folic acid. And my obstetrician has me taking calcium and iron."

"Anything else?"

"No, except when my blood pressure kept going up, he told me to watch the salt. But that hasn't helped."

"Didn't think it would," her mother said. "They told me that, too. No vitamins but calcium and iron—don't know what they're thinking about!"

"It'll take weeks for more protein to really start working, won't it?" Barbara asked. "Am I going to have to take 'water pills' in the meantime?"

"No! Those should never be used. There are two nutrients that will help with that, and rapidly. It's not certain why, but they're probably more closely related to the cause of toxemia in the first place. These two nutrients are magnesium and pyridoxine—also called vitamin B_6."

"Magnesium? That's what they gave me when I had convulsions with the baby I lost. Is Barbara that bad?" Mrs. Johnson was very agitated.

"It's not a matter of that bad. It's likely that if she'd had a little more magnesium all along, she wouldn't have as much of a problem now. In other words, magnesium and pyridoxine are probably part of the prevention of the problem, as well as the cure."

"Do I take vitamin B_6 and magnesium then?"

"Yes. But since your blood pressure is up as high as it is, and you have so much fluid, I think we'd better give you an injection or two, also."

"Is it dangerous for the baby?"

"I've never observed it to do any harm. This treatment is described by Dr. John Ellis in his book, *Vitamin B₆: The Doctor's Report*. Dr. Ellis has used it in many more cases than I, and has also not observed ill effects."

I asked the nurse to give Barbara 10 cubic centimeters of 2 percent magnesium chloride (200 milligrams total) and 6 cubic centimeters of pyridoxine (600 milligrams) intravenously. I also asked Barbara to raise her daily protein intake to 100 to 150 grams daily, and to use 200 milligrams of pyridoxine 4 times a day, along with 500 milligrams of magnesium oxide 3 times a day, for now.

"Isn't that an awful lot of vitamin B₆ and magnesium?" Barbara asked.

"Yes, it is. But it's what's needed, and won't hurt. Later, you'll probably be able to cut back. If you get any diarrhea, then cut back the magnesium. Also, for reasons of stress, I'd like you to use extra B complex and vitamin C, 3 grams a day."

"That's not for toxemia?"

"Not especially. But it's wise under any conditions of extra stress."

"Do I have to eat lots of meat?"

"No, just so it's protein. If you're thinking of becoming a vegetarian, there are techniques of protein combining to get more value from plant protein. One good book on this topic is *Diet for a Small Planet* by Frances Moore Lappé."

"She can't be healthy being a vegetarian, can she?" Mrs. Johnson looked worried again.

"Many people are. But she'll have to do some reading."

I asked Barbara to return the next day. She said she would, right after she saw her obstetrician, who was watching her closely, too.

She was back the next day without her mother. "Mama means well, but, you know. . . ." she said.

"I don't know if I like this treatment," she said. "I was up all night urinating. I weighed 151½ this morning, and my blood pressure was down to 136/90. I told my obstetrician what you did, and he just shook his head and left the room. But he didn't tell me to stop, or not to come here. Now what? Do I need another shot?"

"No, with your blood pressure coming down like that, and 6½ pounds off in 24 hours, I think perhaps one was enough. Looks like you caught it in time. How have you been doing on protein?"

"I've had 4 eggs, 6 ounces of cheese and all kinds of peanuts since yesterday. I didn't ask—do I eliminate carbohydrates?"

"No. Just make sure the proteins stays high."

"Should I keep my B_6 and magnesium the same?"

"For now. As you're doing well, come back in three days next time, unless you start to swell again."

"Yes' That's done really well, hasn't it?" Her ankles were still a little puffy, as were the backs of her hands, but nowhere near as bad as before.

When she returned three days later, she had no edema at all. Her weight was 144, and her blood pressure 130/80. We were both very pleased. I asked her to cut her pyridoxine back to 200 milligrams 3 times a day, and the magnesium oxide to twice daily.

The only sign of Barbara's preeclampsia that remained was a trace of protein in her urine. Not only had she stopped any progression into eclampsia, she really didn't have preeclampsia anymore.

Over the next four to five weeks, she came in at weekly intervals. As her blood pressure continued to drop, her edema stayed away. Apparently, as the extra protein began to raise her own serum albumin levels, she needed less vitamin B_6 and magnesium. Just to be safe, though, I asked her to continue with 100 milligrams of B_6 3 times daily, and 250 milligrams of magnesium oxide twice daily, as a final reduction.

Two days past her due date, she delivered a healthy 8-pound, 1-ounce baby boy.

A Serious Information Gap

The prevention and treatment of toxemia of pregnancy is one of the worst examples of the information gap between nutritional/biochemical research and customary medical practice. As noted above, some of the earliest work on this subject was published in 1935.

Most of the early research in toxemia prevention emphasized the vital role of sufficient dietary protein. Despite the dramatic effects of the pyridoxine-magnesium treatment, as exemplified above, the basis of toxemia prevention lies in enough high-quality protein during pregnancy. In fact, some research on eclamptic (toxemic) and preeclamptic women indicates a very simple protein connection. Toxemic and pretoxemic women are much more likely to suffer from hypoalbuminemia (a shortage of albumin, the major blood protein). As every first-year medical student learns, hypoalbuminemia allows fluid to leak from the bloodstream into the tissues, thus producing edema, which is, of course, characteristic of toxemia.

The best-known pioneer in prevention of toxemia of pregnancy is Tom Brewer, M.D. Dr. Brewer has for years totally eliminated toxemia among his patients by emphasis on proper diet with sufficient protein.

The precise biochemical reasons why pyridoxine and magnesium are specifically therapeutic, as well as preventive, in cases of toxemia are not known. However, considering the much higher levels of estrogenic hormones produced during pregnancy, and the known estrogen-pyridoxine antagonism, it's not a surprise that pyridoxine might be helpful.

Magnesium is a known cofactor with pyridoxine in many enzymatic reactions.

I'm not an obstetrician, and haven't treated many patients for preeclampsia, and I certainly didn't do anything to develop this treatment. The credit for this goes to another pioneer in nutritional/biochemical treatment, John Ellis, M.D.

In his book cited below, Dr. Ellis details his development

and use of pyridoxine and magnesium therapy in toxemia. He found that these elements reduce the elevated blood pressure and edema, before the problem becomes critical. Even in advanced cases, pyridoxine and magnesium are helpful.

I've found that combining the high-protein, pyridoxine, and magnesium approaches is extremely effective. Of course, if started early enough, prevention of the problem is accomplished, and treatment of the actual condition isn't necessary.

So, given the above, why is there more than a miniscule incidence of eclampsia and preeclampsia?

I know you've heard this from me before, but I have no other explanation than the general medical bias against the use of diet, vitamins, and minerals in the treatment of disease. It's "just known that such treatments aren't likely to work." So, not only are they not used, but diet-vitamin-and-mineral treatments are rarely researched. Since most physicians prefer to follow only treatment programs which they believe have been "thoroughly researched" at several university centers, even harmless and extremely effective programs such as this are widely ignored.

During pregnancy, I usually recommend a diet of high-quality protein, and lots of it. I also recommend at least 20 milligrams of pyridoxine and 100 milligrams of magnesium each day. Ordinarily, that is enough. This is, of course, in addition to the usual multiple vitamin, extra iron, calcium, and diet free of refined foods, sugar, artificial flavor, color, and preservatives.

However, for mothers who intend to nurse, pyridoxine should be cut down to 10 milligrams a day or less following the delivery of the infant, as large doses may inhibit lactation.

FURTHER READING

Nutrition and Pregnancy
Brewer, Gail Sforza, with Brewer, Thomas H. *What Every Pregnant Woman Should Know: The Truth About Diets and Drugs in Pregnancy* (New York: Random House, 1977).

Brewer, Thomas H. *Metabolic Toxemia of Late Pregnancy: A Disease of Malnutrition* (Springfield, Ill.: Charles C Thomas, 1966).

Toxemia

Blekta, M. et al. "Volume of Whole Blood and Absolute Amount of Serum Proteins in the Early Stage of Late Toxemia of Pregnancy." *American Journal of Obstetrics and Gynecology*, vol. 106, no. 1, 1970, pp. 10–13.

Brewer, Thomas H. "Limitations of Diuretic Therapy in the Management of Severe Toxemia: The Significance of Hypoalbuminemia." *American Journal of Obstetrics and Gynecology*, vol. 83, no. 10, 1962, pp. 1352–59.

Burke, Bertha S. et al. "Nutrition Studies During Pregnancy." *American Journal of Obstetrics and Gynecology*, vol. 46, 1943, pp. 38–52.

Chesley, Leon C. "Plasma and Red Cell Volumes During Pregnancy." *American Journal of Obstetrics and Gynecology*, vol. 112, no. 3, 1972, pp. 440–50.

Cloeren, S. E. et al. "Hypovolemia in Toxemia of Pregnancy: Plasma Expander Therapy with Surveillance of Central Venous Pressure." *Archive für Gynäkologie*, vol. 215, 1973, pp. 123–32.

Hamlin, R. H. J. "The Prevention of Eclampsia and Pre-Eclampsia." *The Lancet*, January 2, 1952, pp. 64–68.

Kelman, L. et al. "Effects of Dietary Protein Restriction on Albumin Synthesis, Albumin Catabolism, and the Plasma Aminogram." *The American Journal of Clinical Nutrition*, vol. 25, November 1972, pp. 1174–78.

Strauss, Maurice B. "Observations on the Etiology of the Toxemias of Pregnancy: The Relationship of Nutritional Deficiency, Hypoproteinemia and Elevated Venous Pressure to Water Retention in Pregnancy." *American Journal of Medical Science*, vol. 190, 1935, pp. 811–42.

Vegetarianism

Lappé, Frances Moore. *Diet for a Small Planet* (New York: Ballantine Books, 1975).

Vitamin B$_6$

Ellis, John M., and Presley, James. *Vitamin B$_6$: The Doctor's Report* (New York: Harper & Row, 1973).

A 58-year-old woman has spells of a racing, pounding heart for which no clear medical explanation has been found. In addition, she feels nervous and chronically drained of energy. She is found to have hypoglycemia, poor absorption, and weak adrenal gland function. A dietary program leads to considerable improvement. A discussion of adrenal gland dysfunction and the controversy over natural adrenal supplements concludes this case.

A Case of Palpitations

Settling herself into one of the office chairs, the pleasant, grandmotherly lady said: "I'm sure you're not able to help everyone, Doctor, but I've heard so much lately about the importance of good nutrition, vitamins, and minerals that I thought I'd give it a try. It certainly can't hurt!"

Uncertainty about what nutritionally oriented health care can do is quite usual. As experience with this type of health care is new to many, it's hard to guess when it might be vitally important. My first patient that morning, Mrs. Wingate, had apparently decided to give it a try.

"Well," she said, "there are a lot of little things. But the worst are these 'spells' I've been having."

"What sort of spells?"

"It's like I can't get enough air . . . then my heartbeat starts to go fast, and pound. Sometimes it gets irregular for a while."

"Does your chest hurt?"

"No."

"Anywhere else hurt?"

"No."

"How long does each spell last?"

"Well," she paused to think. "The not-getting-air feeling lasts only a few seconds before my heart starts to pound. Then that lasts anywhere from five minutes to an hour or two. I have to sit down. I feel too weak to do anything. Finally it goes away."

"How long have you had spells like this?"

"More than two years now."

"Have they been worse lately?"

"Yes, and more frequent."

"Haven't you checked about this problem before?"

"Yes. I got this medicine. . . ." She rummaged around in her purse. "Here it is."

She handed over a bottle of digitalis tablets, a medication originally derived from the foxglove plant.

"Does this help?"

"Some. I haven't had as many spells since I started it two months ago. But I still have them."

"Did the doctor say what the problem was?"

"No, just that my heart went too fast sometimes, and these pills were important to keep that from happening."

"Did you have tests done?"

"Oh, my, yes! I had several electrocardiograms, and one of those where I got on a treadmill and ran. Those were all normal. I also had lots of blood tests, and stomach, gallbladder, and colon x-rays. Everything was normal. But I still had my problem, so I got these pills."

"Why did you have all those x-rays?"

"Oh, I have some other problems, too, like I said."

"What are those?"

"Well, I have a lot of gas and indigestion. It's especially bad when I eat meat. Sometimes it just seems to sit there like a lump. Other times, I get gas. But that's been getting worse for years, so I just expect that's my age catching up with me."

"Perhaps. We'll come back to that later. What other symptoms have you had?"

"I'm tired all the time, no matter how much sleep I get. I've been more nervous, too. I just don't have the energy I feel I should. I know I'm 58 years old, but I'm too young for *that*." She paused to think. "Oh yes. . . . My memory isn't too good." She smiled. "I get dizzy spells from time to time, too; sometimes I feel shaky inside, even though it doesn't show."

"Do you have allergies?"

"Why, yes, but I've had those for years. I just take my decongestant for my hay fever, and don't even talk about it anymore. I'm sure that doesn't have to do with anything."

"Is there diabetes in your family?"

"I had an aunt who got it when she was older. But I had a blood sugar test, and it was normal."

"I think you should have the glucose tolerance test done over again, but this time for six hours. Can you come back for that?"

Mrs. Wingate looked puzzled. "Do you think I might have diabetes?"

"No, but I suspect you may have hypoglycemia—low blood sugar—which might be setting off your spells. If you do, then you'll have to get that better to get the spells better."

"Oh." Mrs. Wingate paused once more. "Do you think it might be related to the rest of my problems, too?"

"Very likely. But let's just have you do this one test first to see if we're going in the right direction."

My next contact with Mrs. Wingate came unexpectedly the following week. She had come in for her test, which involves drinking a large dose of sugar on an empty stomach. The nurse hurried into my office, saying: "Mrs. Wingate felt faint, and her pulse is 110. But her blood pressure and everything else are normal; she'll be OK. Would you check her, too?"

We went to the examination room. Mrs. Wingate opened her eyes as we came in.

"Hello, doctor," she said. "This is exactly the kind of spell I was telling you about. But I really didn't expect to demonstrate it to you today."

I counted her pulse, which had slowed a little to 100, and listened to her heart, which sounded normal except for its speed.

Everything else was OK., too.

"Would you like to stop the test?" I asked.

"Oh, no. I can tell that this spell will be gone soon; it doesn't feel like a really bad one. I'd like to finish the test if it will help figure out what's the matter. Just so I can do it lying down."

I assured her that would be fine, and that the test could be stopped anytime she wanted.

A few days later, Mrs. Wingate returned to learn the results of her six-hour glucose tolerance test.

Those results showed that her blood sugar level had not gone up very high initially and that after four hours, her blood sugar had gone down to 49 milligrams percent, which coincided with her pulse going up to 110.

"This shows several things. First, it explains your spells. When your blood sugar drops to a level too low for you, it sets off an adrenalin response. You get shaky, sweaty, pale, and your heart beats too fast.

"Second, another part of your adrenal glands, the adrenal cortex, is probably weaker than it should be. When the highest point on a glucose tolerance test is less than 50 percent higher than the fasting level, it's called a 'flat curve.' The majority of persons with a 'flat curve' glucose tolerance test have relatively weak adrenal glands. Of course, another clue to this is your life-long history of allergies.

"Lastly, you do have hypoglycemia. But it's important to know that hypoglycemia is not a disease, but a very important symptom of other problems. For example, one textbook of medicine lists nearly 40 known causes. But most of these are extremely rare. I've found that most hypoglycemia originates from only a few causes. Poor diet is always involved. Chronic stress and lack of exercise are important contributing factors. So is lack of exposure to the sun. And a large number of hypoglycemic persons have weak adrenal glands, called hypoadrenocorticism, which in turn has some of the same causes."

"You said hypoglycemia probably is related to my other symptoms. Which ones?"

"Probably most of them. People who have hypoglycemia almost always say, as you did, that they're tired all the time. They're frequently nervous when there's no reason to be; they have no energy. Often, they're shaky."

"Dizzy spells?"

"Sometimes. But that's more likely related to weak adrenal glands. But that's just theory so far; there's a test for that, a urine collection for 24 hours. And I'd like you to turn in a hair specimen for mineral testing."

"Why?"

"It's very rare to find normal mineral nutrition in a person with hypoglycemia. It's important that any mineral problems be corrected."

"And what about my stomach problems?"

"They're also very common in persons with hypoglycemia. The type you have sounds typical, like a lack of stomach acid production. Many people with hypoglycemia have this."

"Is there a test for that?"

"Well, sometimes a tube is put down into the stomach to draw out the contents and measure the acid. But there's an easier way that usually works. Get some betaine hydrochloride at the health-food store. Take it before you eat. If your stomach feels better, and you have less gas, then it's very likely you don't have enough acid."

"Is taking acid safe?"*

"There wasn't an ulcer on your x-ray?"

"No."

"Then the worst that could happen is heartburn. You can neutralize that right away by drinking a glass of water with about ¼ teaspoon of bicarbonate of soda, or baking soda. But I have an idea it'll help you digest your meals better."

"Speaking of meals, what diet do I follow?"

"A high-protein, low-carbohydrate diet is usually recommended to help overcome hypoglycemia. That sort of program fits traditional American eating patterns best. But you must be

*Precautions for hydrochloric-acid-supplement use are described in chapter 45, "Poor Absorption."

careful not to go too low on the carbohydrates, or you will probably feel worse. Persons with weak adrenal glands can't tolerate extremely low carbohydrate diets.

"If you want to consider more radical dietary changes, you might consider the high-complex-carbohydrate approach. In fact, with the possibility of weak adrenals and lack of stomach acid, it might be preferable in the long run. For most people, this approach is a more difficult adjustment, though." I suggested two book titles covering generally each approach: *Low Blood Sugar and You*, by Carlton Fredericks and Herman Goodman for the high-protein approach, and *Hypoglycemia: A Better Approach* by Paavo Airola, for the complex-carbohydrate approach.

I advised Mrs. Wingate to eat absolutely no sugar or refined foods, especially white flour. Carbohydrates should come from whole foods like fresh vegetables, whole grains, beans, potatoes, and fruits.

"What about vitamins and minerals?"

"For now, a high-potency B complex vitamin 3 times a day. And at least 1 gram of vitamin C 3 times a day. Also, if you get very nervous, niacinamide is very helpful."

"Is that all?"

"For now. Please go ahead with this, and check back in three or four weeks when your tests should be returned."

When Mrs. Wingate returned, her report was encouraging. Shortly after eliminating all sugar and refined food, her indigestion and gas had improved considerably. Once she got her betaine hydrochloride, her gas problem and difficulty with protein digestion had gone completely. "When I remember to take it, of course!" she remarked.

"Unless I'm fooling myself, my nerves are a little better, too. I've had a little bit more energy, and I'm not quite as tired. But I still have my bad days."

I assured her this was very usual at this early stage.

"How did my tests turn out?"

"Your mineral test isn't too good. It's low in calcium, magnesium, sodium, potassium, copper, iron, manganese, and chromium."

"Why is it low in so many minerals?"

"That's very frequent in people who don't make enough acid in their stomachs. Acid seems very necessary for proper mineral absorption."

"Do I need to take all those minerals?"

"Almost all. But don't worry, that can probably be done with a multiple-mineral tablet, instead of separately."

"Did my adrenal gland test come back?"

"Yes, and it was a little low, too."

"What do I do about that?"

"The diet that you're following is just about right. The vitamins that you're using, C and B complex, are very necessary for recovery of the health of your adrenals. There are additional ones that are very important."

I gave Mrs. Wingate a second list that read as follows:

1. Vitamin C (as already recommended)
2. B complex (as already recommended)
3. Pantothenic acid
4. Vitamin A and D
5. Vitamin E
6. PABA
7. A multiple-mineral tablet
8. Tablets made from animal adrenal gland
9. Tablets made from animal pituitary gland

"What are the last two things for?" Mrs. Wingate asked. "I've been reading about this problem. Don't I need shots?"

I replied that there were very useful injections of wholly natural adrenal cortical hormones, but in her case, I'd prefer to use them only if the other things weren't working well. Second, while I could make her a list of nutrients of major importance to her adrenal glands, I couldn't possibly list all helpful nutrients; the knowledge of them just doesn't exist. But if she took tablets made of whole gland substance, the chances were excellent that everything needed would be there, even if only in small amounts.

"That makes sense," she replied. "That's certainly a long list. But I'll do it if it will help."

"Good. But that's not all."

"No?" Mrs. Wingate looked a little surprised.

"Remember I mentioned stress, lack of exercise, and not enough sunlight?"

"Yes. But are they that important?"

"As important as diet and vitamins. Let's take them one at a time."

"First, and easiest in theory: get out in the sun often! And don't put it off; it rains so often here that when the sun's out, you should be, too!

"Second, as soon as you're feeling strong enough, start a regular exercise program. Don't overdo it to start, just do enough to make you a little tired.

"Last, and this is the hardest, you must find some way of reducing the stress in your life, or dealing with it differently. I suspect you've had some chronic stresses."

Mrs. Wingate smiled. "I know, but I've just not gotten around to doing anything about it. I think I will, now."

Three months later, Mrs. Wingate returned. "I'm doing much better!" she announced. "I haven't had another spell for two months now. I've definitely got more energy; my nerves are greatly improved. Even my hay fever was better this summer. I only took a decongestant every once in a while."

Pausing to smile, she continued. "My husband says I haven't been like this for years. Now, he's getting too tired! Isn't that due to my adrenal gland treatment, too?"

I agreed it probably was.

I've seen Mrs. Wingate two or three times in the 2½ years since she first came in. We've talked about reducing her supplements to a maintenance level, about exercise, and as Mrs. Wingate says, "How to stay out of health trouble before it happens!" She continues to feel well.

Although she's done well, as many persons do with her sorts of problems, she's been fortunate. Once she started to recover, she had no setbacks. Of course, once she understood what she had to do, she did everything exactly as she should. For many persons with hypoglycemia, especially those with hypoadrenalism, it isn't always as easy or quick. As Mrs. Wingate said on her first visit, nutrition, vitamins, and minerals don't always solve all health problems. But as we both agreed, they certainly can't hurt, and usually will improve health, overall.

Hypoglycemia and the Adrenal Glands

Hypoglycemia, while causing many symptoms, is usually in turn caused by something else. In Mrs. Wingate's case, whenever her blood sugar dropped too low, she had spells of rapid heartbeat, weakness, and feeling like she couldn't get enough air. Many people with secondary hypoglycemia have similar spells. Also like many others, she was tired all the time, nervous, forgetful, and frequently felt shaky inside. All of these symptoms could be said to be due to her hypoglycemia.

However, once her hypoglycemia was found, a search for its causes turned up weak adrenal glands and poor digestion or absorption of nutrients. Helping to correct or compensate for these problems led to correction of the blood sugar problem and the symptoms it caused.

Mrs. Wingate's digestion problem seemed sufficiently obvious that I simply asked her to try taking supplemental hydrochloric acid for it. Also, she'd had a recent normal (ulcer-free and gastritis-free) x-ray of her stomach.

However, I've given up in most cases the "try it" method of deciding whether more stomach acid is needed, in favor of radiotelemetric testing. This had numerous advantages: it's extremely precise in measurement, doesn't require pumping the stomach, and allows functional testing.

More important, it minimizes the chances of setting off stomach irritation, bleeding, or even ulceration in case of a wrong guess.

Some readers may note that I've used a more old-fashioned test of adrenal gland function in Mrs. Wingate's case: A 24-hour collection of urine to measure the overall production of hormones by the adrenal gland (more precisely the adrenal cortex).

Many more modern endocrinologists favor a single measurement of serum cortisone, usually taken at 9 A.M., as their only screening test of adrenal gland function. Obviously, I'm not an endocrinologist, but I disagree about what test should be used. Cortisone is only one of 30 to 50 hormones made by the adrenal cortex; while it is one of the most important, it doesn't give an overall measurement of adrenal function.

More important, the 24-hour urine test appears clinically to correlate better with other parameters of weak adrenal gland function, such as low blood pressure, or abrupt drop in blood pressure on sudden change to upright position. (These parameters are admittedly also debatable between regular and nutritionally/ biochemically oriented physicians.)

Which brings us right to another controversial area in nutritional/biochemical medicine: the connection between hypoglycemia and hypoadrenalism (weak adrenal glands).

Some 20 to 30 years ago, John Tintera, M.D., an endocrinologist from Yonkers, New York, established and popularized the concept of hypoadrenocorticism (weak adrenal gland function) and its connection with hypoglycemia. Through treatments based on this concept, he helped many individuals back to health.

Even today, the concept of hypoadrenalism is poorly accepted by some health professionals. I've heard statements such as: "Either you have Addison's disease, or you're normal. Addison's disease is extremely rare. So you couldn't have hypoadrenocorticism."

Some brief logic disposes of this argument. Any gland or organ in the body can function at a normal rate, or can overfunction (*hyper*function) or underfunction (*hypo*function). That is especially true of endocrine (hormone-producing) glands such as thyroid, ovaries, pituitary, and adrenals.

Let's take thyroid disease as a good parallel. Besides normal function, there's hyperthyroidism and hypothyroidism. The important point is that there are degrees of overfunction and underfunction. Total absence of thyroid hormone function, or very nearly total, is called "cretinism." As is well known, there are many persons who suffer from hypothyroidism who are not classified as cretin. They're somewhere on the gradient between normal and zero, or near-zero, function, and are generally lumped under the category hypothyroid. Likewise, there's a gradient between normal adrenal function and zero, or the near-zero function called Addison's disease.

There really should be little argument about the connection between hypoadrenalism and hypoglycemia, either. A major textbook of endocrinology (see Williams) points out that insulin and glucocorticoids (the hormones from the adrenal glands that help to regulate blood sugar) have generally opposing actions. Stated briefly, insulin tends to make blood sugar go down; adrenocortical hormones make it go up.

So, in persons with normal (or high) insulin levels and hypoadrenalism with low levels of glucocorticoids, what's likely to happen? The downward pressure of insulin on blood sugar levels is not opposed by the normal upward pressure of adrenocortical hormones: low blood sugar, especially after meals when insulin levels are highest, is the likely result.

Given the above, why have I called the problem of hypoadrenalism controversial?

The reason for the controversy lies mostly in the treatment devised by Dr. Tintera. He used a whole, natural-hormone-containing extract of animal adrenal glands, called adrenal cortical extract, or ACE. He found that by using frequent injections of this material (unfortunately it doesn't work by mouth nearly as well) that persons with hypoadrenocorticism could be helped back to health.

Once again, the parallel with hypothyroidism is clear. Persons with hypothyroidism are given tablets containing small amounts of thyroid hormone as a supplement, or in some cases, replacement. Traditionally, this supplement has been from natural animal sources; along with the modern trend, the natural supplement is now frequently replaced with synthetically manufactured hormones.

The synthesis of cortisone was accomplished in the late 1940s; although synthetic, this product was at least a chemical duplicate of part of the natural hormone. However, since that time, numerous synthetic derivatives of cortisone not found in nature have been developed. Each of these derivatives has its advantages, disadvantages, and proponents, the earliest of whom tend to be the pharmaceutical firm which develops and patents that particular synthesis.

There is no question that synthetic cortisone and its synthetic derivatives are much more powerful than the naturally derived adrenal cortex extract. Synthetic derivatives also can be given by mouth, a definite advantage over injection.

From the nutritional/biochemical point of view, however, these synthetic derivatives are totally unacceptable, except in extreme emergencies, when the slower, natural course of action is simply too slow.

The drawbacks are several. Natural adrenal cortical extract contains the whole spectrum of some 30 to 50 hormones as produced by nature. These hormones are all properly balanced with respect to one another. Even though science may not have found all the functions of all the more minor hormones, or may have dismissed them as negligible, the chances are excellent that almost all of them have important, if unrecognized, biological function. Nature does little that's wasted; even what's thought of as wasted or unnecessary in one era is frequently found to have a function when another generation of scientists takes a closer look.

Synthetic hormones are single hormone preparations, often not even found in nature, and strengthened all out of proportion to nature's balance. It's as if the spectrum of B vitamins found in brewer's yeast was eliminated except for vitamin B_1 and then this B_1 was semisynthesized in dosage strength 500 to 1,000 times greater, or more. To compound the error, this greatly strengthened semisynthetic vitamin B_1 is then presented as more effective than the naturally occurring B complex in brewer's yeast. This scenario is obviously a farce; but it's a good parallel of the situation of adrenal cortical extract versus synthetic cortisone.

The side effects of synthetic cortisone preparations are numerous, potentially serious, and well known. Just a few of them include suppression of immunity to infections, delayed wound healing, peptic ulcer, osteoporosis (thinned-out bones), hypertension, and diabetes. The list could go on, but that's enough for the general idea.

By contrast, whole, natural, ACE has never been found to have even a fraction of the side effects noted above. Even in patients who can't get off it, long-term use is relatively safe. In most persons, with other appropriate support measures, it can in fact be discontinued eventually.

Which brings us to another drawback to synthetic cortisone derivatives. When they're used in long-term treatment, they're so powerful that they can suppress a person's own adrenal function, and make it practically impossible to get off them, despite side effects.

So why all this long-winded explanation? Observant readers have noted, I'm sure, that I didn't ask Mrs. Wingate to take ACE injections as part of her treatment, reserving these for later only if the other treatment didn't work. She was asked to use tablets made of whole animal adrenal substance. These are considerably weaker than ACE itself, containing virtually no active hormone at all. (If it's present, it's in microscopic amounts.) This treatment, not scientifically proven (it's not even been studied), proceeds on the general theory that if some key component of adrenal gland is deficient, and this is important to the individual's own hypofunctioning glands, it will be found, if in only small amounts, in whole animal gland.

Once again, this theory isn't scientifically proven. It does seem to help in clinical practice, though.

Second, Mrs. Wingate would have had to learn home self-injection of ACE, just as diabetics do with insulin. (I discourage coming to the office for long-term injection programs, as long as it's safe to do at home. Active participation in self-care is always preferable.) While many persons with hypoadrenocorticism need and benefit from ACE injections, they are a slightly more radical measure. Most nutritionally oriented physicians, like most physicians of any sort, tend to be conservative in approach whenever possible, even though it may be slower.

The list of vitamins, exercises, stress reduction, sunshine exposure, and good diet is often good enough for milder degrees of hypoadrenocorticism, as it was for Mrs. Wingate.

Actually, this long explanation of ACE was more to explain

its use in the many hypoadrenal patients who need it and rely on it, and for whom synthetic cortisone and its derivatives would be unnecessarily radical. ACE has only a few drawbacks. It's relatively weak, and does take longer to work. It also must be taken by injection, not by mouth.

Oh yes, another drawback . . . ACE has [at the time of this writing] been banned from interstate commerce by the Food and Drug Administration.

Because of dangerous side effects?

No . . . there really aren't any.

Why, then?

Because "It's not been shown to be effective . . . [synthetic] cortisone [and its derivatives] should be used for Addison's disease. . . ." ACE is "considered to be a new drug [and will] require new drug applications. . . ." (see FDA report).

This, despite the facts:

• Adrenal cortex extract isn't even a drug. It's a whole animal extract. Of course, that doesn't impress the FDA, which, believe it or not, has classified your blood and mine as a drug.

• It's not new . . . it's been in use since the 1930s.

• Hundreds of doctors, and thousands of successfully treated patients can testify to its effectiveness.

• It's used by nutritionally oriented physicians for milder degrees of hypoadrenocorticism which have been proven by independent laboratory testing (I have over 100 such patients myself).

The FDA recommendation of synthetic cortisone and its derivatives for the milder forms of hypoadrenocorticism are like killing a fly with the proverbial sledgehammer.

Suffice it to say that in Mrs. Wingate's case, if ACE had been used, it would have aided in her recovery from hypoadrenocorticism, and as textbooks point out, would have helped her hypoglycemia (secondary to hypoadrenocorticism) through the previously cited upward pressure of glucocorticoids, present in ACE, on the blood sugar, without the numerous side effects of high-powered synthetic corticosteroids (preparations of cortisone).

FURTHER READING

Airola, Paavo. *Hypoglycemia: A Better Approach* (Phoenix, Ariz.: Health Plus, 1977).

Currier, W. D. "Dizziness Related to Hypoglycemia: The Role of Adrenal Steroids and Nutrition." *The Laryngoscope*, vol. 81, no. 1, January 1971, pp. 18–35.

Food and Drug Administration. *"Report on Adrenal Cortical Extract."* April 1978.

Fredericks, Carlton, and Goodman, Herman. *Low Blood Sugar and You* (New York: Constellation International, 1969).

Tintera, John W. "The Hypoadrenocortical State and Its Management," in *Hypoadrenocorticism* (New York: Adrenal Metabolic Research Society of the Hypoglycemia Foundation, 1974).

Williams, Robert H., ed. *Textbook of Endocrinology* (Philadelphia: W. B. Saunders, 1974), pp. 271, 635.

Readers interested in further investigation of this subject might contact: Adrenal Metabolic Research Society of the Hypoglycemia Foundation, Inc., 153 Pawling Avenue, Troy, New York, 12180.

Some patients are more aggressive "cooperators" than others. In this case, a complex health problem of 20 years standing was only cleared up after six months of effort. A host of symptoms including colitis, headaches, and sinus infections was eventually traced largely to unsuspected food allergies, complicated by weak adrenal gland function . . . and a deficiency of certain digestive enzymes.

18 A Complex Case of Food Allergy

No matter how knowledgeable or competent a physician is, there is only a limited amount of help he or she can give without the active cooperation of the patient in the process of health improvement. After all, there is no way that anyone else can tell exactly how you feel. No doctor can follow a patient around 24 hours a day, seven days a week, observing and recording everything that happens.

Margaret Shane is an excellent example of a patient who finally got fed up with years of various symptoms, and decided to do something about them herself. In the space of a few months, with only a little help from me, she was able to discover the source of most of her health problems, and clear them up.

On her first visit, Mrs. Shane listed for me several problems.

1. Colitis: duration, 20 years. Symptoms, excess cramping and gas, frequent diarrhea. Three series of gastrointestinal x-rays, "nothing the matter." Diagnosed as "tension," and told repeatedly to relax.

2. Headaches: duration, also 20 years, every one or two

days. Usually relieved by aspirin, so no diagnostic work done. Also dismissed as "tension."

3. Conjunctivitis: duration, ten years. Symptoms, chronically scratchy, tearing, bloodshot eyes. Neither cortisone eye drops nor avoiding makeup had helped.

4. Chronic vaginal infections, started after antibiotic treatment. Despite many creams and suppositories, never cleared.

5. Recurrent sinus infections and congestion: very severe when living in the Midwest. Improved by move to West Coast and increased vitamin C, but not cured.

   Extensive skin tests for allergies had shown trees, grasses, dust, weeds, and cats to be a problem. The only foods which skin tests had shown to be problems were cucumbers and mushrooms.

6. "Neuritis-type" pains and episodes of weakness in the legs, along with weak and shaky spells. These episodes of pain, weakness, and shakiness had been present for two years. Mrs. Shane had been to her family doctor, who made a number of tests, then referred her to a specialist. After many blood tests, the specialist referred her back to her family doctor with the same conclusion: "There is nothing the matter."

At the same point, Mrs. Shane decided that there must be something more the matter than tension. She was tired of being referred to relaxation classes and being told she was overly concerned. After considering alternatives to what she'd already tried to improve her health, she decided to try nutritional medicine.

After going over the symptoms, I concluded it would be best not to run very many tests until I'd had a chance to review the results of the tests that had already been done. We could obtain copies, and go from there.

In the meantime, there were some general support measures that could be taken.

She agreed that that was reasonable. However, despite the reported "normality" of her prior tests, there was one that seemed a bit odd to her. She'd requested and had done a six-hour glucose tolerance test, which had been described to her as normal, but a "flat curve."

She'd done some reading about hypoglycemia since, and asked if a flat curve really was normal. I answered that it was not, but was usually a hypoglycemia variant associated with relatively weak function of the cortex of the adrenal glands, or more rarely, with different types of intestinal malabsorption.

Mrs. Shane was sure she'd not been tested for either of these possibilities. So, to save a little time, we decided to get a 24-hour urine test for adrenal function underway.

The general support measures I suggested were:

1. No sugar, white bread, or refined foods
2. Bran: 2 tablespoons daily to help colitis
3. *Acidophilus* and vinegar, to help vaginal infections, as described in chapter 43, "Surviving Drug Therapy."
4. A product containing animal intestinal substance, again, to help colitis

Mrs. Shane also asked if I could recommend any books for additional reading. Although I didn't think that her problems were primarily psychological, I advised that she read *Psychodietetics: Foods as the Key to Emotional Health* by Dr. Emanuel Cheraskin of the University of Alabama, and Dr. W. Marshall Ringsdorf, for a good overview of the effects of nutrition on health.

At her next visit, Mrs. Shane reported that the addition of bran and animal intestinal substance had not improved her case of colitis at all. Since she didn't seem discouraged by this, I waited for her to continue.

She'd read Dr. Cheraskin's book, she said, and had become particularly interested in the chapter on allergy. In that chapter, the findings of Dr. Arthur F. Coca on self-testing for food allergy are summarized.

In the book *The Pulse Test*, Dr. Coca describes his finding that many allergic individuals have a pulse elevation after eating foods to which they are allergic. He outlines a method of self-testing for these food allergies.

Mrs. Shane had tried this. To her surprise, her pulse rose to 95 after eating her usual breakfast of toast, cereal with bananas, raisins, honey, and orange juice. She'd tried eliminating a few of the foods which she thought caused her pulse to rise, and thought some of her symptoms were a little better.

Understandably, she was still a little skeptical. After all, she'd been through extensive skin testing for food allergies, and as noted before, only cucumbers and mushrooms were "positive." Also, it seemed like too simple an answer after years of unsuccessful medical tests and treatments.

However, I had a feeling she was onto something. I'd seen stranger symptoms disappear when an unsuspected food allergy was finally eliminated. A resting pulse of 95 is not normal, particularly if it is usually lower. Last, Dr. Coca's work seemed quite applicable to food-allergy testing for many people. Even allergists are among the first to point out that skin tests for food allergy are frequently unreliable.

For all these reasons, I encouraged her to continue the pulse-testing for allergies.

Mrs. Shane asked how her adrenal function test had turned out. In her case, as in most cases with flat-curve hypoglycemia tests, her adrenal test was relatively low. Specifically, it was just below the lowest number considered to be normal by the lab.

For this reason, I asked her to make sure the supporting group of vitamins and gland substances for weak adrenal glands was part of her supplement program.

I wrote a list for her that read as follows:
1. Vitamin C
2. B complex
3. Pantothenic acid
4. Vitamins A and D
5. Vitamin E
6. PABA
7. A multiple-mineral tablet
8. Tablets made from animal adrenal gland
9. Tablets made from animal pituitary gland

She asked if this could be part of the *cause* of her problems. I answered that while weak adrenal function could make the effects of allergies worse, and supporting the adrenals would help her feel better, it was very probable that chronic food allergies could "run down" her adrenal function to its present state. In that case, the result of this test would be *effect*, not cause. So continuing the self-test for food allergies was very important. She assured me she'd continue, and left.

When Mrs. Shane returned in four months, her report was very encouraging. However, before telling me of her success, she emphasized that achieving it was no easy job. She'd been working at it for the entire time since her last visit. However, as her first week or two of self-testing indicated that she did have food-allergy problems, she'd become determined to carry the testing through to the end. After all, 20 years of symptoms, and the prospect of eliminating them, were strong motivation. Still, it was no easy effort.

Briefly, she'd determined, by checking symptoms as well as pulse, that honey and orange juice caused the worst headaches. Orange juice was the source of her watery, irritated eyes. Apples, fish, and beef caused colitis and gas. Wheat caused the skin under her rings to discolor.

As she said, her usual breakfast of toast, honey, cereal, raisins, and orange juice was "literally poisoning" her!

No specific food seemed to be causing her neuritis or sinus problems, but when she eliminated all the foods which caused her pulse to rise, these problems disappeared, along with the vaginitis.

Mrs. Shane found that the foods to which she was allergic, those which caused her pulse to rise, could be divided into "major" and "minor" groups. The "major" group caused definitely noticeable symptoms (including bodily discomforts not previously noted). This group included beef, fish, wheat, honey, carob, cranberries, apples, oranges, and coffee.

The "minor" group, which caused a pulse rise but couldn't definitely be associated with symptoms, included pork, lamb, rice, cantaloupe, grapes, raisins, pineapple, cherries, rye, peas, and peanut butter. Although realizing she was allergic to them, she found she could eat them occasionally with no noticeable problem.

Foods which caused no problem at all were chicken, all dairy products (milk, cottage cheese, cheese, yogurt, buttermilk), corn, eggs, potatoes, pears, peaches, tomatoes, lettuce, broccoli, squash, cauliflower, carrots, beets, onions, cabbage, celery, artichokes, ketchup, mustard, pickles, avocados, honeydew melons, and—despite her skin tests—cucumbers and mushrooms.

It appeared that Mrs. Shane had cleared up most of her problems with the help of Dr. Coca's pulse test and her persistence. I congratulated her on her effort.

However, having had such success, she was interested in pursuing nutritional testing further.

We decided to do a mineral analysis using a hair specimen. After going over her self-tests a bit further, she left to return in a month.

When she did, her symptoms were still gone, as long as she ate no offending foods. The only thing left was a minor amount of excess gas that she couldn't trace to any foods eaten.

Her mineral test offered a possible explanation. She was abnormally low in nearly every mineral tested.

The vast majority of similar tests, with nearly all minerals low, are due to insufficient stomach acid. As this can also be responsible for gas and bloating, I asked her to try using betaine hydrochloride (a source of hydrochloric acid) to see if it helped. This time a brief trial would tell, so I asked her to return in two weeks.

Once again, Mrs. Shane didn't respond to the usual remedy, as she hadn't to my first general support measures. As she said, she'd never been a "usual case." The betaine hydrochloride had given her heartburn, so, wisely, she'd given it up.

We decided to try again. As the minor gas problem remained, I asked her to get a blood test for pancreatic enzymes. As she was still faced with the problem of mineral deficiencies, I drew up a list of supplements to help correct this.

When her pancreatic enzyme test returned, it was "low normal." Since it wouldn't hurt, I asked the nurse to advise her to try pancreatic digestive enzymes before meals, to see what would happen.

When she returned next, she reported that this time my recommendation had been just what was needed. With the pancreatic enzymes, the last trace of her gas problem was gone. Her colitis, headaches, conjunctivitis, sinus congestion, vaginitis, and spells of neuritis and weakness were gone. She'd deliberately tested a few of the foods she'd found herself to be allergic to previously, and symptoms had returned. She said she was now convinced; in fact she felt better than she had in years. She'd lost her feeling of chronic tiredness, as well as 8 pounds of retained fluid (also noted by Dr. Coca to be a frequent allergic symptom). The months spent in self-testing had been worth the effort. After all, it had been a little more than six months since her first visit, and she'd alleviated problems she'd had from 2 to 20 years.

While pulse-testing worked well for her, it is only one of several allergy-diagnosis systems, and doesn't work for everyone. Individuality in health care is underlined again.

Mrs. Shane had previously been found to have hypoglycemia. Her case emphasizes the complexity sometimes involved in nutritional medicine: her hypoglycemia was caused in large part by her food allergies, and only cleared up when these were removed.

Several publications have appeared outlining the possibility of the reverse course; getting rid of allergies by controlling hypoglycemia. One of these, *Goodbye Allergies* by Judge Tom R. Blaine, emphasizes allergy relief by control of hypoglycemia and hypoadrenalism (which Mrs. Shane also had). It certainly could be asked "Why not cure these, and the allergies will go away?"

Sometimes this works, but in Mrs. Shane's case, considering the specificity of many of her allergy symptoms, it was my opinion that her hypoglycemia and hypoadrenalism were probably secondary to her food allergies, rather than the other way around. This proved to be so.

This case required much hard work on the part of the patient herself, more so than in the usual health problem. My own suggestions directed toward the "usual answer" didn't work in the expected manner. But the outcome was good and illustrates well the principle that for many problems, there's only so much a physician can do to help. The rest is often up to you.

FURTHER READING

Blaine, Tom R. *Goodbye Allergies* (Secaucus, N.J.: Citadel Press, 1968).

Cheraskin, Emanuel, and Ringsdorf, W. Marshall, Jr., with Brecher, Arline. *Psychodietetics: Food as the Key to Emotional Health* (New York: Stein & Day, 1974).

Coca, Arthur F. *The Pulse Test* (New York: Lyle Stuart, 1967).

After psychiatry (for the whole family) and antibiotics fail to help the bed-wetting of a 10-year-old boy, allergy tests are carried out. Three days after his allergenic foods are eliminated, he stops wetting the bed for the first time in his life. Curiously, food allergy was named as one cause of enuresis as early as 1931, but its importance is usually downplayed or ignored altogether.

19 A Case of Allergic Bed-Wetting

"We've tried everything," Mrs. Crosby said, "but nothing seems to help. We took him to a urologist, who ran kidney and bladder x-rays. He said his bladder was a little small, and tried stretching it, but that didn't help. The pediatrician tried him on a drug that's supposed to stop it, but that didn't help either. The whole family's been to a psychiatrist, for a year and a half, but we stopped that when he didn't improve. We got one of those alarm devices finally, even though the psychiatrist didn't like it. But that's no good either. No matter what we do, Everett still wets the bed nearly every night. And he's almost 11 years old!"

Everett shifted uncomfortably in his chair. Even though he'd been to several clinics, Everett's problem was still embarrassing.

"He's been checked over and over for infection, but usually there isn't any," Mrs. Crosby continued. "He had antibiotics several times anyway, but they didn't help. He can't go to camp or visit with any friends because of this. I thought maybe some vitamins and minerals might help, so I brought him here."

"I'm sure that a few vitamins might be good for him," I replied, "but I don't think that's the answer to his problem." Both Everett and Mrs. Crosby looked disappointed. "Oh," Mrs. Crosby said. "We hoped. . . ."

"Hold on. I didn't say there wasn't a nutritional answer. I just said that adding vitamins and minerals isn't it. What you probably need is to subtract something, not add something."

"Subtract something? What do you mean?"

"Many cases of bed-wetting are caused by food allergies. If that's Everett's problem, then all he needs to do is stop eating something."

"Allergies? Is that a new discovery?"

"Not at all. It goes back years."

"But Everett doesn't have any allergy symptoms. He's never had asthma, hay fever, or breaking out."

"If he has enuresis—bed-wetting—he might very well have an allergy symptom. That's the symptom! Any organ in the body, including the bladder, can react to an allergy. Sometimes it's just one organ, sometimes several. Please get a book called *Eating Dangerously: The Hazards of Hidden Allergies* by Dr. Richard Mackarness. I think you'll be surprised at the incredible number of mental and physical problems that allergy can cause. But, back to Everett. I'd like him to get checked for food allergies, before we do anything else."

"Skin tests?"

"No, blood tests for antibodies to specific foods. It's called radioallergosorbent testing, or RAST for short."

"Which foods?"

"I have a short list of what might be called the most likely foods. This includes milk, wheat, eggs, corn, citrus, tomatoes. But I'd also like you to make a list of Everett's favorite foods."

"Why's that?"

"Unfortunately, our favorite foods are frequently among the ones we're likely to be allergic to."

"That's easy, Mom" Everett said. "I like peanut butter, chicken, and milk."

Mrs. Crosby laughed. "I could feed Everett peanut butter sandwiches, chicken, and milk for months and he'd never get tired of them."

"You mean I might have to stop eating peanut butter?" Everett asked. He looked upset.

"Don't know yet. If it turns out you're allergic to it, and you want to stop bed-wetting, you'll have to."

Everett thought for a minute. "Not even a little?"

"Probably not. But why don't we wait until the tests are done."

I turned to Mrs. Crosby again. "Does anyone else in the family have allergies, as far as you know?"

"Well, my brother had asthma when he was younger, but it's gone now. That's all, as far as I know."

"Does Everett have any other health problems?"

"Not as far as I know."

Mrs. Crosby took her son to the nurse to have the blood tests drawn.

After the tests returned, Everett and his mother came in to discuss the results. They had decided to test him for milk, wheat, eggs, corn, oranges, tomatoes, peanuts, chicken, apples, beef, Cheddar cheese, and carrots.

Everett sat on the edge of his chair. "Can I eat peanut butter?" he asked.

"Not if you want to stop wetting the bed. Your test shows you're very allergic to peanuts."

Everett looked depressed. "OK. But I told Mom if it doesn't work, I'm going to eat the whole jar later on."

"Let's give it a fair try, Everett. What else does the test show?"

"He's allergic to milk. That seems to be the most common allergen in cases of enuresis. However, he has one favorite food left: there's no sign of allergy to chicken."

"All right!" Everett declared.

"Your test showed you're also allergic to corn and carrots. That's all."

"Carrots?" Nobody's allergic to carrots!" Mrs. Crosby said.

"Everett is. But try it and see."

"What about Cheddar cheese?"

"No, no significant antibody levels there."

"Even though he's allergic to milk?"

"That happens sometimes."

"How about other milk products?"

"It's probably best to stop ice cream and cottage cheese. However, you should be able to tell. If he stops wetting the bed almost completely by not eating peanuts, milk, carrots and corn, you should be able to identify other causes by elimination on the few occasions when bed-wetting recurs."

"That's true," Mrs. Crosby said, "I certainly hope this works." She got up. "When shall we come back?"

"Give it two or three weeks. You'll need some time to experiment."

A month later, Everett and his mother returned to talk over how he was doing.

"His father and I couldn't believe it. Three days after Everett stopped eating the foods his test showed, he stopped wetting the bed. He's only wet twice since. Once was when I let him have a carrot; I couldn't believe anybody was allergic to carrots. Well, he wet the bed that night. The other time, we had beets; we don't have them very often. That caused a problem, too. Everything else was food Everett doesn't have trouble with."

"Yuk, beets," Everett mumbled.

"It's just as well; he doesn't like them anyway."

"Hate them," Everett said, "but I sure miss peanut butter."

James C. Breneman, M.D., has been trying to get the attention of the medical community and the general public about the relationship between bed-wetting and allergy for over 20 years. Despite his publications, as well as those of others, I didn't come across this information in four years of medical school or in subsequent internship-residency training in family practice.

Instead, we were advised that the cause of the problem was

unknown; that kidney and bladder x-rays should be done as well as screening tests for infections. If this all proved negative (as it generally did) then drugs, psychotherapy, or nothing were the alternatives. Yet Dr. Breneman's first article was published in 1959; Dr. Bray's in 1931.

Even though not all bed-wetting is related to food allergy, a conservative approach to treatment would dictate that allergy be excluded first, before proceeding to procedures with more risk, such as kidney x-rays, or drug management.

FURTHER READING

Bray, George W. "Enuresis of Allergic Origin." *Archives of Disease in Childhood*, vol. 6, 1931, pp. 251-53.

Breneman, James C. "Allergic Cystitis: The Cause of Nocturnal Enuresis." *General Practice*, vol. 20, December 1959, pp. 85-98.

————. "Primary Nocturnal Enuresis (Bedwetting)." *Basics of Food Allergy* (Springfield Ill.: Charles C Thomas, 1978), pp. 54-66.

Gerrard, John W., and Zaleski, Anne. "Functional Bladder Capacities in Children with Enuresis and Recurrent Urinary Infections." *Clinical Ecology*, edited by Lawrence D. Dickey (Springfield Ill.: Charles C Thomas, 1976), pp. 224-32.

Mackarness, Richard. *Eating Dangerously: The Hazards of Hidden Allergies* (New York: Harcourt Brace Jovanovich, 1976).

Zaleski, Anne; Shokeir M. K.; and Garrard, John W. "Enuresis: Familial Incidence and Relationship to Allergic Disorders." *Canadian Medical Association Journal*, vol. 106, January 8, 1972, pp. 30-31.

Removing an allergen—wheat—from the diet helps a 5-year-old boy but does not eliminate his enuresis. Physical examination reveals a curvature of the spine, not severe, but definite. With the suspicion of nerve compression the boy is referred to a chiropractor, who makes an adjustment and solves the problem. . . . With an extended discussion of the role of chiropractic as the author sees it.

A Case of Bed-Wetting from Nerve Compression

20

Jamie McDowell and his mother were in for a follow-up visit about his bed-wetting. Jamie's mother was a friend of Mrs. Crosby's. When she'd heard about Everett's success with stopping wetting, she'd brought Jamie in for allergy tests.

Jamie was only 5, and like many 5-year-olds, let us know quite loudly what he thought of having his blood drawn. But the test had turned up a problem with wheat. After Mrs. McDowell took all the wheat out of his diet, his enuresis improved, but wasn't gone entirely.

"I'm happy and disappointed all at once," Mrs. McDowell said. "He's about 50 percent better—that's certainly a help—but I was hoping his problem would clear up entirely, like Everett's. We've checked him for allergy to everything he eats, too.

"Isn't there anything else we can do? I don't want to put him on drugs, but I can't stand him wetting the bed until he's 10 or 11, or whatever."

"Most frequently, I've found enuresis will clear up by allergy elimination. But there are other causes, too. Let's take Jamie to the examination room."

I had Jamie's mother remove his shirt and his outer pants. I asked him to stand up and turn around facing his mother.

Jamie had an evident scoliosis, or curvature of the spine. It wasn't severe, but definite. He was distinctly tender over the lower parts of the spine, the sacral and lumbar regions.

"I've been told that scoliosis just runs in our family, and doesn't really make any difference," Mrs. McDowell said. "I had him looked at once; the doctor said he didn't need a brace or anything, and he never complains of pain. Do you think it has anything to do with his bed-wetting?"

"Yes, I do, but there's only one way to find out. Have it corrected and see."

"But how could a spinal curve make him wet the bed?"

"Remember, the nerves that help control bladder function come from the spine. If one or more of these nerves is compressed by bone due to his spinal curve, it might not function properly. That can lead to poor bladder control and bed-wetting. I'd like you to take Jamie to see a friend of mine, a chiropractor."

"A chiropractor?" Mrs. McDowell looked very surprised. "I thought medical doctors and chiropractors hated each other. They always told me in nursing school to stay away from them."

"I was told that, too. Old prejudices die hard. But most chiropractors these days are extremely well trained. You should see the curriculum from chiropractic school.

"Leaving that aside, there are some areas of health care that only a chiropractor or osteopathically trained physician can help. This is probably one of them. I'm sure you'll get a careful examination and explanation of proposed treatment for your approval before it's done."

Mrs. McDowell thought for a minute. "Considering the way Jamie's back looks, you're probably right. I'll talk it over with my husband. Jamie is wetting less now that he's off wheat, but I'd like it to stop completely."

I didn't see Mrs. McDowell for several months, when she came in for her annual checkup. She told me that after a short series of adjustments, Jamie's remaining bed-wetting had stopped. It returned only occasionally, when Jamie accidentally ate wheat, or once when he fell off his bicycle, hurting his back. A return visit to the chiropractor quickly solved that.

Chiropractic is one of the most emotion-charged subjects among medical doctors. Usually it is not possible to hold a rational discussion on the topic. Nonthinking, automatic condemnation of chiropractic health care is so inbred into medical students that the mere mention of the word makes tempers flare. Most of the time, it's like attacking church, home, and flag, all at once. Yet most medical doctors have never bothered to investigate chiropractic with the same scientific objectivity and methods of observation they're taught to use when investigating any unknown topic.

When I wrote my observations on chiropractic in *Prevention*, I received a comment from a colleague that he hoped it didn't mean "an across-the-board endorsement." Of course not. I don't make a wide-ranging, uncritical endorsement of chiropractic, its philosophy or practice . . . or of "modern scientific medicine" or nutritional biochemistry, either.

Chiropractic does have a place, however, in the prevention of illness and the treatment of disease. As with many other things, that place lies somewhere between the 100 percent applicability claimed by its very early advocates, and the 0 percent cited by detractors.

Let's take Jamie's case. The "usual and customary" treatment would have been a drug to stop bed-wetting, or perhaps psychotherapy, or under some circumstances, an alarm device. The most frequently used drug is also used in adults as a rather powerful antidepressant. Also, infection and any congenital malformation would be looked for, and some metabolic screening would probably be done.

The nutritional/biochemical approach would be to screen for food allergy and to look for any possible metabolic problems that might contribute to bed-wetting. Treatment would involve removing any offending allergens, and nutritional/biochemical treatment for any metabolic problems (although this is unusual).

The chiropractic approach is to look for an abnormal irritation of the nerves that control bladder function, and if found, to remove the disorder essentially by manipulation.

In Jamie McDowell's case, it required a combination of two approaches: removing food allergy and chiropractic manipulation, to clear up his problem.

Looking back at the three approaches, it's obvious there's value in all of them. I certainly advise looking for chronic infection or congenital malformation. When these problems are present, and solved or at least properly treated, bed-wetting is helped. Removing allergens where they occur and removing pressure from nerves are both things to consider.

Some cases will be helped by one approach, some by another, some by a combination. If the cause can be found, then usually treatment appropriate to the cause will help.

In Jamie McDowell's case, the only thing that cleared the remainder of his problem was chiropractic treatment. Which led me to the statement that sometimes chiropractic is the only treatment which will help. Sometimes—not always.

As I understand it, one of the underlying principles of chiropractic is that if the function of a nerve serving a certain organ or group of organs is impaired, then the function of that particular organ or group of organs will also be impaired to some degree.

Another principle is that frequently nerve function is impaired by an abnormal condition of the spinal bone segment, ligaments, or muscles if the bone is out of proper position, exceeds its normal range, or is fixated. The nerve involvement usually occurs where the nerve exits from the spinal column.

A study of an anatomy book, combined perhaps with an anatomical specimen or model, makes it obvious that this can happen.

To digress for a moment to a different, but analogous situation recognized by "scientific medicine," I'd like to mention

Bell's palsy. This is a condition of fairly rapid paralysis of either half of the face, lasting usually several weeks, with (usually) eventual recovery.

This condition is caused by pressure on the facial nerve as it passes through a channel of bone on its way out of the skull. The pressure is not because the bone "slips," but because (it's thought) a virus makes the nerve swell up causing it to be compressed where it's entirely surrounded by bone. (If that's not clear, imagine putting a long, skinny balloon halfway through a keyhole, and trying to blow it up. It can't blow up in the middle due to pressure from the surrounding metal.)

Under these circumstances, the facial muscles are paralyzed, droop, and sag, until the nerve recovers.

One treatment that's been used for this condition, although it's certainly not the usual one, is surgery to enlarge the bone channel so that pressure is off the nerve. This treatment, called "decompression," can be effective but isn't very much used. The usual treatment is cortisone to try to suppress the swelling. I find vitamins B_{12} and B_1, injected as for sciatica, to be much more effective.

What's this got to do with chiropractic? It's an obvious example of a malfunction caused by nerve compression. Most malfunctions caused by nerve pressure aren't so obvious, but they're real, all the same. If they can be relieved by manipulating a vertebra back into its proper position, an essentially conservative approach, then the more radical treatments involving potentially toxic drugs or surgery should not be used.

Of course, there are several questions to be addressed, such as: "Won't I get hurt? I heard someone had his back broken in half. How do I find a good chiropractor? How do I know if chiropractic can help my problem or not?"

All of these questions, in slightly varied form, could be asked of any health profession. Certainly, some persons have been injured by chiropractic care, as well as by scientific medicine. In fact, medical students are regularly warned about iatrogenic, or doctor-caused illness, so the problem is not just limited to chiropractic, but is a general problem in finding a competent practitioner of anything. As usual, indirect means are usually all that are available, such as talking to friends, neighbors, or others who have been under treatment. If you're really lucky, you may find a medical doctor who's able and willing to advise you with more than a blanket negative.

I don't want to exclude osteopathic physicians, D.O.'s, from this discussion. Many D.O.'s provide excellent manipulative therapy for their patients when it's needed. For reasons unknown, this is more acceptable to many medical doctors than chiropractic manipulation, even though the same sort of thing is being done.

Often, it is impossible to decide whether or not a problem can be helped by chiropractic without actually going over the problem with a chiropractor and evaluating the advice given. A second opinion in this, as well as other in fields, can't hurt.

Most competent chiropractors are very aware of the limits of their field, and will refer patients back to medical doctors or other health-care practitioners when it appears that chiropractic won't help, or isn't working out.

Before I conclude, I should note, emphatically, that chiropractic or other manipulative therapy is totally inappropriate treatment for some problems, too, just as it's the best for certain others.

I realize I'll probably get it from both sides for this discussion. I'll probably be condemned by medical doctors for the "mistaken belief that chiropractic can help anything" and looked upon questionably by chiropractic physicians for presuming to judge their art with no training in the field. So, why do I bother? Wouldn't it be safer, and maybe make this whole book more "acceptable," to tiptoe lightly around the topic, saying nothing?

In this book, I report what I've observed in everyday practice, with as much explanation and reference material as possible and practical. Among the "nonnutritional but natural" therapies most valuable to many of my patients has been chiropractic (and osteopathic) care. I've seen examples over and over again. It would be a disservice not to report a case or two of the most common problems along with the rest.

After months of heavy aspirin consumption to control the pain of osteoarthritis, a woman has a nutritional/biochemical analysis. Vitamins prove to be of no help. Blood tests, however, reveal allergies to several common foods, and a stomach-acid test shows the likelihood of very poor digestion and absorption. When B_{12} injections are given, further improvement comes rapidly. . . . Admittedly, there are several factors in this case which cannot be easily explained—a situation not all that unusual.

A Case of Allergic Arthritis

21

Flora Dunn was frightened. Her voice was controlled, but a small edge of fear showed through. "The main problem is that no one can tell me exactly what's the matter," she said. "My family doctor said it was osteoarthritis. One doctor at the referral clinic said it was probably rheumatoid arthritis; another said it wasn't that, but he couldn't tell exactly what it was. He ran tests for lupus, which were negative, but then said sometimes they are in the early stages. He wanted me to come back to repeat the tests in six months when they might turn positive."

She looked distressed at this. Her words continued to pour out rapidly. "In the meantime, all anyone tells me to take is aspirin. It doesn't really help, and this . . . this whatever it is, just continues to spread and get worse. It got so bad last month I couldn't even pick my baby up! I went over to my friend's house for help, and just cried. She told me to call over here; she thought changing my diet and taking some vitamins might help. She's always believed in that kind of thing. I've always been healthy and thought she was being silly, but I'm willing to try anything, especially after the referral clinic couldn't tell me what the matter was. . . ." Her flood of words and emotion trailed off just a little.

"Let's go back to the beginning. I'd like you to tell me where this started, and what's happened since."

"Well, about eight months ago my left index finger started to swell, mostly the middle joint, but the whole finger swelled above and below it, too. I didn't remember injuring it but figured it must be some kind of sprain, and it would go away.

"Then we went to the ocean for a vacation. The water was cold, but I went in for a swim anyway. That night my finger hurt much worse; I couldn't bend it. My neck started to hurt, and my ankles got stiff. They all hurt worse the next day so I didn't go swimming the rest of the time we were there. Since it didn't go away, I saw the doctor when we got home.

"He ran tests for rheumatoid arthritis and had x-rays taken. They were negative. He told me to take aspirin. I just kept getting worse so he sent me to the referral center. By then, my wrists were aching and hurt to move. My ankles were worse, and my left knee was swelling. Well, I saw several doctors; they ran lots of tests and x-rays, and they all came out negative. And all they told me to do was take aspirin, too!"

"Did you have any symptoms other than the joint pains?"

"Not one. They asked me that at the clinic too, but there really hasn't been anything else. Just joint problems."

"If it's OK with you, I'd like to have copies of those records sent here so I can see exactly what the tests showed. There's no point repeating what's already been done."

She nodded. "That's fine."

"I'd like you to come into the examination room so I can have a look at the problem myself."

I found nothing different from what Mrs. Dunn had described. Her left index finger was swollen and difficult to bend. Her left knee appeared slightly swollen, as did both ankles. Both wrists were tender, but not swollen. Physically, everything else appeared normal.

"Before I can make any recommendations, or even try to tell you what's the matter, I'd like you to get some tests done. I know you've had tests and x-rays, but not from a particularly nutritional/biochemical point of view.

"In all cases of arthritis, it's helpful to have a look at mineral status. I'd like you to turn in a specimen of hair for mineral analysis. Also, some cases of arthritis are associated with food allergy as well as other allergy. I'd like you to get a serum antibody test for a basic group of highly allergenic foods."

"I understand you need tests, but isn't there anything I can do in the meantime? I'd like to try anything if you think it might help."

"There are things you could try, but without a better diagnosis, I can't say I have a lot of hope they'll work. However, I think we'd better talk about basic good diet first."

I asked Mrs. Dunn for details of her diet. Unfortunately, like many others, hers was laden with sugar-added products and refined flours, and laced with synthetic chemicals.

"Even if it doesn't help your arthritis, changing to a good diet will keep you healthier in the future," I observed. "I want you to eliminate all the refined sugar from what you eat. Also, no refined flour, and please get rid of any artificial colors, flavors, or preservatives. On the positive side, eat as many fresh, raw, whole foods as possible. Use whole grains. Cooking foods when necessary, such as meats or potatoes, is fine, but anything you can eat raw, do."

"I've heard that from my friend, too." Mrs. Dunn managed to look hopeful and doubtful all at once. "Do you really think it will take this away? Aren't there some vitamins I can try, too?"

"Even if a good diet doesn't cure your problem, it'll help you otherwise," I repeated. "Now, I'd rather wait until after your tests are back, but if you'd like. . . ." I gave her a list of supplements including vitamin C, niacinamide, pantothenic acid, calcium, and cod-liver oil. After some brief discussion, she left to have her tests done.

Before Mrs. Dunn's next visit, her records arrived from the

referral clinic. Her "rheumatoid factor" test, uric acid levels, sedimentation rate, blood count, urinalysis, and a complete set of x-rays were all negative.

When Mrs. Dunn arrived, she appeared more dejected than frightened or nervous. "It's been a month, and it's gotten no better," she said. "The pain and stiffness are just the same. I did exactly what you said, too. It's really been a problem finding food to eat with no sugar in it."

"Has the pain worsened or spread?"

"No."

"Wasn't it steadily worsening before?"

"Yes."

"Well, don't feel too bad. Maybe you've slowed it down a little. Besides, I told you I was just guessing at what supplements you might need until we got your tests back. It looks as if we may have found something."

Mrs. Dunn brightened. "What?"

"It appears you're allergic to beef and wheat."

"Beef and wheat? I eat those every day, and have for years! I've only had these joint pains for nine months. Why should that cause me trouble now?"

"I can't answer that. I can't even say for sure that these allergies are the problem; it's likely, but not certain. What I'd like you to do is eliminate beef and wheat entirely for now, and see what happens. If that helps, I want you to check through the rest of your diet for any further allergies."

"Is that all?"

"No. I'd like you to stop taking all those supplements except vitamin C."

"Why?"

"As you said, they don't appear to be helping. However, more important, your hair mineral test gives a strong indication that you're not absorbing minerals, and probably much of the rest of your diet, as well as you should."

"What do you mean?"

"Calcium, magnesium, iron, manganese, zinc, chromium,

and selenium are all low. When this happens, it usually indicates a problem with assimilation. However, I'm surprised you haven't had any symptoms."

"What sort of symptoms?"

"Nothing major, but usually people who aren't assimilating have some sort of digestive-tract symptoms such as excess gas, bloating, constipation, occasionally diarrhea."

"I haven't had any of that at all . . . what's causing the poor absorption? These allergies?"

"Sometimes allergies do lead to that. But I'd expect more gastrointestinal symptoms. I'd like you to get checked for digestive enzymes and stomach acid."

"How do I do that? Have my stomach pumped?"

"Not anymore. The enzymes are checked by a blood test. To check the stomach acid we have you swallow a little capsule containing a radio transmitter. It's sensitive to pH and radios out to a receiver what your stomach acidity is. Then we give you test solutions to see what your stomach does. It's called gastric analysis by radiotelemetry."

"Is there a wire or string attached?"

"No. It just goes on through."

"So, no supplements except vitamin C until after that?"

"Right, because it doesn't look like they'll be absorbed."

Mrs. Dunn came in for her pH test a few weeks later. I had a spare minute, and went in to see how she was doing. When I came into the room, she sat up excitedly.

"I have to tell you," she started with a rush. "It must be allergies. I haven't had any beef or wheat since I left, and my pains are definitely less. I can walk better and use my wrists and arms more. . . ."

"Hold on," I said. "Lie back down on your left side. We don't want that capsule to slip out of your stomach any sooner than it has to."

She lay back down.

"I'm glad to hear it's working for you," I said. "You really should get checked for other allergies."

"Oh, I am. I've already turned in a list to the receptionist."

The nurse came back into the room. "I was about to let Mrs. Dunn go," she said. "Look at the recording."

I looked at the printout, then checked the machine to make sure there was no malfunction. The recording had been going for 30 minutes, and showed a pH of 5, indicating virtually no acid at all. (Normal pH is 1.8 to 2.3. The lower the number, the greater the acidity.)

"Are you sure you don't have any stomach symptoms?" I asked Mrs. Dunn.

"The nurse asked me that too. She thought sure I would have gas or something, but I don't."

I had Mrs. Dunn take two crushed hydrochloric acid tablets. Three minutes after she swallowed them, the recording indicated the pH dropping to 1.6, showing that the machine was working, and that the capsule was in her stomach.

"Why don't I have symptoms if I don't have any stomach acid?" Mrs. Dunn asked.

"I don't know. Most people do, but you're a good example of an exception to the rule. Oh, before you go, I'm going to ask the nurse to give you a vitamin B_{12} injection. Most people who don't have enough acid in their stomachs also don't assimilate vitamin B_{12} very well. We always try an injection to see what happens, since it's harmless."

The next day the nurse came into my office. "Mrs. Dunn called back this morning," she said. "She said four hours after her vitamin B_{12} shot her joints began to feel funny. This morning, her pain is almost gone. What's going on? We don't usually give vitamin B_{12} for arthritis. And I looked up her blood count again; she's not anemic."

"Pernicious anemia is an end-stage of vitamin B_{12} deficiency; a lot of other things can go wrong before it happens. I know we don't usually give vitamin B_{12} to help with arthritis; it usually doesn't work. But Mrs. Dunn is apparently different; her lack of stomach acid was a clear enough indication she needed at least a try with B_{12}."

Mrs. Dunn needed to come back only twice. I had her take

hydrochloric acid supplements before meals,° learn how to give her own B$_{12}$ injections, and take the supplements she needed. She also had to stop eating potatoes, Cheddar cheese, and lettuce as well as beef and wheat. Despite the vitamin B$_{12}$, hydrochloric acid, and other supplements, her arthritis starts to return if she eats these or other foods she's allergic to.

Probably the reason allergic arthritis caused by food is not diagnosed more frequently is that many physicians are still not used to the idea of foods or individual nutrients being more than marginally important in either the cause or cure of more than a very limited number of diseases.

Food allergy-caused arthritis is sufficiently frequent that no evaluation of arthritis is complete without testing for it in one way or another.

Mrs. Dunn's case illustrates this fact, as well as two other common findings. The first is that there often is an overlap between poor digestion/absorption and food allergy. Some authorities suspect that poor digestion is part of the cause of food allergy; of course, it usually can't be proven causative in any one particular case.

Second, her case shows once again that when absorption is poor, it's always worth trying vitamin B$_{12}$ injections to see if any symptoms are relieved. While Mrs. Dunn's response was more spectacular than most, no harm is done in trying.

Medically sophisticated individuals might be inclined to ask what Mrs. Dunn's blood count showed. Traditional medical teaching holds that achlorhydria should be accompanied by macrocytic (large red blood cells) anemia, or pernicious anemia, which are key indicators of vitamin B$_{12}$ and/or folic acid deficiency. Mrs. Dunn's blood count was normal, yet vitamin B$_{12}$ helped. That is not contradictory, but shows the value of early,

°Precautions for hydrochloric-acid-supplement use are described in chapter 45, "Poor Absorption."

preventive-type therapy before end-stage problems appear.

Mrs. Dunn, like many others, having found what appeared to be the cause of her problem, began to add sugar and other toxic substances back into her diet. After further symptom recurrences, she's finally decided to drop these permanently, too.

FURTHER READING

Breneman, J. C. "Allergic Arthritis." *Basics of Food Allergy* (Springfield, Ill.: Charles C Thomas, 1978), pp. 84-91.

Childers, Norman Franklin, and Russo, Gerard M. *The Nightshades and Health* (Somerville, N.J.: Horticultural Publications, Somerset Press, 1977).

Another case in which hypoglycemia and food allergy intertwine to create a knotty problem. The final kink in the case—headache—is not smoothed out until two very common foods are removed from the patient's diet. . . . A special discussion of hypoglycemia, and the not surprising reason why most physicians refuse to accept it as a "legitimate" health problem.

A Case of Headaches, Tiredness, and Hidden Food Allergy   22

Sara Weiss was a teacher, and very well organized. As she came from the waiting room, she put away a stack of papers from her fourth grade's last English test, which she'd been correcting.

"I have to make the best use of my time," she explained. "With 3 children of my own, and 33 in the class this year, I never get everything done. Which brings me to one of my problems: the last two or three years, I've had less energy to get through the day. I know I'm getting older, but 34 is no age to be as worn out as I am."

As she talked she looked through her purse, and finally pulled out a slip of paper. "I hope you don't mind. I wrote everything down, so I wouldn't forget. I always keep lists; it helps me get things done."

She began to go over her list. "First, I'd like to get rid of these headaches, if nothing else. I've had them for years. I've analyzed them and found they occur most frequently at 10 A.M., 2 P.M., and 4 P.M. I used to drink (she named a heavily advertised soda), as the advertisement mentioned those times. I thought it was made for me. It seemed to help, but less with time. I've been doing some studying, though, and have decided I have hypoglycemia." She paused for a breath.

"I want a glucose tolerance test, one of the long ones. I've read that the short ones aren't so good to diagnose low blood sugar." She looked almost as if she were expecting an argument. Not getting any, she continued.

"Second, my continuous tiredness. I think that's low blood sugar, too, but I want to make sure.

"Third, my muscles ache a lot when I haven't been exercising or using them especially much. Also, they seem weaker than they should be, particularly my legs. Sometimes it seems I can't stand in front of my class another minute.

"Last, I've had premenstrual problems for several years: bloating, weight gain, and irritability. I used to take 'water pills' for that, but they gave me backaches, so I stopped. I heard that vitamin B_6 will help. Will it?"

She looked at her list again. "That's everything."

"I'll answer the last question first. Vitamin B_6 will probably help you get rid of premenstrual problems. Start with 100 milligrams 3 times a day. You can adjust the dosage up or down as needed, as it's nontoxic.

"Your first two problems, tiredness and headaches, *could* be associated with low blood sugar. The timing of the headaches is particularly suspicious. Are those between-meal times for you?"

"Yes. Since I'm teaching, I can't get to food then, as I can in the evening. I've noticed that eating does help them go away."

"Any symptom that can be made better by eating or drinking something has to be suspected of being associated with hypoglycemia. Don't forget, though, there are other causes of headaches and tiredness."

"Oh, I know that. I saw my chiropractor. He says I have no spinal cause for headache. I thought of seeing a neurologist, but the pain isn't that bad, just regular, and annoying until it goes. Besides, after I decided it must be low blood sugar, I stopped eating sugar, and that's when the headaches got a little less. Then I thought I'd come in to see if I was right."

"It sounds like you're on the right track. Let's get you scheduled for a six-hour glucose tolerance test, to settle it.

"Now, about your tiredness. How much sleep do you get? How about exercise? Are you under any extra strain?"

"I get too much sleep, eight to ten hours a night. I have to go to bed early, I'm so tired. That's another reason I can't get anything done. My husband can't understand how I can be so worn out with all that sleep. I can't understand it myself.

"I don't get much exercise, except on weekends. If I try, I feel even worse. And, no, I don't have any unusual emotional strain. My marriage is fine, the kids are healthy. . . ."

"All right, what about physical causes? Have you been checked for any common problems such as anemia or weak thyroid function?"

"Not in the past three or four years. Go ahead and check, but I'm sure that's not what the problem is."

"Just to be sure, let's do a blood count and thyroid function test. OK?"

She nodded agreement.

"That leaves your muscle problem. How long have you had the aching and weakness?"

"The weakness is only the last couple of years. The aching has been for much longer, on and off. I haven't been able to find a pattern for it. Don't get me wrong about weakness, though. I can walk around, run when I have to, and do what I need to. It's more a feeling of fatigue, like I have to force my muscles to work. Maybe it's just lack of exercise, but it wasn't that way two years ago."

"When did you stop taking the diuretics?"

"What?"

"The 'water pills.' "

"Oh, those. About a year and a half ago, when I started getting backaches, like I told you. I took a little potassium until they went away. You don't suppose my muscular weakness is due to that, do you? Now, why didn't I think of that? I read about it, too. Can I get a blood test for potassium, please?"

"I was going to suggest that. Also, we should get a mineral analysis done on a hair specimen."

"Whatever you think. I don't mean to tell you what to do. I

just want to get better as fast as I can, now that I've got it figured out."

"Let's wait to see. I think those are enough tests for now. Perhaps there'll be others later. But let's talk about those later.

"Before you go, though, I need to ask you a few questions. Since this is the first time you've been here, I need a little background. We don't have much time left, but could you tell me if you have any health problems you didn't mention? Have you had any operations or been in the hospital? Are there any illnesses in your family?"

"Let's see. My grandmother had diabetes. But that's all, except one of my sisters has hay fever really bad. You know I forgot to mention that. I should have written it down. I get hay fever just a little for two or three weeks every spring. I haven't been in the hospital except for babies and to have my tonsils out when I was 6."

"Thanks. That's all I need for now."

Mrs. Weiss gathered her things together, and after checking her list once more, went to the office nurse to schedule her tests.

Her next visit was to see about the results of her tests. "Well, what do we do now?" she asked.

"Your blood count was normal, and so was your thyroid test. But the serum potassium was very close to the lower end of the normal range, and your glucose tolerance test wasn't normal at all."

"It wasn't? I got the results from the nurse and showed them to my younger brother. I didn't tell you he's a medical student, did I? He said it looks normal to him. It doesn't go low enough to be hypoglycemia; besides, he says that's a very rare disease. But after all the reading I did, I was so convinced. . . ."

"I'll agree to one thing. The whole subject of hypoglycemia or low blood sugar is very confusing. Primary hypoglycemia, which is usually thought to be due to an insulin-secreting tumor, is very rare. But secondary hypoglycemia is quite common."

"Secondary? What does that mean?"

"That's the type that most books on hypoglycemia are describing. Secondary means that the hypoglycemia is due to something else. Overconsumption of sugar and refined foods, mineral deficiencies, emotional stress, lack of exercise, food allergies, weak adrenal glands—all of these, by themselves or in combination, can cause hypoglycemia. Then, the hypoglycemia causes most of the familiar symptoms. In your case, tiredness and headaches. So it's somewhat a matter of semantics; we could skip calling it hypoglycemia altogether, and focus on the primary problem *causing* the hypoglycemia, which in turn causes the other problems.

"Actually, though, secondary hypoglycemia is a fairly accurate description, as all of these primary causes can lead to a common metabolic problem: a derangement of the body's energy control systems, which we call hypoglycemia or low blood sugar. But let's get back to your particular case.

"Your blood sugar test is abnormal by three criteria. First, the lowest number is below 55. Second, one number is more than 25 below the fasting level. Third, the nurse noted several symptoms which happened at the same time as the lowest point on your test."

Mrs. Weiss looked at her notes. "Yes, I did get a rather bad headache at 2 p.m., when the low point on my test occurred. By the way, where can I find the criteria you use for judging blood sugar tests?"

"Most doctors specializing in a nutritional/biochemical approach use their own individual criteria. But many are very similar to those published by H. L. Newbold, M.D., in his book, *Mega-Nutrients for Your Nerves.*"

"Could this be responsible for all my symptoms?"

"Probably many of them. Since your mineral analysis hasn't returned, why don't you go ahead with a program for hypoglycemia in the meantime, and see how you do?"

I asked Mrs. Weiss to go onto a high-protein, low-carbohydrate diet, along with B complex vitamins, vitamin C, and vitamin E. Of course, she should eliminate all refined sugars, refined carbohydrates, and all artificial colors, flavors, and preservatives. Briefly we discussed the alternative high-complex-carbohydrate, plus more-raw-food approach favored by many physicians, but she decided that at present it didn't fit her lifestyle. I requested that she return after one month. Her mineral analysis would certainly be back by then.

"Well, how are you doing so far?" I asked, when Mrs. Weiss came in for her appointment a month later.

This time she had her notes out and ready. "About 50-50. My biggest disappointment is that my headaches aren't much better. My tiredness is definitely less, though. I'm not any ball of fire, yet, but still there's a difference.

"My muscles still ache and feel weak. No change there. My premenstrual bloating and irritability were much less this month, though, with the vitamin B_6."

"That's some progress anyway."

"Yes. I wanted to ask you about something you said last time, that my serum potassium test was very close to the low end of normal. You didn't ask me to do anything about it. Were you waiting for my hair mineral test?"

"In fact, I was. Let's look at it."

Her hair test showed a level of potassium only 50 percent of the lower limit of normal.

"Why is my hair test abnormally low, when my serum test was only low normal?"

"Radioisotope studies have shown conclusively that a person's total body storage of potassium can be depleted as much as 10 to 20 percent before the serum potassium becomes abnormally low."

"That'll probably help my muscles, anyway."

I agreed. The rest of Mrs. Weiss's mineral analysis showed a need for zinc (an almost universal hypoglycemic finding) as well as low copper and manganese. I asked her to add these supplements to her list, stay with her previous program, and check back in another four to six weeks.

There'd been a minor office emergency before Mrs. Weiss's next visit, so I was a little behind time for her appointment. However, she'd brought her usual stack of papers to correct, and was putting them away as she came in.

"My headaches aren't any better," she said. "I still get them when I haven't eaten. My tiredness is about the same. One good thing though, I don't feel the same degree of muscle weakness. I'm sure the potassium helped."

"What about the muscle aching?"

"That's still there."

"You're not really doing as well as I'd expect at this point. Most people with hypoglycemia related strictly to poor nutrition show more relief from symptoms after eight to ten weeks of good diet control, with appropriate supplementation. We'd better look a little more for other problems. . . . You once mentioned a minor problem with hay fever, didn't you?"

"But I don't have that now. Besides, hay fever doesn't cause low blood sugar, does it?"

"No, it doesn't. But having hay fever does indicate that you have allergies. You may well have more of them than you suspect. Did you know that food allergies are a frequent major contributing cause, or even a primary cause of hypoglycemia?"

"No, I didn't. Should I get skin tests done?"

"Those aren't very accurate for food allergies. I used to do them, but I don't bother anymore."

"What do I do, then? I've read about pulse testing for food allergies, but with my job and family, I just don't have the time. I don't have the time to go on a fast, either."

"Those are both good methods, and certainly inexpensive. I've seen them work well. There's another method available that's relatively new, but clinically very useful and highly accurate. It's a blood test."

"A blood test for allergies? What's it called?"

"It has a horrendous name. It's called a radioallergosorbent test, or RAST test for short. The principle is much simpler than the name. It's a way of detecting antibodies in your blood serum. If a person is allergic to something, his or her system will produce antibodies to it. This test can determine if you have antibodies to specific foods, and if you do, what level of antibodies. That is, it can tell what you're allergic to, and how bad the allergy is."

"That sounds like a very good test. There must be a drawback, though. What is it?"

"Aside from having to have blood drawn, the only one I know of is the relative expense. Pulse testing and fasting followed by food 'challenges' cost only the time involved."

"Are they as accurate?"

"If done properly, they can be just as accurate."

"But I really don't have the time. Let's do the blood test. Besides, as I said before, I want to get better as fast as possible."

She gathered her things together, and went to have the blood specimen drawn.

The next (and last) time I saw Mrs. Weiss was five months later. School was out, but she was carrying as many papers as ever. This time they were her own, part of a master's degree program she was working on.

"I just came in to ask if I shouldn't get a follow-up on some of my tests. I don't want to be taking supplements I don't need anymore."

"That's a good idea. But, tell me, what's happened to your various symptoms?"

"Oh, yes, I made sure to write down everything to tell you. I've never been so amazed. My blood test came back highly positive for antibodies to beef and eggs; I've been eating beef all my life, and eggs are practically my favorite food. Of course, there's a lot of both on a high-protein diet like I was on.

"Well, I decided to see what was what, so I stopped eating beef first. You know, my muscle aches cleared up and haven't been back since. When I stopped eating eggs, I was even more surprised. My headaches went away in 48 hours. I've had only two in four months. Also, my tiredness is gone completely. I feel more energetic than I have in years.

"You know, I think for me beef and eggs are every bit as bad as sugar. I've tried a little of each just to see. The sugar makes me feel bad, but the eggs and beef are worse. Those are supposed to be good foods, too. Is that really possible?"

I answered that it obviously was: she had proven it to herself. As a general rule, refined sugars and refined foods should be in no one's diet. But for sensitive individuals, allergy-causing foods can be nearly as bad. In Mrs. Weiss's case, as in many others, food allergies were one major cause of her hypoglycemia, and its consequent symptoms.

The Hypoglycemia Controversy

Hypoglycemia is presently one of medicine's most controversial subjects. A small but vocal minority of physicians say the problem is widespread; the majority say hypoglycemia is a medical oddity, a rare condition. These physicians indicate that most persons who think they suffer from hypoglycemia are just tense or worried, needing a psychiatrist or a tranquilizer or two.

Perhaps "controversial" is the wrong word. Most physicians who don't believe in hypoglycemia don't argue about it, but just try to cover the whole subject under a blanket of silence. If it isn't talked about maybe it'll go away.

As noted in Mrs. Weiss's case, "primary" hypoglycemia is extremely rare. In these few cases, there is an overproduction of insulin by a usually nonmalignant tumor of the pancreas. In even more rare cases, tissue outside the pancreas has been found to be overproducing insulin. Of course, just like an overdose of injected insulin, internally overproduced insulin drives the blood sugar too low, producing hypoglycemia (low blood sugar) symptoms.

Secondary hypoglycemia is a rather common problem. As also noted in the case above, secondary hypoglycemia means exactly that: the hypoglycemia is due to other causes, such as too much sugar in the diet, emotional stress, food allergies, weak adrenal gland function, thyroid or ovarian problems, nutrient malabsorption, food allergy, vitamin and mineral deficiencies, no exercise . . . and, I'm sure, many factors I haven't listed. Therefore, I often de-emphasize the term *hypoglycemia*, and try to focus the person's attention on correcting the *cause* or causes of the secondary hypoglycemia. If these are taken care of, the hypoglycemia will go away.

You might ask then, why spend any time at all on secondary hypoglycemia? Why not just get to the cause of it, and throw the term away altogether?

An excellent parallel can be drawn with another usually secondary problem, anemia. Anemia, like hypoglycemia, is usually caused by something else: iron deficiency, gastrointestinal bleeding, hemolysis (excess breakdown of blood cells), deficiencies of copper, folic acid, vitamin B_{12}, vitamin B_6, and many other less well known causes. Sometimes there is more than one cause.

Before the cause or causes of the anemia can be discovered, it is usually necessary for a physician to find the anemia in the first place. As in most mystery stories, the villain or villains are not found, or sometimes not even suspected, in the early stages. Medical diagnosis likewise proceeds a step at a time. As with anemia, hypoglycemia has to be suspected and diagnosed before its causes can be further investigated.

Since a normal level of blood sugar is critical to the function of the brain, it's not surprising that many of the effects of hypoglycemia, lowered blood sugar, show up as mental or emotional symptoms. I do not intend to present anything like a complete discussion of hypoglycemic symptoms here (for excellent discussions, please see Further Reading). I'll just mention that in cases of unexplained tiredness, shakiness, foggy mind, extreme forgetfulness, depression, fits of anger, crying spells, headaches, and other mental symptoms, I always include testing for hypoglycemia as part of the evaluation.

This brings us back to the "which came first—the chicken or the egg?" problem. As noted above, mental/emotional stress can upset the body's blood sugar control systems sufficiently to cause hypoglycemia. So: does the hypoglycemia cause the mental upset, or does the mental upset cause the hypoglycemia? That question cannot be answered with a definitive general rule. For some people it's one, for some the other, and for most, somewhere in between, or perhaps a kind of vicious circle. Individual problems require individual answers. With hypoglycemia, as with other health problems, I try to keep as many factors in mind as possible, and help the patient deal with all of them, referring to other health-care professionals when necessary for help I don't have the expertise or time to provide.

Why isn't hypoglycemia more often diagnosed by most physicians? Once again, there are many answers.

Many organs, including the pancreas, liver, adrenals, thyroid, brain, and pituitary, are involved in blood sugar control. In hypoglycemia, these and other organs are involved in varying degrees. Likewise, hypoglycemia cuts across various organ systems—gastrointestinal, nervous, endocrine—involving each to varying degrees. Much medical training involves thinking in "single-disease single-cause" terms. While this type of training and thinking is valuable sometimes, unless a physician can also think in "whole-person multiple-cause" terms when necessary, multifactorial problems like secondary hypoglycemia just aren't considered.

Medical training over the past few decades has emphasized the mental causation of physical symptoms, or psychosomatic disease. There's practically no emphasis on somatopsychic problems. Since hypoglycemia has so many prominent mental symptoms, many physicians almost automatically assume the problem is psychosomatic, investigate no further, and prescribe tranquilizers, a psychiatrist, or tell the patient, "It's all in your head" or "Nothing's the matter."

Traditional medical training also neglects nutritional factors almost entirely. Since much of the treatment of hypoglycemia, whatever the cause, is nutritional or biochemical, many physicians wouldn't be able to help patients with the problem even if willing to make the diagnosis.

So the failure of a non-nutrition-oriented physician to diagnose and treat hypoglycemia is not entirely his fault. The whole of his background and training is stacked against it.

FURTHER READING

Abrahamson, E. M., and Pezet, A. W. *Body, Mind, and Sugar* (New York: Avon, 1977).

Buehler, Martin S. "Relative Hypoglycemia: A Clinical Review of 350 Cases." *The Lancet*, July 1962, pp. 289-92.

Cheraskin, Emanuel, and Ringsdorf, W. Marshall, Jr., with Brecher, Arline. *Psychodietetics: Food as the Key to Emotional Health* (New York: Stein & Day, 1974).

Conn, Jerome W., and Seltzer, Holbrooke S. "Spontaneous

Hypoglycemia." *American Journal of Medicine,* September 1955, pp. 460–78.

Fredericks, Carlton, and Goodman, Herman. *Low Blood Sugar and You* (New York: Constellation International, 1969).

Newbold, H. L. *Mega-Nutrients for Your Nerves* (New York: Peter H. Wyden, 1975).

A man with severe headaches seeks alternative treatment. He has already undergone years of expensive testing, including a brain scan and spinal tap, taken huge quantities of painkillers and has psychiatric help. A brief examination reveals that nutritional therapy isn't what he needs either. Instead, he is referred to a chiropractor, and his suffering ends in short order.

A Headache for a Chiropractor   23

Ray Harper looked well. I thought perhaps he'd come in for a routine check and a discussion of staying well, as people who practice preventive self-care do. But that wasn't the case.

"I have headaches all the time, every day," he said. "Sometimes small ones—I have one now—and frequently bad ones. They hit me at any time of the day or night, and last from a few hours to a few days. I've looked and looked for a cause, and can't find any. My mother's been after me for years to try natural health care, but I couldn't believe that modern scientific medicine couldn't cure me. Then I saw what happened with a friend of mine when he changed his diet and took some vitamins. He's a patient of yours, so I thought I'd come in."

"How long have you had headaches?"

"Several years, but really bad the last two or three. When I say really bad, I mean it. I've had to stay home from teaching classes pretty often. Luckily, I've been able to keep my job, but I don't know how much longer I can with the amount of time I've missed.

"Now, before you ask me if my headaches are due to the academic rat race, I've been to see a psychiatrist already. I was sent there after having every test imaginable done, and everything came up negative. The psychiatrist decided I was no more neurotic than anyone else but since my headaches were so bad he tried me on antidepressants and then tranquilizers, anyway. I gave each drug a try for a few weeks, but none of them helped."

"So what do you do for your headaches?"

"I've taken more aspirin than I want to remember. That takes care of the minor ones, but most of them aren't minor. If the aspirin doesn't work, I usually put up with them and wait for them to go away. I get irritable and grouchy, but that beats being all doped up. For the really bad ones I take codeine or Demerol, or go to the emergency room for a shot."

He reached into his pocket. "Here, I thought you'd want a list of the drugs I've taken at one time or another."

I read over the list. It contained the names of every pain-reliever available, as well as antimigraine drugs, and an impressive array of tranquilizers and antidepressants.

"Have any of these worked at all?"

"The painkillers do stop the pain, but it always comes back. The rest haven't done any good at all."

"I assume you've had a variety of tests done?"

"I've been hospitalized for testing twice. I've had blood tests, urine tests, and x-rays. I've had skull x-rays, two EEGs [brain-wave tests], a brain scan, and a spinal tap. They did one of those CAT scans. I've been seen by neurologists, neurosurgeons, and several other doctors. They finally all decided I needed a psychiatrist. But I told you what came of that. I've had my eyes checked and glasses changed. That didn't help."

"I assume your blood pressure is normal?"

"That was one of the first things they checked."

"Do your headaches get worse if you don't eat?"

"No, they don't. But after I'd been through a lot of negative tests, I insisted they do a six-hour glucose tolerance test. I'd read about headaches due to low blood sugar, so I thought it was worth a try. That was negative, too, but I know those are inter-preted differently by different physicians, so I brought a copy along." He handed me another slip of paper.

I studied it for a minute. Mr. Harper was right; nutritionally oriented physicians generally apply different interpretive stan-dards to glucose tolerance tests than conventional physicians do. However, Mr. Harper's test was perfectly normal by any stan-dards.

"That's quite normal," I said. Mr. Harper nodded.

"Do your headaches go in cycles?"

"Not at all. I tried plotting them on a calendar for nearly a year. Couldn't find any pattern."

"Do they occur more at home, or when you're out?"

"Neither, really. I have noticed they happen more often when I'm particularly active. I had to give up jogging because it seemed to make them worse. But nobody's been able to put that together with anything."

"Is there anything else that makes your headaches worse?"

"Driving on the freeway at rush hour. But then that gives a lot of people headaches."

"Do you wake up at night with headaches?"

"Yes, I do. That always had the psychiatrist puzzled. He said if it was worry, I wouldn't go to sleep in the first place and wouldn't wake up from a sound sleep with one."

"Does that happen often?"

"Fairly frequently."

"Describe a typical headache for me."

"They're not always the same, but usually they start at the back of my head. Sometimes they stay there; other times they spread over my whole head. Occasionally they start in my fore-head."

"Are they entirely on the left or right side of your head?"

"No, both sides, but usually worse on the right, particularly in the back of my head."

"Have you ever been hit on the head?"

"Several times. I had a concussion playing intramural football when I was a graduate student. A scaffold accidentally fell on my head, luckily not from very far up, about four years ago. My really bad headaches got much more frequent after that. I thought there could be a connection but the doctors said no, not this long after."

"Do your neck muscles get sore or tight with headaches?"

"With headaches, and without. I get a crick in my neck a lot. Those muscles stay tight a lot. Just tension, I guess."

"Maybe not. I want you to sit up straight in your chair, square your shoulders, then relax."

Mr. Harper did. "Now, without moving your shoulder, rotate your head as far to the right as you can."

He turned his head. Using the middle of his chin as a reference point, it appeared he could turn 50 to 55 degrees from center. I asked him to try the same thing to the left; he could rotate at best 45 degrees. I asked him to try both rotations again, with the same results.

"That explains your difficulty on the freeway," I said.

"What do you mean?"

"Apparently you haven't noticed; many people with your problem don't. You can't rotate your head to either side as far as normal. Most people can turn approximately 90 degrees; the best you can do is 50 to 55 degrees to the right."

"That gives me headaches?"

"No, the same condition that prevents neck rotation can cause headaches." I got up, and went to the side of his chair. "Excuse me, but this might hurt." I pressed on one of the vertebral spines in his neck.

Mr. Harper winced. "That hurt. But doesn't everyone hurt if you push them like that?"

"No, and I check routinely." I pressed on several other vertebral spines. Almost every one of them hurt. "Your problem is right here. Your cervical vertebrae are out of alignment. All the diets and vitamins in the world won't do you any more good than what you've been through already. What you need is help from another branch of natural health care, manipulative therapy. You need chiropractic or osteopathic care. I'd like to refer you to a chiropractor I know. Without this type of care, your headaches will stay with you."

"A chiropractor? I always thought chiropractors were, well, you know . . . sort of fringy, kind of like faith healing or voodoo. I'm surprised to hear you making that kind of recommendation."

"Mr. Harper, like any physician, I've been trained to try to achieve for my patients the best possible results with the least possible risk. I've learned since leaving medical school that in cases like yours, that means competent chiropractic or osteopathic manipulation."

"What will that do to relieve my headaches?"

"I think your headaches are caused by abnormal pressure on nerves that serve various structures around your neck and head: muscles, joints, ligaments, and so on. That pressure varies as you move your head and neck, so the headaches vary."

"Are you sure?"

"Considering all the negative tests you've had, and your physical findings, I'm fairly sure. But keep in mind; this is just a theory until proven."

Mr. Harper thought for a minute. "I've tried everything else . . . why not?"

Eight weeks later, Mr. Harper was back at my office. Since we'd only talked once, I'd almost forgotten that he'd been in.

"I came back to talk about preventive health care," he said. "But before that, I want to tell you I haven't had a headache in two weeks. The chiropractor said I corrected as rapidly as anyone he's seen. And I can turn my head clear around to the left to see the freeway traffic, and not get a headache." He demonstrated a 90-degree rotation in both directions.

"That is rapid. I'm glad it worked out that well for you."

"I want to ask something. I went through all kinds of tests—a spinal tap, brain scan, EEG, two hospitalizations—and nobody even thought to recommend a chiropractor. Why? After the chiropractor examined me, took x-rays, and explained the anatomy of the neck bones and nerves to me it was obvious. He couldn't be sure, but said it was likely those blows to my head had a lot to do with it. Thinking back, that makes sense too. So, why?"

"Remember what you said when I first recommended manipulative treatment? Unfortunately, that kind of attitude is encouraged by a few of my medical colleagues and is taught in medical schools.

"Like many other physicians, I decided to look into manipulative care for myself, particularly after some of my patients told me what had happened to them. I found that in some cases manipulative therapy by a competent practitioner is the only treatment that works."

———— • ————

Due to irrational opposition, or perhaps ignorance of the proper place of manipulative therapy, Mr. Harper was exposed to both unnecessarily risky treatment and testing. Most important, he suffered from headaches much longer than necessary.

In a general or family practice, headaches, as well as neck pains or backache, are a common complaint. A substantial proportion of persons with these problems are best helped by an osteopathic or chiropractic practitioner, and not by drug therapy (or by nutritional/biochemical therapy). That is because manipulative treatment gets at the cause of the problem; drugs simply treat the symptoms, which usually keep returning until the causes are removed.

Please don't take this wrong, or too far. I didn't say all headaches, backaches, and neck pains are helped this way, just a substantial proportion. But since manipulative therapy is essentially conservative, carrying less risk than long-term drug treatment, and less risk than some advanced medical testing, logic says it should be tried early. If it doesn't help, or especially if a problem grows worse, then further testing and other forms of treatment should be employed in turn.

All of the medical procedures mentioned and therapies tried for Mr. Harper have an important place in modern medicine. When necessary, I'll recommend them. But the bias of scientific medicine irrationally suppresses an important and relatively safe technique which should at least be looked into for persons with headache, neck pains, and a variety of backaches and pains.

Editor's note: A more extensive discussion of Chiropractic is included in chapter 20, "A Case of Bed-Wetting from Nerve Compression."

A woman who is otherwise in extraordinarily good health at 90 is bothered by failing energy and tingling sensations in her fingers and toes. Maturity-onset diabetes is suspected but tests show her blood sugar metabolism to be normal. Although she's been taking vitamins for years—even injections of B_{12}—it's suspected her requirement for these nutrients is unusually high, or her utilization of them is faulty. When other B vitamins are added to her injections, her symptoms improve markedly.

24 A Case of B Vitamin Deficiency in a Healthy 90-Year-Old

Ethel Watson had been in only once before. When I saw her name on the appointment schedule, I thought she must be new, as I didn't remember who she was. Then I noticed her record on top of the stack, with a sticker indicating she'd last been in three years before. I opened her record to review it briefly.

According to my notes, we'd talked about diet and vitamin supplements, and I'd given some minor advice. Apparently she'd not been ill, as there was no notation about any symptoms, or any clue about why she'd made today's appointment. As I put her record down, one other thing caught my eye: her birth date, 1888.

I went out to the waiting room to get her. As she got up quickly from her chair, I noticed she was carrying a cane. Any notion that she really needed it was quickly dispelled by her quick walk down the hall to my office. She appeared to use the cane to clear her way of possible obstacles.

As she sat down, she remarked: "I really don't need this

stick, you know. It's just to beat off those neighborhood dogs when I go for my walks twice a day. Before I got it, one of them nearly took my leg off. Now they've all learned what it's for and keep their distance." She put it down with her purse.

"I'm sure you don't remember me." she continued. "I didn't get into any real problems when I was in last, mostly because I just wanted to see what you'd say. Most of what you told me I knew already. I wanted to find out if I could talk to you about vitamins and diet and staying healthy. Most of the young doctors, nothing personal of course, but most of you young doctors think someone my age is just lucky to be alive. I'll be 90 in a few weeks, you know."

She paused. "They just take a look at my age and tell me that whatever aches and pains I have just go with getting old. I should take some aspirin, pay my bill, and wait for the undertaker. I don't look at it that way: I intend to stay as fit as I can until I get ready to go and that won't be for a few years yet.

"Now, let me tell you what's bothering me. I don't feel as perky as I think I should; I know I can have more energy. I'm getting too sleepy in the afternoon. My Lord! I've got too much to do to sleep away my days. I'm much too forgetful. My joints are aching; my bowels are sluggish, and the way I eat they should go like clockwork.

"What's really got me bothered in the past few years has been these tingly feelings I get in my fingers and sometimes my toes. They just come and go, but they've been more frequent since I turned 85. My arms and legs have been going to sleep on and off. I know that comes from needing B vitamins, but I eat right and take my B, and it doesn't help."

She thought for a minute. "Is that all? That memory of mine! I'm going to have to write everything down, even the way to the bathroom if this keeps up. Oh yes: my eyes. At my age, I need glasses for close work and reading. I get my glasses checked every six months; the eye doctor says my prescription's fine. I even checked with another one to make sure, but she told me the same thing. But my eyes are still getting blurry on and off. It's like working through water sometimes. It comes and goes like the numbnesses and tingling. It's not predictable.

"Now, I've done enough reading to know that sometimes those are early signs of maturity-onset diabetes so many of us old folks get. Heaven knows, I'm mature enough. I want a test for it, but I don't want one of those sugar tolerance tests. I haven't had any refined sugar since 1951 and I don't want any now." Having apparently arrived at her major worry, she stopped.

"That's easy enough to get around," I said. "Since you don't intend to eat any more refined sugar, you can just be tested with a high-natural-carbohydrate meal. We'll do a fasting blood sugar test, then have you go eat breakfast with lots of natural carbohydrates. For example, you could have oatmeal with honey on it, whole-grain toast with honey or jam with no sugar, juice, and fruit. Then two hours after you're done, we'd do another blood sugar test."

"Would that be accurate?"

"For your body, and the way you live, yes. There's no point testing you with refined sugar, glucose, unless it's part of your living pattern."

"Do you think I have diabetes?"

"I can't say for sure . . . but you're right, occasionally symptoms like you have are early warning signs of diabetes: the numbnesses, tingling, and eye problems. It's wise to check. Also, while we're at it, I'd like you to get another test. It's barely out of research stages, but looks like an excellent screening test for diabetes, particularly since it represents a summation of abnormally high blood sugar over weeks to months, even if the fluctuation is erratic. It's called a 'hemoglobin $A1_C$' test."

"Do I have to do anything special for that?"

"No, just take a blood test."

"Alright."

"Before you go, I want to talk to you a bit about diet and especially nutrient absorption. You know that as we all get older, our stomachs don't make as much acid and sometimes we don't make enough digestive enzymes. Sometimes all that's needed is supplementation of acid or enzymes to improve absorption of nutrients and make symptoms go away. This is especially so after age 80."

"You're getting more forgetful than I am," Mrs. Watson scolded. "I'm way ahead of you there. That's one reason I came back to talk to you, because you mentioned that to me last time I was in. I hadn't heard that from a doctor since the 1930s."

I looked at her record. Although I'd recorded her diet, which was excellent, and a good group of supplements, I hadn't put anything down about digestive aids.

"I'm sorry, looks like I didn't note that. I will this time."

"Not your fault. You can't record every word an old lady tells you. Back in, I think it was 1938, I'd developed a case of gas. I went to old Dr. Samuels; he died the next year. He just told me to take hydrochloric acid; it came in drops in those days. I've taken it so long it's automatic. Maybe I didn't tell you. Later I added enzymes and before you mention it, vitamin B_{12} injections I give myself from time to time. I couldn't get a doctor to give them to me, so I talked my pharmacist out of them. He's 74, and old enough to know they help people our age."

I had nothing further to say at this point. Mrs. Watson was indeed ahead of me. After a word or two more, she went off to get her tests done.

She was as chatty as before when she returned. This time she was carrying a newer, heavier cane.

"Darn dog, excuse my French, a big Labrador ran off with my last one," she said. "Now, do I have diabetes or not?"

"I'm glad to report your fasting blood sugar was 95 milligrams percent, and two hours after eating it was 137 milligrams percent, both within normal. Also your hemoglobin $A1_C$ was 5.8 percent, also well within normal."

"Good. So what's the matter with me? Do you think I'm getting multiple sclerosis or something?"

"No, I don't. And before you go any further with testing I'd just like you to add to your vitamin B_{12} injections, to see how you feel."

"More B$_{12}$? I've already tried that."

"No, not more B$_{12}$. I'd like you to add in the other B vitamins, especially niacin, B$_6$, and folic acid."

"I already take those. I take B complex tablets and extra folic acid."

"I know. What I mean is to inject those vitamins right along with the B$_{12}$."

"Why? I thought they worked just fine by mouth, and only B$_{12}$ needed to be injected."

"That's usually so, but practicing physicians have observed over the years that some people, especially older individuals, respond much better to B vitamin injections of various sorts than to swallowing them. I was told in medical school that was 'quack' medicine, but I've learned differently since."

"But why do you want me to try them?"

"Because your symptoms, especially the tingling and numbness that comes and goes could be due to something as simple as B vitamin deficiency. And after all these years, researchers have finally investigated and found that in fact B vitamin injections maintain normal vitamin levels in some older persons much better than oral vitamins. And cheaper, too, especially if you give your own shots."

Mrs. Watson looked quite interested. "That part about cheaper just sold me," she said. "I'll try it; I know it can't hurt. I'm certainly an older individual. If it works for me, I can stop buying B complex pills. On my pension every little bit helps. If it doesn't work, I'll be back."

I wrote out her prescriptions. Swinging her cane, she left the office.

A month or two later, I heard that she'd called in to say her B vitamin shots were working just fine. Her tingling and numbness were gone, her eyesight cleared, and her bowels were back to working "like clockwork." Only her joints still hurt; she'd be in about that when it was bad enough to worry about. Right now, since her energy was back to par, she had "too much to do to bother seeing doctors!"

———

The "index of suspicion" about nutrient malabsorption must rise with age. After age 70, it's important to prove it *doesn't* exist, rather than the other way around. Much ill health can be treated and prevented by nutritional means if this point of view is adopted.

I can't say why niacin (B_3), B_6, and folic acid are frequently found deficient in older individuals who eat reasonably well. It's probably not associated with any of the currently known absorptive defects. All that can be said is that it goes with aging.

A case like this always brings to mind my medical school days, when various scientific professors would denounce to the students the completely useless procedure of B complex vitamin injections to help elderly persons feel better. Any help was attributed to placebo effect; the implication of "financial rip-off" was heavy.

FURTHER READING

Chope, Harold D. "The Nutritional Status of the Aging." *California Medicine*, vol. 74, no. 2, February 1951, pp. 105–10.

———. "Relation of Nutrition to Health in Aging Persons." *California Medicine*, vol. 81, no. 5, November 1954, pp. 335–38.

Elsborg, L.; Lund, V.; and Bastrup-Madsen, P. "Serum Vitamin B_{12} Levels in the Aged." *Acta Medica Scandinavica*, vol. 200, 1976, pp. 309–14.

Fisher, S. K. et al. "Assessment of Multiple Dietary Nutrient Deficiencies for Elderly Men and Women." *Federation Proceedings*, vol. 36, no. 3, March 1, 1977, p. 1093.

Frank, O. et al. "Superiority of Periodic Intramuscular Vitamins over Daily Oral Vitamins in Maintaining Normal Vitamin Titers in a Geriatric Population." *The American Journal of Clinical Nutrition*, vol. 30, no. 4, April 1977, p. 630.

Jansen, Coerene, and Harrill, Inez. "Intakes and Serum Levels of Protein and Iron for Elderly Women." *The American Journal of Clinical Nutrition*, vol. 30, September 1977, pp. 1414-22.

Krehl, Willard A. "The Influence of Nutritional Environment on Aging." *Geriatrics*, vol. 29, May 1974, pp. 67-76.

Morgan, A. G. et al. "A Nutritional Survey in the Elderly: Blood and Urine Vitamin Levels." *International Journal for Vitamin and Nutrition Research*, vol. 45, 1975, pp. 448-62.

Pollitt, Norman T., and Salkeld, Richard M. "Vitamin B Status of Geriatric Patients." *Nutrition and Metabolism*, vol. 21, no. 1, 1977, pp. 24-27.

Thornton, William E., and Thornton, Bonnie P. "Geriatric Mental Function and Serum Folate: A Review and Survey." *Southern Medical Journal*, vol. 70, no. 8, August 1977, pp. 919-22.

Todhunter, E. Neige, and Darby, William J. "Guidelines for Maintaining Adequate Nutrition in Old Age." *Geriatrics*, June 1978, pp. 49-56.

A woman with arthritis in her hands has been taking 16 aspirin daily to help control the pain and stiffness. Her hands display nodules on the fingertip joints and are sore, stiff, and weak. In many cases, this particular form of arthritis responds well to large doses of vitamin B_6. That proves true in this case as well. . . . The patient also learned she was allergic to eggs, and improvement was even greater when she eliminated them from her diet.

A Case of B_6-Responsive Arthritis

25

Abigail Baker came in with two large shopping bags. One of them rattled and banged at the slightest movement; the other made no noise except a convincing thud when it hit the floor.

She proceeded to empty the contents of the noisy bag onto my desk. Out of it came bottles and containers of every size and description. Each was filled to varying degrees with pills of many colors and shapes.

As she took the bottles out, one by one, Mrs. Baker went over them, half to herself, half to me. "Butazolidin," she said. "Indocin, Ascriptin, Motrin, Valium (pulling out a particularly large jug), giant-economy-size aspirin, Prednisone . . . I wouldn't take that . . . Percodan, Empirin with codeine, APCs. . . ."

The next group of bottles to issue from her bag had more colorful labels, but apparently didn't impress Mrs. Baker much more than the first set. She continued her recitation: "Vitamin C, vitamin E, multiple mineral, zinc, cod-liver oil, wheat germ oil, dolomite, alfalfa, brewer's yeast, pantothenic acid, desiccated liver, kelp, lecithin, B complex . . . at least that one did me a tiny bit of good. . . ."

As she worked unloading her sack, I noticed she was having a definite problem with her hands. She dropped a bottle or two; she winced with pain when lifting the largest and heaviest.

As she finished, my desk top had disappeared under her impressive collection of drugs and vitamins. There were 27 different varieties, "and there are just as many at home," she said.

I wished she had brought in a listing on paper; it would have been easier to work with. I told her so.

"I'm sorry, I should have done that," she said. "But I was so discouraged and fed up. However, if it's paper you want. . . ." With that she turned to her second sack.

She started to stack sheaves of paper of varying thicknesses on the only remaining space on the desk. "Here's Dr. Jones's reports. He's my family doctor. Dr. Anderson, the arthritis specialist. One from an internist. These two I forget . . . and (bringing out the thickest piles) the university and the ———— Clinic," she said, naming a major local referral center.

Now that her sacks were empty, I hoped we could get to the problem. I asked her where she'd like to start.

In answer, she held out both hands. "I'd like some relief for this arthritis," she declared. "I don't seem to be able to get it. Right now I'm taking 16 aspirin a day. That does better than anything else, but I still have pain and stiffness. But, if I take more than that, my ears ring, and my stomach gets more irritated than it already is."

Mrs. Baker's hands showed severe arthritis of a fairly common type. All but one finger had enlarged nodules ("knots," she said) on either side of the end joints. These were all acutely tender to pressure. The middle joints of her fingers had no nodules, but were enlarged, stiff, and slightly sore. The rest of her finger joints (adjacent to the palms) and her wrists weren't enlarged, but hurt slightly to move. (Technically, the swollen, hard nodules on her fingertip joints are called Heberden's nodes, after an eighteenth-century British physician.)

She also mentioned that her shoulders, knees, and hips hurt "on and off," and that she had "some kind of rheumatism" in her muscles. This produced varying soreness and stiffness. "But the worst is my hands; if I can just get rid of this pain, I can stand the rest," she repeated.

Her arthritis had started when she was 53, just when her menstrual periods were coming to an end. She'd first noticed the eruption of one of the Heberden's nodes, on her left ring finger. It had swollen and become acutely painful for two or three weeks. However, over the next year or two, her hands became more stiff, she got more Heberden's nodes, and she'd begun to visit doctors to see if she could get it stopped.

After two or three years, with only steadily worsening arthritis to show for her search, she gave up on drug treatment entirely, except aspirin. She'd then begun to visit health food stores, working her way through various vitamins and minerals, and changing her diet.

That hadn't particularly relieved her arthritis either, but had some benefit. She reported that "except for this arthritis, I haven't felt as good in 30 years." Her energy levels were much better, her tiredness gone. Her hair had stopped thinning, and dandruff disappeared. Her digestion improved. So she kept on with the vitamins and minerals.

I took a few minutes to go through her medical reports. She'd had blood tests several times for rheumatoid arthritis and gouty arthritis. These were all negative. X-rays showed "slight to moderate osteoarthritis" in her finger joints. All other tests were negative. Despite the variety of drugs tried, final recommendations were usually for aspirin.

"Well, I suppose you're going to want further tests and examinations," she said.

I replied that I didn't; her tests to the present looked quite satisfactory. It was time to start doing something about her problem, as the answer was quite apparent in her hands.

Mrs. Baker looked extremely skeptical. "You mean to say you can tell what I need just by looking at my hands?"

I replied that she had a characteristic sub-type of arthritis that I'd seen many times before. It really wasn't uncommon: she simply had a more severe case than most. Although the entire cause of the type of arthritis isn't known, it responds so reliably to treatment that my "in-office" diagnosis of it is named after the remedy: I presently identify it as pyridoxine-responsive arthritis.

Almost everyone with this arthritis sub-type improves with treatment centered around pyridoxine, or vitamin B_6. As her hands were typical in appearance, I saw no reason why she shouldn't improve as others had.

Mrs. Baker picked up her bottle of B complex tablets from the midst of her collection and handed it to me. She remarked that she thought that it might have done her a little good, but not much. "Didn't it contain pyridoxine?"

The label listed the pyridoxine content of each tablet as 10 milligrams. She said she'd taken three a day. I replied that the doses required were often much higher than that; in a severe case, several hundred milligrams were often needed. Also, sometimes other nutrients were necessary to aid the action of the vitamin B_6. Last, in many cases of pyridoxine-responsive arthritis, food allergy seemed to play a part. If necessary, this could be tested later.

However, for now, I asked her to start with 200 milligrams of pyridoxine 3 times daily, backed up with a B complex tablet including 50 milligrams of each of the Bs, 3 times a day.

"Is that all?" Mrs. Baker asked. "What about all the rest of this stuff?"

"Save it for now, but don't take any. We need to know how well the B_6 and B complex work by themselves. If they work as I expect . . . well, for the nonnutrients, your wastebasket is a suitable spot. The vitamins and minerals you can take later, if you wish."

Mrs. Baker shook her head, and surveyed her collection of bottles. "If it's that simple . . . ," she started to pile the containers and papers into their respective shopping bags.

I wrote out my recommendations as a reminder, and asked her to check back in a month.

Precisely one month to the day later, Mrs. Baker reappeared; this time I couldn't hear her coming. She was much more cheerful.

She reported that "better than 50 percent" of her pain had subsided. What remained was in her hands, particularly the nodular end joints. Her "rheumatism" was gone; her shoulder, knee, and hip pain, likewise. Even the pain in her hands was "more than 50 percent" better; she was down to 6 aspirin daily, from 16.

She inquired if the "knots" (Heberden's nodes) were likely to go away. I advised that they wouldn't. The best that could be done was to take the pain out of them. The only time I'd ever seen a Heberden's node disappear was in someone who'd started to take lots of vitamin B_6 as soon as the node appeared.

I advised Mrs. Baker that she'd done well for one month's time; it appeared the vitamin B_6 was definitely doing its job. At this time, I wanted her to add on the other nutrients that work with vitamin B_6, and also to get an antibody test for food allergies, as they were frequently involved in arthritis.

Magnesium and essential fatty acids were the other nutrients I had in mind. I recommended dolomite tablets (3, twice a day) as a magnesium source in her case, as I suspected she had a need for calcium, also. For essential fatty acids, 1 tablespoon daily of a mixture of safflower, sunflower, and soy oils should do.

Mrs. Baker took these recommendations and went to get her blood test.

She returned in six weeks. This time, she reported she'd been able to stop her aspirin entirely. The pain in her hands was down to a negligible level; "quite tolerable," she said. As she demonstrated, her hands were becoming much more flexible.

I pressed on her Heberden's nodes. The same pressure that had previously brought considerable pain didn't even get a wince. "It hurt just a little," she said, "but not enough to complain about."

Her allergy test showed negligible levels of antibodies to all foods tested but one: eggs. The antibody level here was extremely high.

"I've been eating eggs all my life," she exclaimed. "But if it might make a further difference in my arthritis, I'll stop."

We talked about her supplement program. I recommended that she maintain the initial levels for five to six months, and then try to taper down to a "maintenance" level that would keep pain away. I also recommended adding in vitamin E, which should always be taken when essential fatty acids are being used in therapeutic doses. For general good health, she should add back vitamin C.

I didn't see Mrs. Baker again for eight months. She reported that one week after stopping the eggs, the last of her pains and stiffness had gone. Also, she'd been able to cut the vitamin B_6 to 400 milligrams daily. Currently, she was using 300 milligrams daily "and more when it flares up occasionally," which controlled it, promptly. She took the oil every other day, and the dolomite regularly. "At my age, I figure I need it," she said. Her hands were much more flexible and usually pain-free.

"I took your other advice, too," she said.

"What's that?"

"I dropped my entire collection of drugs in the garbage."

Once again, I'm indebted to Dr. John Ellis for the findings leading to the remedy described in this case. He's also been a key clinical observer of the use of vitamin B_6 in the carpal tunnel syndrome and the treatment of toxemia of pregnancy, as well as many other uses of vitamin B_6. His book, *Vitamin B_6: The Doctor's Report,* is a storehouse of B_6 information.

Quite obviously, the amount of pyridoxine (vitamin B_6) recommended for pain relief in Mrs. Baker's arthritis is well beyond that needed to correct any vitamin deficiency. My best guess at present is that pyridoxine in large amounts either stimulates or slows an enzyme system or in some way "modulates" the production of a hormone in the body. Of course, there may be another explanation: once again, the clinical observation precedes the understanding of all the biochemistry.

After using pyridoxine for this particular condition for several years, I've come to the conclusion that although it's a major part of the treatment, it works much better if combined with other cofactors, particularly magnesium and essential fatty acids. While the biochemical actions in this type of arthritis aren't at all clear, these are frequently observed pyridoxine cofactors in other known biochemical interactions, as well as other clinical situations.

Mrs. Baker's pain relief was quite good. While this is a frequent result, for others there's only partial improvement. Occasionally it doesn't help at all, but in my experience that's unusual.

As I've mentioned before, I prefer to have as much documentation as possible for any nutritional/biochemical treatment. In this instance, Dr. Ellis's book is the only documentation I'm aware of at present. However, so many of my patients have furnished "living documentation" that despite an occasional failure, I always recommend trying pyridoxine with its cofactors for the type of arthritis/rheumatism described in Mrs. Baker's case.

As long as I'm going over largely unexplained results, I should mention that I have also no explanation for the connection between most nonrheumatoid, nongout types of arthritis and food allergy. This is such a common overlap that I include allergy screening routinely in almost all cases of degenerative osteoarthritis, or nonspecific arthritis. (All of these terms are more or less interchangeable descriptions of arthritis not associated with gout and not rheumatoid arthritis.)

Quite often, food allergy is uncovered. Its importance in the arthritis is demonstrated without a double-blind, controlled study, by the simple measures of stopping the food and observing for pain relief, then restarting it and watching for pain to return.

Once they've cleared their diets of significant allergens, patients frequently report they can really tell when they occasionally slip and eat an allergenic food.

The involvement of food allergy in arthritis doesn't seem to be very widely publicized. A recent textbook by J. C. Breneman, *Basics of Food Allergy*, does give a brief, but very enlightening discussion of the "arthritis-allergy connection."

Last, I should mention that this type of arthritis does make an occasional appearance in men and pyridoxine therapy (along with its cofactors) is usually successful for men, too. However, women with pyridoxine-responsive arthritis outnumber men by a great proportion.

FURTHER READING

Breneman, J. C. "Allergic Arthritis." *Basics of Food Allergy* (Springfield, Ill.: Charles C Thomas, 1978), pp. 84–91.

Ellis, John M., and Presley, James. *Vitamin B_6: The Doctor's Report* (New York: Harper and Row, 1973).

A man with arthritis learns from his brother about a new dietary program. Developed by a botanist, it calls for the elimination of potatoes, peppers, tomatoes, eggplant, and tobacco products. Trying it on his own, he discovers it works. Some other patients of mine—but not all—who subsequently tried this diet found it helped considerably. Apparently, these individuals are sensitive to solanine and other substances in the plants.

The 'Nightshade' Elimination Diet for Arthritis

26

I frequently learn things from my patients. Sometimes only a little, occasionally a lot, but always something. I first heard of nightshade-induced arthritis from one of my oldest patients, Anthony Vessalo. As further reading, time, and experience has convinced me that this is potentially a very important discovery about degenerative arthritis, I thought I would pass along this information to you just as Mr. Vessalo did to me, in describing his own case.

Mr. Vessalo had been one of my first patients when I began my practice in Kent, Washington. He'd come in with osteoarthritis, particularly bad in his knees. By applying niacinamide therapy, as developed by William Kaufman, Ph.D., M.D., he'd been able to get his symptoms under good control and resume pain-free walking again.

As Dr. Kaufman had pointed out, the niacinamide acted as a control, not a cure. When Mr. Vessalo tried to discontinue its use, his symptoms would return in a few weeks; when he restarted it, they subsided once more.

"Remember you told me niacinamide wasn't a cure for degenerative arthritis, just a less harmful control?" he asked. "And I should use it until someone found a cure? Well, at least in my case, I think someone has. Have you got a minute?"

"I've always got a minute to learn something. Tell me about it." (Mr. Vessalo had come in that day for a minor eye irritation.)

"Well, it all started last winter when I went back to visit my brother Joe in Philadelphia. He's seven years older than me. He's been really crippled up with arthritis; had to walk with a cane. I wrote him about how I did with niacinamide, but I never got any answer. Well, I had to go back East anyway, so I thought I'd drop in on him back in Philly.

"Was I surprised! When he came walking downstairs, he came right along, no cane and not bent over. He looked ten years younger than the last time I saw him. I figured he'd been taking niacinamide. But he said, no, he hadn't.

"I asked him what he did, take cortisone or something? He said no, one of his friends had heard that some university professor in New Jersey was saying tomatoes caused arthritis. That sounded so crazy that he thought he'd go find out about it. Joe always ate a lot of tomatoes, anyway.

"Turns out this professor said there was some chemical . . . let me see. . . ." He fumbled in his wallet for a scrap of paper. "It's in tomatoes, potatoes, peppers, eggplants, and tobacco. Grows in them."

I'd known in a vague way that solanine was one of the naturally occurring toxins in the so-called deadly nightshade. I also had known that the above plants were all members of the nightshade family. So what Mr. Vessalo was saying made sense.

He continued. "It seems some people with degenerative arthritis are particularly sensitive to even small amounts of solanine and other substances in regular food like tomatoes.

"Now, Joe wasn't sure if he believed it, but our family being Italian, we always ate a lot of tomatoes, eggplant, and peppers. On top of that, Joe chewed tobacco. Had for years. The only thing he didn't like was potatoes.

"Well, he was really hurting bad, so he decided to just go

'cold turkey.' He'd heard sometimes it took a year to find out if it worked. Joe always was stubborn; he figured he'd wait two years to see if it helped. Of course the hardest thing to do was give up his tobacco. But he did it all just like that.

"He said in six months he was much better. By nine months, he'd given up his cane, and was getting around just fine. Some of his muscle aches and pains were gone, too. He wasn't saying he was cured, probably had some permanent damage left, but what a difference.

"You can imagine what I thought. Sure the niacinamide had helped me, but every time I went off it, my pain came back. And look at my own brother!

"I'd always eaten lots of Italian food, too. Only thing I didn't do was chew tobacco. I smoked a pipe. I know you told me to stop, but I just hadn't. So I decided to try it.

He looked wistful. "You know, the hardest thing for me was the tomatoes. Every year for 50 years I've grown the most beautiful tomatoes in my garden. I knew I was going to miss them this year, if it worked.

"I didn't want to hurt, so I kept on taking my niacinamide for three months. Came off it this spring. I waited for the knee pain to come back, but it never did.

"It worked for my brother, and seemed to work for me, but I wanted to be sure. So a couple months ago, I ate a few tomatoes. My knees started to hurt in two or three hours, and my back let me know, too. The only other time I've had any problems is when I accidentally had a piece of pepper when I was out. Aside from that, my arthritis has hardly hurt. No niacinamide, either. I wanted to ask: What's the connection between niacinamide and the nightshade plants?"

"I don't know. I can't say for sure that there is or isn't any. Sounds like there was in your case, but it might have been a coincidence. It certainly seems you're a nightshade-sensitive person, though."

"You never heard about tomatoes, potatoes, and arthritis before?"

"Only from the viewpoint of allergy, like any other allergy-induced arthritis. But this isn't allergy, it's toxicity, just like a slow poison."

"I wonder how many people are sensitive to this nightshade stuff in food and tobacco."

"No way of knowing. Considering the biochemistry behind what you've described, the potential sounds high. There are probably many sensitive individuals. But I'm fairly sure no wide-scale testing has been done yet to find exact percentages."

Just then, the receptionist tapped on the door. "Your next patient has been waiting," she said.

Mr. Vessalo got up to go. "I'm sorry to take up so much time," he said. "I really only came in about my eyes."

"I wanted to hear what you had to say. Thank you for letting me know. I certainly intend to look into it further."

Since Mr. Vessalo came in and told me about his arthritis, I've asked others with degenerative arthritis to try the "No-Nightshades Diet" (as it's been named by its originator, Professor Norman F. Childers of Rutgers University). There have been some disappointments, where it just didn't seem to work. However, there have also been some very happy people whose arthritis pain has cleared up as they stayed away from the nightshade plants.

It appears that nightshade-caused arthritis isn't allergy in the usually accepted sense, but toxicity, or poisoning. The distinction between toxic and allergic problems isn't always clear. Generally speaking, allergic substances are ones that the body reacts vigorously against, with antibodies, white blood cell reactions, and other tissue reactions.

Toxins in general don't seem to evoke this vigorous response. They simply invade cells and tissues, silently causing symptoms only when there's enough poison accumulation to interfere with the functions of various cells or tissues significantly.

At present, it appears that nightshade-solanine-caused arthritis is in this latter category.

The answer lies in the dose or amount of toxin taken in. A

large amount of solanine and other toxins from the nightshade plants will kill, like a large amount of cyanide, or nitrite. Very small amounts may not cause obvious problems, and the body may be able to get rid of them. If not, they'll cause varying degrees of chronic disability.

At present, there is no blood test or other quick test to discover who is nightshade-sensitive, and who isn't. Abstaining for at least three months, and in some cases up to twelve months, is the only way to figure it out.

It's very possible that there may be other toxins in other foods or food families that may cause problems for some individuals and not others, like the nightshade family. With the present relative lack of scientific interest in the relationship of food to disease, it may be some time before researchers other than Dr. Childers even look into this general area.

This case—and the others in this section—underline the point made so many years ago "One man's meat is another man's poison." Despite the simplicity and antiquity of this observation, it is up-to-date and extremely important in nutritional medicine.

FURTHER READING

Childers, Norman Franklin, and Russo, Gerard M. *The Nightshades and Health* (Somerville, N.J.: Horticultural Publications, Somerset Press, 1977).

Kaufman, William. *The Common Form of Niacin Amide Deficiency Disease: Aniacinamidosis* (Bridgeport, Conn.: Yale University Press, 1943).

———. *The Common Form of Joint Dysfunction: Its Incidence and Treatment* (Brattleboro, Vt.: E. L. Hildreth, 1949).

Some 30 years ago, Dr. William Kaufman documented the usefulness of large amounts of niacinamide in the symptomatic treatment of osteoarthritis. Generally ignored because of the advent of cortisone, this treatment—which must be monitored by a physician—is nevertheless useful, particularly in degenerative arthritis affecting the knees.

27 A Case of Degenerative Arthritis

"I'd like some help for my knees," Mrs. Arthur said. As this was the first time we'd met, I asked what the problem was.

"They hurt all the time unless I take medicine," she replied. "Sometimes even then. Especially my left knee."

"What medicine are you taking now?"

Mrs. Arthur named a powerful drug sometimes used in cases of arthritis to reduce swelling and inflammation, thus controlling pain.

"I'd like to get off this; it must be dangerous since I have to get a white blood cell count every month. The doctor who gave it to me said I'd have to stop this drug if my white blood cell count went down too low."

"Have you taken other drugs?"

"Yes, everything but cortisone. I've heard too much bad about it." She named several other widely used drugs for arthritis pain, including aspirin and two new ones.

"How did they work?" I asked.

"Oh, they all worked a little, even the aspirin. One or two

worked fairly well. But they all had possibly serious bad effects. I just don't like the idea of taking a synthetic drug that's not natural for my system. Isn't there anything else I can do?"

"Before I can recommend anything, I need to get some other information, and examine your knees. When did they start to hurt?"

"Let me see. I'm 52 now, and they first got noticeable . . . seven years ago now . . . I was 45. At first it was only every once in a while, but maybe three years ago the pain got bad enough that I went to see the doctor about it."

"When did they start to swell?"

"About three years ago, too. It was just a little every few months at first and went away on its own. But I was in an automobile accident nearly two years ago. I banged both knees pretty bad. The left one had a chip taken out six months after that. Now they swell a little every few weeks. Of course, it's worse if I don't take medicine."

"Do any other joints hurt or swell?"

"Every once in a long time one or another finger joint aches for a day or two. But none ever swell, it's always a different one, and it always goes away by itself. So I don't think it's a problem."

"Do you have any other health problems you know about?"

"Well," Mrs. Arthur thought for a minute. "It's not really a health problem, but I do get tight muscles fairly often. I think that's just nerves and tension, though."

"Do you have much problem with your nerves?"

"I've always been high-strung. My mother was, too. I take a nerve pill every once in a while."

"Have you had any tests or x-rays done?"

"Yes, both blood tests and x-rays."

"What did they show?"

"I don't remember exactly, except I didn't have a positive test for the crippling kind of arthritis."

"Can you think of anything in your lifestyle that might have led to this problem?"

"I've always thought it was what one of my doctors called 'wear and tear' arthritis. I played on a volleyball team for ten years, until I was 36. I stopped because my left knee started to hurt. The pain left, though, as soon as I stopped. So I figured it was just a sprain or something."

"Have you had any other injuries besides the auto accident?"

"Yes. When I stopped playing volleyball, I decided to ski to stay in shape. I've twisted both knees a number of times, and tore the ligaments in the left one several years ago."

Mrs. Arthur stopped and looked directly at me. "I hope you're not going to tell me to stop skiing, too, like my last doctor. I know it hurts, but I just take my medicine and go anyway. I'm not ready for a rocking chair yet!"

"I'd like to check your knees, and have tests done before I recommend anything."

Mrs. Arthur's knees didn't appear swollen. Tests for ligament strength were normal. She had no tenderness over either joint. There was no evidence of a torn interior cartilage. However, like many persons with degenerative arthritis of the knees, her knees had a characteristic grating sensation when compressed over the kneecap and then moved. She also had slight tenderness at the attachment of one of the major ligaments of the left knee.

"I agree that this is probably degenerative arthritis or osteo-arthritis in your knees," I told Mrs. Arthur. "Since no tests have been done in over a year, though, I'd like you to have them done to make sure, before I ask you to do anything."

She agreed that this sounded reasonable. After we discussed these tests, she got up to go, then stopped.

"I don't know how I forgot. I take a pill every day for hyper-tension. That's just my nerves, though. I've been checked for all the other things. Besides, it never goes up very high, and gets better when I relax."

I made a note of that, but as our time was up indicated we'd best talk about it at another visit.

When Mrs. Arthur returned, we went over her test results. Her uric acid test (for gout) was quite normal. The blood test for rheumatoid arthritis was negative. The test for inflammation was normal, although it could have been affected by the drug she was taking. Her x-rays, though, were positive: the radiologist had found early but definite signs of degenerative arthritis in both knees.

"Well," she said, "that just confirms what we both thought. Now, what do we do about it? What about the mineral test you had me bring in some hair for?"

"The mineral analysis hasn't yet been returned from the lab. I'm sure that will give additional clues about what to do. But for now, I'd like you to start with:
1. Niacinamide: 1,000 milligrams (time-release), 3 times daily
2. Vitamin C: 1,000 milligrams, 3 times daily
3. Vitamin D: 2,000 units, twice daily"

"I understand about the vitamin C," she said. "I've read it helps stop joint deterioration, and the vitamin D; that has something to do with calcium, doesn't it? But what about that niacinamide? What's it for? Isn't that an awful lot? I know one time I took 100 milligrams of niacin and turned red all over."

She looked uneasy.

"There are several questions here. First, don't confuse niacinamide with niacin. They're both forms of vitamin B_3, and both prevent vitamin B_3 deficiency. Chemically, though, they're different molecules, and have varying biological activity. Practically speaking, niacin will cause a 'flush' or 'blush' reaction; niacinamide won't.

"Second, that is a large dose of niacinamide, so I'd like you to start out at a lower dose—1,000 milligrams a day—and build up slowly toward the full amount. If you have any nausea, reduce the dose. Niacinamide seems safe in most people, even in large doses, unless they're nauseated by it.

"Last, and most important, it's to help control your arthritis, along with the other things."

Mrs. Arthur was still curious. "But I never heard of taking niacin—I mean niacinamide—for arthritis. Is that something new?"

I sighed a little, inwardly. "No, it's not new at all. Niacinamide therapy for arthritis was first described in 1943 by Dr. William Kaufman, who was then a practicing internist in Bridgeport, Connecticut. In 1949 he published an extremely careful, detailed analysis of hundreds of cases of arthritis treated with niacinamide. This book, *The Common Form of Joint Dysfunction: Its Incidence and Treatment*, along with Dr. Kaufman's earlier book, *The Common Form of Niacin Amide Deficiency Disease: Aniacinamidosis*, is still the most valuable and comprehensive clinical study of the uses of niacinamide aside from the area of mental health."

"Can I get a copy at the health food store?"

"Unfortunately, no. I first located a copy after eight months of searching, in Washington, D.C., at the Library of Congress."

"Oh, well, that's OK as long as it works. Does it cure the arthritis?"

"No. One of the things Dr. Kaufman discovered was that pain from arthritis decreased, and mobility of the joints involved improved, sometimes greatly, starting two to six weeks after the patient began to take niacinamide. Generally, the improvement continues unless the niacinamide is stopped. Then the whole problem starts to return, generally in the same two to six weeks."

"So, it's a control, not a cure?"

"Exactly. But you don't have to stop there. As Dr. Kaufman pointed out, degenerative arthritis is an overall problem of abnormal metabolism. So, while taking niacinamide to control the pain, you should still work as much as possible on general health and returning your body metabolism to as normal as possible."

Mrs. Arthur thought for a minute.

"Even if it just controls it, it's still better than taking drugs. Should I stop those now?"

"Taper off as the niacinamide takes over. You should know."

"You said something about nausea. Can I have other side effects from niacinamide?"

"Yes, although they've never proven dangerous. In some persons niacinamide causes the results of certain liver function tests to rise. Most doctors who use niacinamide monitor this from time to time, although it's completely reversible when the niacinamide is stopped, and has never proven dangerous—unless the warning sign of nausea is ignored."

"I'll watch out for that," she said. "When should I come back?"

"In about a month. We should be able to tell something then."

When Mrs. Arthur returned in six weeks, there was a visible difference. Most notably, she smiled several times in the first few minutes, something she'd not done once in her first two visits. Her face, which had been tense, rigid, and almost unchanging in expression, had become more relaxed and animated. In fact, her overall attitude was much more relaxed and pleasant than before. I knew before she started to speak that the niacinamide was at work.

"I can't believe my knees, doctor," she started. "They haven't hurt for three weeks, and no drugs. No swelling, either. But, the best thing is my nerves. I haven't felt this calm in years. I've even been laughing at my husband's jokes, and I haven't done that for years."

She paused. "You know, I didn't know how tense I was. But my husband keeps me right on my vitamins. When I forget to take them, he can tell. He tells me, 'Go take your arthritis vitamins.' He says he's glad my knees are better, but he likes the improvement in the rest of me even more. I haven't taken a nerve pill since I started my vitamins.

"Even my blood pressure is better. My neighbor, who's a nurse, has taken it for me for years. This month it's been lower than it's been for five years. The last time was 130/70. I haven't taken my blood pressure pill, either. Does niacinamide cure high blood pressure, too?"

"It usually doesn't. But if the source of the high blood pressure is entirely 'nerves,' then it usually helps."

Mrs. Arthur's mineral analysis had returned. It showed deficiencies in several minerals, so I asked her to take supplements. And, of course, I recommended a diet free of sugar, white flour, refined foods, and artificial colors, flavors, and preservatives.

"All of this should restore more normal metabolism, and help your health overall, as well as your degenerative arthritis."

"Oh, I understand that," she said. "I started an organic garden three years ago; this is the first month I've been able to dig in it without my knees hurting. And by the way, what about that and my skiing?"

I encouraged her to continue with her exercise.

"I'd like you to come in to have your knees checked periodically. If it looks like the degenerative arthritis is worse, we can talk about exercise then."

Mrs. Arthur agreed this seemed reasonable and agreed to come back for the rechecks on her knees, as well as the liver-monitoring tests as long as she took niacinamide. With that, she left.

I've seen Mrs. Arthur many times since then. Her knees have remained pain-free, and they've not swollen again. They've gotten a little stiff when she reduced her niacinamide dose "just to see." But the stiffness leaves when she raises it again.

Her case of nerves has never returned. Of course, this was not a surprise to me, as niacinamide is the mainstay of megavitamin treatment for nervous diseases, also.

Her blood pressure has remained normal.

The original problem of degenerative arthritis of the knees even seems to be improving, although very slowly. Each time I've checked her knees, the internal grating is less.

Her case furnishes an excellent example of a basic principle of nutritional or preventive medicine; that a symptom in one part of the body is frequently just a localized expression of an overall disturbance in metabolism. Thus, when the correct measures are taken, not only does the most bothersome symptom get better, but so do other supposedly unrelated problems.

Niacinamide and Osteoarthritis

Dr. Kaufman has been one of the least-recognized pioneers on nutritional/biochemical medicine. In a 200-plus-page book, he detailed his painstaking work using niacinamide for osteoarthritis (also called degenerative or wear-and-tear arthritis), and the excellent results he frequently obtained. His work is a classic of clinical investigation.

Unfortunately, his book is generally unavailable; it's distribution was apparently not wide.

Although I'm just speculating, there are probably two reasons why niacinamide therapy has not been more widely used. First is of course the general medical apathy/antagonism toward the use of vitamins to treat anything other than end-stage deficiency disease. Second, and probably as important, is that cortisone became generally available for use at about the time when Dr. Kaufman's book was published. Initially, cortisone therapy appeared to be *the* cure for arthritis. By the time the initial overuse of cortisone had died down, and the drawbacks of cortisone therapy became apparent, Dr. Kaufman's volume was passed by.

As noted, niacinamide therapy controls much of the pain and swelling in osteoarthritis. It does not cure it. In my own work, which is of course not as extensive as Dr. Kaufman's, I've observed that niacinamide is the most effective for degenerative arthritis in the knees; in this use, it practically never fails. Of course, I always try it for osteoarthritis elsewhere in the body, too, where results are usually good.

In the doses necessary to help arthritis, niacinamide is being used in "beyond vitamin" amounts, and probably compensates for an as-yet-unidentified metabolic defect in persons with degenerative arthritis.

Caution is therefore necessary: if possible, niacinamide should be used under the supervision of a physician familiar with its effects.

Niacinamide is preferable to niacin in almost all cases, as there are fewer side effects.

If nausea occurs with the use of niacinamide, the dosage is in excess and should be reduced.

In the range that's therapeutically effective (1,000 to 4,000 milligrams daily), the results of certain liver function tests may in some persons become elevated. Although this does not necessarily appear to be harmful, liver function tests should always be monitored in anyone who plans to use niacinamide over a period of time.

As with many other therapies, the benefits of arthritis treatment must be weighed against the possible risks.

If you find that niacinamide helps you, biochemical monitoring is essential, for the reasons noted above.

An observation attributed to Thomas Spies, M.D., another early vitamin worker, is that individuals who are deficient in or whom could be benefited by niacinamide therapy frequently are humorless and unsmiling. According to Dr. Spies's observation, they seem to have no sense of humor. As Mrs. Arthur's case illustrates, this does seem to be the case sometimes.

FURTHER READING

Kaufman, William. *The Common Form of Niacin Amide Deficiency Disease: Aniacinamidosis* (Bridgeport, Conn.: Yale University Press, 1943).

————. *The Common Form of Joint Dysfunction: Its Incidence and Treatment* (Brattleboro, Vt.: E. L. Hildreth, 1949).

————. "Niacinamide Therapy for Joint Mobility: Therapeutic Reversal of a Common Clinical Manifestation of the 'Normal' Aging Process." *The Connecticut State Medical Journal*, vol. 17, no. 17, July 1953, p. 584.

————. "The Use of Vitamin Therapy to Reverse Certain Concomitants of Aging." *Journal of the American Geriatrics Society*, vol. 3, no. 11, November 1955, pp. 927–36.

A weakness and tingling of the hands, known as carpal tunnel syndrome, and often the cause of surgery, is traced to a dietary deficiency of B vitamins—particularly B_6 or pyridoxine. Although observations published years ago suggest that B_6 in these cases should at least be tried, it rarely is. . . . Is this indifference to vitamin therapy scientific caution—or inexcusable bias?

A Case of Weak, Tingling Hands

28

Mrs. Erickson was depressed. She'd been told she had to have an operation to relieve the problem in her hands, which was rapidly becoming worse. She'd resigned herself to this, and was only in today because, "My best friend, Millie Clark, kept after me that maybe vitamins and diet would help. So I finally decided to come."

Her symptoms had begun three to four months previously. She'd noticed a peculiar numbness in both hands, worse on the left than the right. For a while, she thought it was due to "sleeping wrong," because it was particularly bad when she woke up, and after massaging, her hands became better.

However, shortly after the numbness started, she also developed tingling, once again worse on the left than the right. Like the numbness, her tingling sensation was variable, coming and going, but worse in the mornings. Like the numbness, she decided to ignore this symptom too; "I'm 72 years old and thought it was poor circulation, like many people my age."

Unfortunately, after nine or ten weeks of varying symptoms, the condition became continuous, lasting all day. No matter how much massaging she did, it never left completely. Another problem she'd been trying to ignore became so serious that her husband had noticed it, too; a weakness of both hands and forearms.

This weakness had become glaringly obvious one morning when she tried to serve breakfast. While carrying eggs from the stove to the table in an iron skillet, her grip had weakened. She couldn't hold the pan, and was unable to grab it with her other hand holding the serving implement. Skillet, eggs, and spatula had all gone crashing to the floor.

"My husband wasn't angry," she said. "He'd been watching my weakness without telling me. He'd noticed I wasn't playing my piano lately. But when I dropped that pan, he insisted I see a doctor."

So she'd gone to see a doctor in a nearby town. This doctor told her she had carpal tunnel syndrome and referred her to a surgeon. The surgeon had confirmed the diagnosis, and advised her that surgery would be necessary to clear up the problem.

That had been three or four weeks ago. She'd decided not to have the surgery right away, hoping that her hands would start to improve on their own. Instead, they'd become worse. "I don't even try to carry heavy objects or do fine work with my fingers." She'd also developed "shooting pains" from her shoulders to her wrists. When these pains started, she'd gotten very depressed and decided then that surgery was inevitable.

"Carpal tunnel syndrome" is a medical description of a varying group of symptoms arising from compression of the median nerve in its course through the wrist. The immediate cause of the compression is usually a thickening of the ligament that joins the two forearm bones at their further ends, just one to two inches from the palm of the hand. The symptoms coming from this nerve compression are many, but to make a positive diagnosis of carpal tunnel syndrome, they must include three things: impaired feeling in the hand(s), a tingling sensation radiating out into the hands, and a worsening of the numbness and tingling when the wrist is flexed as hard as possible for 30 to 90 seconds.

Mrs. Erickson had all three of these problems as well as weakness and shooting pains. Other people with this problem have had a variety of other symptoms, but always including the above three.

Over the past 30 years, orthopedic surgeons have found that cutting the ligament that compresses the nerve relieves the symptoms. That is what was proposed for Mrs. Erickson.

Examining Mrs. Erickson's hands and wrists confirmed that she had an advanced case. We stopped the wrist-compression test after only 40 seconds as the tingling got much worse. Her grip strength was poor. She had a slight puffiness of both hands, especially noticeable on the backs where the tendons were not standing out as they should. Further clues were small, tender nodules over the furthest joints of three of her fingers.

Last, she could not perform what I call (for reasons to be explained below) the "Ellis test." This test is done by keeping the joints where the fingers join the palm *straight,* and *fully flexing* the next two (outer) finger joints until the fingertips curl around and touch the palm of the hand, at the base of the fingers. All four fingers on each hand are tested at once.

This test, if failed, is a reliable sign of a moderately advanced pyridoxine (vitamin B_6) deficiency. It was discovered by Dr. John Ellis and described in his book *Vitamin B_6: The Doctor's Report.* In this book, Dr. Ellis reports on his many years' work with a nonsurgical cure of the carpal tunnel syndrome and other related conditions. He also outlines, in simple terms, more of the basic biochemical reasons for this problem.

But back to Mrs. Erickson. When I advised her that her problem could probably be cured by vitamins, she was quite skeptical. She said she'd thought her friend Millie was "just a vitamin nut." And besides, her own doctor had told her that vitamins were just a fad, and had nothing to do with health, except in a minor way. However, when I mentioned Dr. Ellis's book, that cases like hers had been cured before without surgery, and that the vitamins were nontoxic, she agreed to give it a try.

I recommended that she take pyridoxine, 200 milligrams, 3 times a day. I also asked her to obtain a high-potency B complex tablet and take this at the same time as the B_6, 3 times a day. She asked if all those B vitamins weren't dangerous, or at least "way too much." I advised her that even excess B vitamins are harmless, and that for now, she needed an excess to "get her out of the hole" that past long years of vitamin deficiency had caused.

When Mrs. Erickson returned in three weeks, she scolded me because "all that B_6 made me too sleepy. I had to cut back to 100 milligrams 3 times a day." But she scolded with a twinkle in her eye: her symptoms were definitely clearing. She reported that the numbness and tingling were gone from her fingers, and remained only in the center of her palms. She was no longer stiff in the mornings, and her hands didn't feel nearly as "tight."

I asked her to try the "Ellis test" once more. Her performance was definitely improved, although not yet perfect. She had better grip strength; the tendons on the backs of her hands were now clearly visible.

"I'm beginning to think Millie was right," she said. I agreed, and asked her to continue the same program, and check back in a month.

When she returned, her improvement was continuing, but at a slower rate. The major gain was in grip strength, which was much better. Mrs. Erickson thought "perhaps it's not improving as fast because of my age." I told her that might be so, but maybe the B_6 needed a little help. So I asked her to add some magnesium oxide (250 milligrams twice a day) and an oil containing essential fatty acids (in this case, a mixture of pressed soy, safflower, and sunflower oils), 1 tablespoon twice a day. Both magnesium and essential fatty acids are well-known B_6 cofactors. I suspected that these nutrients were also deficient in her past diet.

This time, Mrs. Erickson returned in two months. "Thought I'd give it a little extra time," she said. Her problem was nearly gone. She could flex her hands as much as she wanted. There was no more numbness, tingling, or shooting pains. She reported she could "grab onto anything just fine" and could play the piano a little again. She admitted, "Maybe there's something to this vitamin thing after all."

Now that she was convinced, I decided it was time to talk about basic eating habits. I asked her to tell me what sort of things she usually had to eat every day.

As I expected, she was by now a little embarrassed about it, but told me as follows:

Breakfast: waffle (white flour), egg, coffee with sugar, juice, toast (white bread)

Lunch: soup and sandwich (white bread)

Dinner: white bread sandwich, tea and sugar (usually)

Snacks: cakes from mixes, and other white flour products

Few salads and salad oils, and cooking with no-stick pans, so little use of oils.

She said she'd eaten this way "for years." I advised her that the white flour products she used had most of the B vitamins and minerals removed; not using vegetable oils also contributed to her problem.

However, the key factor was the mostly missing pyridoxine, or vitamin B_6. To keep her problem from returning, I asked her to use only whole-grain products in the future, and to use more oils. Also, to be on the safe side, I asked her to continue to use at least 50 milligrams of vitamin B_6 each day.

"Well," she said, as she gathered her things to leave, "I think I'll go have a long talk with Millie. Looks like she saved me an operation." Then she paused. "Oh, I forgot to show you this time, Doctor," she said. Putting down her coat and bag once more, she demonstrated a nearly perfect "Ellis test" with both hands!

A Time Lag Filled with Surgery

This case illustrates well only one of the myriad health problems traceable to food processing and refining. Innumerable studies have shown that more than half of the B vitamins, as well as large proportions of trace minerals, are removed by refining whole grains into white flour. In this case, the lack of vitamin B_6

almost led to surgery for Mrs. Erickson.

Her case also illuminates well the inevitable lag between clinical observation and the discovery of the scientific reasons behind the clinical case result. Nearly 20 years ago, Dr. John Ellis observed that his patients with carpal tunnel syndrome were cured with vitamin B_6. (This actually was only one of many clinical observations made about vitamin B_6 by Dr. Ellis.) Unfortunately, but typically, his work was ignored.

Within the last five years, research biochemists at the University of Texas have demonstrated clearly that pyridoxine deficiency is a fundamental biochemical problem in carpal tunnel syndrome. As this gives pyridoxine therapy "scientific respectability," it may in fact start to be used more widely. But obviously, in the years between Dr. Ellis's initial observation and "scientific proof," thousands of persons have undergone surgery which was preventable by simple vitamin therapy.

It is of course argued that science must proceed slowly, proving or disproving by experiment in stepwise fashion. Otherwise, faulty conclusions may be formed and knowledge not advanced. So the time lag between initial observation and scientific proof and acceptance is regrettable, but necessary. Therefore, most practicing physicians will not proceed with a new therapy until it is "proven."

While this is perhaps appropriate with a potentially toxic drug therapy, or other dangerous procedure, it's inexcusable when the proposed therapy is, like vitamin B_6, almost completely nontoxic. Those physicians who treated their carpal tunnel syndrome patients with pyridoxine years prior to the scientific proof were gratified with the results.

Unfortunately, the still-prevailing bias in medicine is that nutrient therapy is of very little importance, or at best marginally helpful. Many of the other cases illustrate nontoxic nutritional therapies, both general and specific. While most of them are not as rigorously proven as in this case, there is usually either clinical or experimental observation behind them. Particularly when nothing else is working, there is usually no harm done in trying.

Of course, given my particular bias, I usually try nutritional and nutrient therapy before employing more radical, dangerous, and potentially toxic drug or surgical therapy.

FURTHER READING

Ellis, John M., and Presley, James. *Vitamin B₆: The Doctor's Report* (New York: Harper & Row, 1973).

Ellis, John M. et al. "Survey and New Data on Treatment with Pyridoxine of Patients Having a Clinical Syndrome Including the Carpal Tunnel and Other Defects." *Research Communications in Chemical Pathology and Pharmacology,* vol. 17, no. 1, May 1977, pp. 165-77.

————. "Vitamin B₆ Deficiency in Patients with a Clinical Syndrome Including the Carpal Tunnel Defect. Biochemical and Clinical Response to Therapy with Pyridoxine." *Research Communications in Chemical Pathology and Pharmacology,* vol. 13, no. 4, April 1976, pp. 743-55.

Folkers, Karl et al. "Biochemical Evidence for a Deficiency of Vitamin B₆ in the Carpal Tunnel Syndrome." *Acta Pharmaceutica Suecica,* vol. 14, supplement, 1977, pp. 38-39.

The symptoms of hepatitis are highly distressing and usually last two to six weeks. Very large doses of vitamin C can dramatically hasten recovery from this virus. . . . A discussion of the unusual human need for vitamin C (most other creatures manufacture their own internally) and why taking vitamin C during illness is a kind of compensation for a missing enzyme . . . which leads to the answer to the question: Why does one vitamin do so much for us?

29 A Case of Hepatitis

Mr. Schmidt had other-than-usual problems on his mind when he came in for his appointment. "Excuse me, but I'd like to talk about my daughter, Ingrid," he said. "She thinks she has hepatitis. How serious is that? There isn't any treatment for it, is there?" A very worried frown creased his forehead.

"Why does she think she has hepatitis?" I asked.

"She started having flu symptoms a few days ago. Mostly hurting all over and throwing up. She just stayed home; we weren't upset. But yesterday the whites of her eyes began to turn yellow, and today she's yellow all over. Besides, she was exposed to someone with hepatitis about five weeks ago."

I agreed that this certainly sounded as if it were hepatitis. As Mr. Schmidt appeared to be even more worried, I made sure to explain that though a very rare or unusual case of hepatitis could be fatal, the vast majority of patients recovered. While there is, of course, no "average" case of hepatitis, the usual duration of the illness is from two to six weeks, at least for symptomatic illness. Some authorities state that the time for biochemical recovery (based on blood-test evaluation) is about six months.

With this, Mr. Schmidt became a little more relaxed. He sat back in his chair. "It looks like she just will have to wait it out. It's too bad, because she's such an active girl."

He paused. "Well," he said, "even if we can't help Ingrid, can the rest of us come in for a protective shot? I got one of those when I was in the Army, and I guess it worked. I never got hepatitis, anyway."

I suggested to Mr. Schmidt that he and the rest of his family return that afternoon for gamma globulin injections. (These are thought to give some protection against hepatitis.)

"But don't give up on treatment for Ingrid. There is a treatment available which will help her get over her illness—if it is hepatitis—much more quickly than usual. Bring her along this afternoon, too; we can go over the details then."

Mr. Schmidt looked surprised. "I thought you said there wasn't any treatment for hepatitis. I read a magazine article just two or three months ago that said there isn't anything to do for it, either. Is there something new—a new drug, or something?"

Before I could answer, he got up to go. "I guess we'd better talk about this when Ingrid is here," he said.

Later that day, the entire Schmidt family arrived, and all but Ingrid were given injections of gamma globulin. Ingrid was placed in an examination-treatment room; both her parents waited with her.

Ingrid was 19, tall and attractive. That day, though, her attractiveness was diminished by bright orange yellow eyeballs, a deep yellow orange brown cast to her skin, and a generally ill appearance.

I asked Ingrid to describe her symptoms.

"Five days ago I got a chill and fever," she said. "Then I got nauseated. My nausea's been getting worse all the time. It's continuous now. Yesterday and today I've thrown up 11 times. I've been having diarrhea. It's been watery, but not the usual color—it's whitish yellow. I thought it was just the flu, until I started to turn color."

I asked if she'd noticed anything different about her urine.

"Well, yes, that started to get brown one or two days ago," she replied.

254 · *Nutritional and Natural Therapy*

I asked about her reported contact with hepatitis.

She hesitated. "Well, I was staying with this bunch of people in a house, and I just found out that four of them have hepatitis, too, that they just got. So we must all have been exposed to somebody there who had it. . . . I think I have to throw up again," she finished.

The rest of her examination was consistent with a diagnosis of hepatitis. She had some swollen lymph glands and slight to moderate tenderness in the stomach area between the ribs. The tenderness was acute below the rib cage margin on the right side. She had slight liver enlargement.

Clinically, the diagnosis of hepatitis appeared inescapable. However, I explained to Ingrid that before treatment was started, a blood test would be drawn, both as an index to how much her liver was affected, and as another aid in following the effects of treatment. She agreed.

Mr. Schmidt asked, once again, "Is this some type of new drug treatment?"

"No," I answered, "it's not a drug at all. It's just vitamin C. But it has to be given in large doses—25 to 50 grams a day—and intravenously in a form known as sodium ascorbate. Ingrid will probably need from 3 to 5 intravenous treatments [IVs] to get over this. I can't say for sure right now. She'll have to be at the clinic for three to four hours each time."

Ingrid asked, "In my vein? Won't that hurt if it takes hours?"

I assured her that it hurt no more than a shot—she'd had those before.

Mrs. Schmidt had a more serious concern. "Is there any danger in taking that much vitamin C? Twenty to 50 grams is 20,000 to 50,000 milligrams, isn't it? Aren't there problems with that much?"

I agreed that any substance given intravenously had to be used with caution. Vitamin C, unlike most drugs, has been shown to be remarkably nontoxic. There is just one important precaution with doses that large. It acts as a chelating agent and seems to bind or remove calcium (and probably other minerals) from the bloodstream. If this process goes too far, abnormal muscle contractions (called "tetany") can occur. To prevent this, extra calcium is put into the intravenous solution.

"That sounds OK," observed Mr. Schmidt. "Tell me though, has this type of treatment been in use very long? Have you used it for anyone with hepatitis before?"

I replied that I certainly had, and that the results had been excellent. Intravenous treatment of hepatitis and other viral illnesses with sodium ascorbate was by no means new. It originated with Frederick Klenner, M.D., of North Carolina, in the 1940s. Its use has been sporadic elsewhere; most recently, its successful use has been reported by Akira Murata, M.D., of Saga University in Japan.

To give Ingrid and her parents some time to talk it over, I told them I'd return in a few minutes. When I did, they'd decided to give it at least one try.

"Considering how I'm feeling, even if it only helps a little, I'm for it," Ingrid said.

So, that afternoon she was given intravenously 25 grams of sodium ascorbate, 1 gram of calcium, and 10 cubic centimeters of vitamin B complex to support the stress of illness. I told her to come back the following afternoon, and to take as much vitamin C as she could orally in the meantime.

Ingrid and her parents were also advised of the usual isolation procedures for cases of hepatitis. She should not be out in public, especially eating or using public bathroom facilities. Even at home, it would be wise for her to keep her own utensils separate from the rest of the family's, and, as far as possible, to follow scrupulous sanitary precautions. Ingrid promised that she would do this.

I also asked Ingrid's parents to take extra oral doses of vitamin C as an additional preventive, even though they'd had their shots. They should give appropriate doses to the rest of the children; 50 milligrams per pound of body weight per day would be adequate.

When Ingrid returned the next day, accompanied this time

by only her mother, it was apparent that some change had occurred. Her eyes were slightly less yellow, and the jaundice was diminished. However, the principal change was that, aside from the jaundice, she no longer appeared ill. Her movement, attitude, and behavior were no longer those of an acutely ill person, as they had been the day before.

Ingrid confirmed this impression. "My nausea is almost gone," she reported. "I haven't thrown up once—and yesterday and the day before I threw up 11 times!" She also noted that shortly following the sodium ascorbate infusion, she'd had a feeling of "warmth" and "aching" under the ribs on the right side, in the area of her liver.

When I asked her about her other symptoms, she reported that the whitish diarrhea was still present, and her urine was still brown, although less so than previously.

"What about the blood test?" Mrs. Schmidt asked.

I answered that the laboratory had found this test—called "SGOT"—highly abnormal, at 4,580 units, compared to a normal of 25 to 70 units. This test is usually abnormal in acute hepatitis.

That afternoon Ingrid received another intravenous treatment identical to the first. Due to family financial considerations, and Ingrid's excellent initial response, Mrs. Schmidt and I decided to skip a day of treatment, and also to do a follow-up blood test before her next treatment two days later. Of course, Ingrid was to continue taking vitamin C by mouth.

When Ingrid returned two days later, she was by herself. I asked her where her mother was. She replied: "I've been doing so well that she just dropped me off and went to do some shopping."

This time, Ingrid reported that she felt entirely well. She had "lots of energy" and wanted to know if she could go out and do things. I advised her it was yet too soon. She reported that her diarrhea was gone and her stools were brown once more. Her urine was no longer brownish, but clear. She'd felt no further nausea since her second treatment. Her yellow eyes and skin color were still present, but once again, less obvious.

"Will I have another blood test today?" she asked. I said she would.

"I just don't like needles," Ingrid replied.

I thought that this would perhaps be a good time to inquire into Ingrid's hepatitis exposure once more.

"You know," I said, "it's unusual for several people to get hepatitis all at once, unless they're all exposed at the same time. When you were staying with the people you mentioned. . . ."

"I know what you're going to say," Ingrid interrupted. "I guess you figured it out and I know I shouldn't have done it. I know I won't ever again. I've learned my lesson."

"What did you do?"

"Don't you know?"

"Yes," I said, "but I want you to tell me."

"Well," she said, "I shot up some 'speed' with a bunch of kids. I knew it was risky, but I guess I thought it would never happen to me. But we all got hepatitis from the same needle, I guess. . . ." Her voice trailed away.

Ingrid received her third treatment that afternoon. Once again, it was the same composition as the first one. Before the treatment was given, another SGOT test was drawn to be sent to the laboratory.

When Mrs. Schmidt arrived to pick Ingrid up, she had a little bit more to add to what Ingrid had said.

"I can't believe how fast she's gotten better," she said. "One day sick, vomiting, lying around, glassy-eyed, in the bathroom all the time. The next day—wham! No more whining, not throwing up anymore, can't hold her down. And she can't seem to take enough vitamin C. In 3½ days she's gone through almost 100 grams at home. Is it OK for her to take that much more in addition to the IV?"

I answered that it was not only OK, but very important to her getting well as rapidly as possible, and it probably helped prevent liver damage. Ingrid should definitely continue.

Since she was taking lots of vitamin C orally, and doing quite well, Mrs. Schmidt and I decided to skip three days this next time, before another treatment.

The first thing Ingrid wanted to know on her return was, "How was my blood test?" Getting out her record, I told her that the SGOT from the last visit was 1,442 units.

"What was it before?" she said.

I replied, "4,580 units."

"I guess it's really better," Ingrid said, "and that was only four days after the first test. But I shouldn't be surprised; I could tell just by how I was feeling."

Another blood test was drawn, and the IV given for the fourth time. I advised Ingrid I'd wait for the result of the blood test before deciding for sure whether or not she should have another IV treatment, but that probably she wouldn't be needing any more.

"Oh, good," she said. "Since—what I told you—I've really developed an aversion to IV needles."

When the SGOT test returned the next day, it was only 337 units. So I telephoned and asked Mr. Schmidt to bring Ingrid back in ten days. In the meantime, of course, she should continue taking 20 to 30 grams of vitamin C by mouth. Mr. Schmidt assured me that she would: "She says it makes her feel so much better!"

Ten days later, Ingrid arrived with both parents. She was obviously almost completely recovered. Her jaundice was completely gone. Her eyeballs were white once more. She reported her symptoms had entirely disappeared "a week ago," her energy was much better, and she felt entirely well.

Further examination confirmed this. Her lymph nodes were no longer swollen. She had no abdominal tenderness. Her liver was no longer enlarged.

I advised Ingrid that another blood test would be necessary before she could be considered cured. (This SGOT test later was reported at 154 units.) Also, even though she no longer needed massive IV doses of ascorbic acid, she should keep on taking large oral doses. These should be tapered down from 20 to 30 grams a day to 4 or 6 grams a day, and continued for several months.

"I've already started to do that," Ingrid told me. "A few days ago, I noticed that ascorbic acid was starting to give me gas and a little diarrhea. I figured that meant I didn't need as much, so I cut it down to 15 grams, and it went away."

"That's exactly right," I said.

Mr. Schmidt asked, "What are the possibilities of a relapse?"

"Practically zero," I answered, "as long as she keeps taking her ascorbic acid. Dr. Morishige, a Japanese physician, has found ascorbic acid to prevent nearly all cases of hepatitis after blood transfusion. It should also work to prevent a relapse for Ingrid."

"You said sodium ascorbate intravenously worked against other viruses, too," Mr. Schmidt said. "Which ones are those?"

"Practically any virus it's been tried against," I replied. "I've seen it work well against mumps, mononucleosis, and influenza type A, among the common ones. Dr. Morishige has used it with good effect against measles, mumps, virus pneumonia, herpes zoster, and some types of meningitis. Dr. Klenner has used it against encephalitis, poliomyelitis, and pericarditis of the types caused by viruses."

Mr. Schmidt looked very surprised. "Some of those are very serious diseases," he said. "I had a cousin die of virus encephalitis. Why isn't this treatment used or at least tried at all our universities? Are you sure it's not dangerous?"

I answered—once again—that as long as calcium was included in the treatment, it was usually quite safe. There had been exactly one reported case of toxic reaction in a person with a red blood cell disease (called glucose-6-phosphate-dehydrogenase deficiency), but this is rare, usually found only in black people, and can be tested for in advance. Also, it is not certain that vitamin C caused the problem (see Campbell and Mengel).

But, overall, vitamin C is incredibly nontoxic, and is very effective.

"So if it's nontoxic, and works so well against so many serious viruses, I still don't understand why it isn't used!" Mr. Schmidt said. "Ingrid's doing fine."

Once again, I replied that I didn't know. But even in Ingrid's case, I'd run into an example of what might be the problem. I'd saved part of each blood test to submit to the virus research lab of our local university. I'd spoken to a doctor there, describing the case, and the doctor had agreed it certainly seemed like a case of hepatitis. I wanted to send these blood specimens to him. But when he heard of the treatment and Ingrid's response to it, he decided that it couldn't possibly have been hepatitis, and that I shouldn't send in the specimens. "Vitamin C couldn't possibly work for that," he'd said.

"It's too bad people don't have more open minds," Mr. Schmidt observed. "So many more lives could be saved."

I couldn't help but agree.

Why Does Vitamin C Do So Much?

Earlier, I made what might seem overreaching statements about the usefulness of ascorbic acid, or vitamin C, in the detoxification of harmful substances. Now I've extended these remarks to the area of viral illness. I'm sure some readers are starting to wonder how a single vitamin can do so many jobs. Isn't this a little too much?

So, before specifically discussing Ingrid Schmidt's case, an explanation of the place of vitamin C in the human system.

Very few members of the animal kingdom need a dietary source of ascorbic acid. Dogs, cats, cows, horses, elephants, birds . . . practically any animal you can think of manufactures its own ascorbic acid internally. Only humans, other primates (gorillas, chimpanzees, monkeys), guinea pigs, an Indian fruit-eating bat, certain shrimp, and possibly the coho salmon don't synthesize their own vitamin C.

Researchers have found that the reason we humans do not make our own ascorbic acid is because a key enzyme normally present in the liver is missing. This enzyme, l-gulonolactone oxidase, performs the final step in ascorbic acid synthesis. We are missing only this one enzyme: all the other enzymes are present.

Actually, there are many "single-missing-enzyme" conditions. Phenylketonuria (PKU), which all newborns are screened for, is one. Albinos (persons without normal pigmentation) are missing skin, eye, and other color because they're born without the final enzyme in melanin (pigment) synthesis.

These conditions are usually called genetic diseases or inborn errors of metabolism. In fact, the human need for ascorbic acid is, unlike the need for other vitamins, a human genetic disease, an inborn error of metabolism that we all have.

Well, so what? Why bother with this enzyme explanation or

worry about the rest of the animal kingdom? We know we can prevent death from scurvy (total lack of ascorbic acid) with just a few milligrams of ascorbic acid. Scientists who study nutritional requirements have set the Recommended Dietary Allowance (RDA) for ascorbic acid at 45 milligrams daily. Won't that do? Why use so much more for treatment of such a wide variety of health problems that "obviously" have nothing to do with scurvy?

To answer this we need to change our perspective and start treating scurvy as the genetic disease it is. We need to examine the possibilities of fully correcting (or compensating for) the genetic error we all have. We need to combine this approach with careful observation of the biochemical responses of animals who do synthesize their own ascorbic acid.

Under practically any stress, ascorbic acid production skyrockets in animals that produce it. Carcinogens (cancer-causing substances) cause this response. Given drugs, most animals produce much more ascorbic acid. A virus challenge is met by the same response: increased ascorbic acid production. Nature has built the "ascorbic acid response" into the animal kingdom as response to practically any stress or biochemical challenge. Apparently, the only reason humans don't do the same is because of our missing enzyme: we just can't.

In applying ascorbic acid therapy to such a wide variety of illnesses, nutritionally and biochemically oriented physicians are simply "doing as nature does," and finding that it helps.

As a sidenote: researchers have found that under drug stress, the human liver does produce extra amounts of all the chemical precursors of ascorbic acid (see Goodman and Gilman). Our livers are trying to do just as animals do; because of a missing enzyme they can't. So the extra ascorbic acid has to be supplied from the outside.

The nutritional/biochemical approach to the therapeutic use of ascorbic acid is thus to fully correct for the genetic error we all share.

Now, back to virus diseases, including hepatitis. The real pioneer in the ascorbic acid treatment of viral ailments, including very serious ones such as polio and encephalitis, is Dr. Klenner.

As stated before, Dr. Klenner has been successfully helping his patients ward off serious viral illness by the use of massive doses of sodium ascorbate (a buffered form of ascorbic acid) intravenously.

His articles point out that calcium must be used with high doses of vitamin C intravenously or tetany (spasm of muscles caused by lack of calcium) can result. I presently use 1 gram of calcium gluconate per 10 grams vitamin C under most circumstances; more needs to be added for a few patients.

The hepatitis virus (there actually is more than one) seems to affect the liver particularly. When the liver is inflamed, it releases substances normally found within the liver cells such as enzymes and bile. The enzymes are then measured as part of diagnostic testing. The bile (bilirubin) is responsible for the characteristic yellow skin color and brown urine.

In intravenous treatment of hepatitis with sodium ascorbate, the levels of both enzymes and bilirubin drop toward normal much more rapidly than is usual. Clinically, the yellow skin, brown urine, and toxic viral symptoms clear up faster too.

Ingrid Schmidt's case was not unusual, but a routinely expected response to sodium ascorbate therapy.

FURTHER READING

Campbell, G. Douglas; Steinberg, Martin H.; and Bower, John D. "Ascorbic Acid-Induced Hemolysis in G-6-PD Deficiency." *Annals of Internal Medicine,* vol. 82, no. 6, June 1975, p. 810.

Goodman, Louis S., and Gilman, Alfred, eds. *The Pharmacological Basis of Therapeutics* (New York: Macmillan Publishing Co., 1975), p. 1676.

Klenner, Frederick R. "Observations on the Dose and Administration of Ascorbic Acid when Employed Beyond the Range of a Vitamin in Human Pathology." *Journal of Applied Nutrition,* Winter 1971, pp. 61–87.

Mengel, Charles E., and Greene, Harry L. "Ascorbic Acid

Effects on Erythrocytes." *Annals of Internal Medicine,* vol. 84, no. 4, p. 490.

Murata, Akira. "Virucidal Activity of Vitamin C: Vitamin C for Prevention and Treatment of Viral Diseases." *Proceedings of the First Intersectional Congress of IAMS,* edited by Takezi Hasegawa, 1975, pp. 432–36.

Murata, Akira; Kitagawa, Kazuko; and Saruno, Rinjiro. "Inactivation of Bacteriophages by Ascorbic Acid." *Agricultural and Biological Chemistry,* vol. 35, no. 2, 1971, pp. 294–96.

Murata, Akira, and Uike, Motoko. "Mechanism of Inactivation of Bacteriophage MS2 Containing Single-Stranded RNA by Ascorbic Acid." *Journal for Nutritional Science and Vitaminology,* vol. 22, 1976, pp. 347–54.

Stone, Irwin. *The Healing Factor: "Vitamin C" Against Disease* (New York: Grosset & Dunlop, 1972).

The patient has a long history of passing kidney stones. Urine tests show high levels of oxalate excretion, indicating calcium oxalate stones, the most common type. Based on extensive research, the therapy suggested focuses on supplements of magnesium and vitamin B_6 (pyridoxine). Subsequently, three years passed without any further stones.

30   A Case of Kidney Stones

Jim Cox had passed 15 kidney stones over the past nine years. "In a way, I've been lucky," he said. "They've all passed on their own. I haven't had surgery for any of them, but I'm afraid sooner or later I will. I've been hoping all along they'd just go away; I guess I've just been fooling myself. My grandfather died after surgery for a kidney stone. I know modern surgical procedures are improved, but I'd still like to find a way to avoid both surgery and making any more stones, if possible."

Mr. Cox was a quiet, soft-spoken man who appeared to be in his late thirties. His wife and children had been in from time to time, but she hadn't been able to persuade him to take time off from his business to come in about what appeared to be his only health problem. As Mr. Cox explained: "It's not that I'm sick, I just get these stones every so often." However, during his last bout with a stone, which took him to a hospital, he'd promised his wife he'd come in.

"I asked my urologist about preventing kidney stones. He didn't know any method that worked for sure, but said to go ahead and try. He's so sympathetic you'd think he was having the stones himself."

"Do you know what type of kidney stones you've had?"

"No, I don't. Is it important?"

"It's an important clue in determining what type of treatment might be effective."

"One or two of the first few I passed were analyzed. I think they were the same, so the rest weren't analyzed."

"Were you advised to follow any sort of diet or other program?"

"Just to cut out milk and dairy products—I guess to minimize calcium intake. I did that for five years, but it didn't seem to make any difference . . . does that mean my kidney stones were made of calcium?"

"Most common types of kidney stones contain a high proportion of calcium. There are many other components possible . . . many stones are mixtures of various sorts. The proportions can vary widely. That's why it's important to know specifically what type you form."

"I hope I don't have to wait until I pass another one to have it analyzed."

"No, that's not necessary. Urine analysis sometimes shows what type of stone a person is likely to form."

Mr. Cox looked puzzled. "I've had lots of urine tests done. Practically every time I go to the doctor. But nobody ever said anything about preventing kidney stones, based on those tests."

"That type of urinalysis is important. It's for the presence of bacteria or white blood cells indicating possible infection. It's also for red blood cells, sugar, protein, and degree of acidity or alkalinity. This can be useful information for some people who form stones. For instance, chronic infection or the wrong degree of acidity-alkalinity can predispose to forming stones. We'll do that here, too. I assume, though, that these tests have been normal for you in the past."

"That's what I was told."

"Have you ever had a 24-hour collection of urine done?"

"What are they supposed to find?"

"Calcium. Also, phosphate, uric acid, magnesium, and oxalate. Speaking of tests—I suppose you've had kidney x-rays done?"

"I've had them done three times—twice when I was in the hospital, and once just to see if I had a large stone stuck near one of my kidneys, I think. The last one was done the last time I was there. It showed only a small stone that would probably pass, and it did."

I made a note of that. "Also, to complete the mineral picture, I'd recommend you have mineral analysis done on a hair specimen, and blood specimens drawn. The hair analysis is helpful not only for the minerals themselves, but it also gives an excellent clue about whether minerals are being assimilated well from your diet."

"Whatever you say. If it'll all help to get to the bottom of the trouble, I'm ready to get it done."

"I can't guarantee that these tests will do that. There's a good chance; otherwise I wouldn't recommend them. But remember that large-scale statistics don't necessarily apply in each individual case. They're only useful as guidelines, not as firm rules."

"I know that. Not everything that's supposed to work in my business does, either. But even if there's only a small chance, it's worth it."

I'd marked the tests to be done for Mr. Cox on a slip of paper. I asked him to give it to the nurse to get things underway. I also asked him to sign a release, so that we could obtain a copy of one of his previous kidney stone analyses.

It took three weeks to get back all of the laboratory reports. Mr. Cox's follow-up appointment had been timed accordingly; only two days after the last lab report came in, he was back at the office.

"Did we find anything?" he asked.

"Let's go through your reports . . . first of all, it appears your tendency is toward the formation of the most common form of kidney stone: calcium oxalate. Your 24-hour urine tests showed 124 milligrams of oxalate: the normal is only up to 40 milligrams."

"Was there too much calcium, too?"

"No, actually your calcium excretion was on the low side of normal."

"But I could still make calcium oxalate stones?"

"Yes. Even if calcium is normal, excess oxalate will still tend to precipitate with it, causing stones. In fact, most people who form calcium oxalate stones don't have high oxalate levels either. Normal quantities of calcium and oxalate precipitate in their urine. Fortunately, this is usually preventable.

"The level of phosphate is also normal, although on the high side. Uric acid was normal, but your magnesium excretion was low."

"Is that bad?"

"It increases the tendency toward stone formation. However, even if the magnesium was perfectly normal, the oxalate level means trouble. In your case, low magnesium only makes it worse."

"What about my blood tests?"

"Normal calcium and phosphate . . . but that's not a surprise, these are almost always normal. Also, normal uric acid. Magnesium is low again, even though not by much.

"Now, your hair test; first, there's no sign of poor absorption of nutrients. That's very important as nutrition and supplement programs may fail due to poor digestion and absorption. Second, calcium and phosphorus levels are within normal, although on the high side. On the other hand, the magnesium level is quite high: 270 parts per million [ppm] compared to normal, 25 to 75 ppm."

"High? I thought my blood and urine tests showed I was magnesium-deficient."

"You are. Hair mineral analysis is not as easy to interpret as it looks. Some minerals, particularly magnesium, calcium, and zinc, give false elevations. Extremely high levels of these or other minerals on a hair test should always be followed with blood and 24-hour urine studies. More often than not, these very high levels indicate deficiency, although in some cases toxicity is confirmed."

"Then the hair test isn't especially reliable, is it?"

"That's not so at all. For example, if we'd just had your hair test, it still would have pointed to which mineral or minerals needed further study. We'd still have come to the conclusion of deficiency in your case, even though in another case it might be toxicity.

"More generally, it's important to remember that a laboratory test is no better than the laboratory doing it or the doctor interpreting its meaning. False elevations occur in many other tests, too, not just hair tests. Medicine is still just as much an art as a science; no lab test can be trusted 100 percent.

"But back to your particular case. Even if all your magnesium tests had been within normal, not deficient, I'd still ask you to use magnesium as part of the treatment. Researchers have found that taking magnesium makes calcium oxalate more soluble in urine, so it has less tendency to precipitate and form stones. Your apparent magnesium deficiency simply makes this tendency worse.

"The next part of the treatment is pyridoxine or vitamin B_6. Researchers in stone prevention recommend small quantities of this vitamin. In your case, though, since you're making larger than usual amounts of oxalate, it's necessary to use larger quantities to cut that down.

"The last part of the treatment is what *not* to do. Since you make too much oxalate, it'd be best not to eat foods with lots of oxalate in them. Second, more than 2 to 3 grams daily of ascorbic acid, or vitamin C, is likely to aggravate this."

"What about calcium—milk and so on?"

"Once you've been on the pyridoxine-magnesium treatment for a few weeks, it's probably not necessary to control it."

I wrote it down in summary for Mr. Cox:

1. Magnesium, chelated: 100 milligrams, twice daily, or magnesium oxide, 100 milligrams, three times daily
2. Pyridoxine (vitamin B_6): 50 milligrams, twice daily
3. No more than 2 to 3 grams vitamin C daily
4. Eliminate high-oxalate foods, especially spinach and rhubarb
5. Calcium limitation not necessary after a few weeks

Mr. Cox read over the note. "Let me see if I'm clear on this: because of my high oxalate level it's likely I make calcium oxalate stones, even though it's not necessary to be high in either one for this to happen. I have a magnesium deficiency, which will make calcium oxalate less soluble in my urine; however, even if I wasn't magnesium-deficient, additional magnesium would make the calcium oxalate more soluble, so it wouldn't be as likely to precipitate into stones. Did I get that right?"

"Yes."

Mr. Cox thought for a minute. "That doesn't make any sense. What that all adds up to is even though I had abnormal tests, I could have had all normal tests, and still have a kidney stone, which isn't normal!"

"In your case, you're quite right. All that means is that the tests aren't individualized enough, or that we simply don't have the tests invented that would pick up the abnormality. Remember what I said about medicine being still as much art as science."

"So how do you know this is going to work?"

"Two ways: first, I've seen it work before. Second, competent researchers have reported success with this treatment. However, it doesn't absolutely prove it in your case. We'll know for sure if you get no further stones. And we'll get an early indication by repeating your abnormal tests to see if they become normal."

"That seems reasonable. Which tests should I repeat, and when?"

"Blood and urine tests for magnesium, urine test for oxalate in 60 to 90 days. Hair test, especially for magnesium, in six to eight months."

Mr. Cox's tests for magnesium and oxalate were all normal three months later. His false elevation for magnesium on his hair mineral test had gone *down* to nearly normal after six months. Even though his tests were improved, I recommended he continue his treatment to prevent further trouble.

Three years later, he'd not had any further stones. Even though three years is sometimes considered not long enough to prove anything, Mr. Cox's previous history plus his normalized tests probably indicate he will remain stone-free if he continues his pyridoxine-magnesium treatment.

The copy of the several-years-old analysis done on one of Mr. Cox's first stones took over two months to arrive. It showed that as his urine tests predicted, his stone was the calcium oxalate type.

———————

At first glance, Mr. Cox's case does seem confusing. As he so aptly summarized it, his tests were abnormal, but even if they'd been normal the treatment would have been the same: magnesium and pyridoxine.

But his conclusion was only true because his tests showed overproduction of oxalate, and therefore a high probability of calcium oxalate stone, which is specifically preventable with pyridoxine and magnesium. If his tests had shown high levels of uric acid or a different mineral pattern, the suggested treatment would have differed. Of course, if a stone analysis had been available from his prior stones, he might not have needed any further testing.

Last, since calcium oxalate stones are the most frequent type, and neither magnesium or pyridoxine treatment is likely to be harmful, especially in the doses suggested, he could have "just taken it" anyway with a fair chance of success. Of course, this is not my preferred method of approach, as determining causes as closely as possible makes chances of successful treatment better.

Drs. Stanley F. Gershoff and Edwin L. Prien have been working on the pyridoxine-magnesium treatment for prevention of calcium oxalate kidney stones since at least the early 1960s.

Yet even with their proven record of successful treatment, their work is generally ignored in the medical community, at least that part of it in my area. I've grown used to patients (with calcium oxalate stone history) telling me that their urologists have told them there's no "proven" method of kidney stone prevention.

Dr. Gershoff is said to have remarked (in a round-table discussion) that if he'd developed a new antibiotic or other new prescription drug for prevention of kidney stones, every doctor in the country would know about it.

He's right. The unfortunate medical bias, except in a few isolated instances, against vitamin/mineral treatment has kept this valuable and proven treatment largely unknown. If that weren't bad enough, imagine all the kidney stones (oxalate-type only, of course, but this is the major type) that could have been prevented since the sixties, along with all the pain, suffering, hospital days, and economic loss.

Maybe I'm wrong. Maybe my area is different from most of the rest of our country, and this simple preventive measure has established itself in most other areas. Maybe I'll get hundreds of indignant letters from practitioners I've implicitly and unfairly criticized by writing these last few paragraphs. I sincerely hope so; I'll send each an apology. Maybe. . . .

Maybe I should quit dreaming, and get busy on the next chapter.

FURTHER READING

Gershoff, Stanley F., and Prien, Edwin L. "Effect of Daily MgO and Vitamin B$_6$ Administration to Patients with Recurring Calcium Oxalate Kidney Stones." *The American Journal of Clinical Nutrition*, vol. 20, no. 5, May 1967, pp. 393-99.

Lyon, E. S. et al. "Calcium Oxalate Lithiasis Produced by Pyridoxine Deficiency and Inhibition with High Magnesium Diets." *Investigative Urology*, vol. 4, no. 2, 1966, pp. 133-42.

Prien, Edwin L., and Gershoff, Stanley F. "Magnesium Oxide-Pyridoxine Therapy for Recurrent Calcium Oxalate Calculi." *The Journal of Urology*, vol. 112, October 1974, pp. 509-12.

Zinsser, Hans H. et al. "Urinary Organic Acids Found in B$_6$-Deficient Rats and Calcium Oxalate Calculus Patients." *British Journal of Urology*, vol. 43, 1971, pp. 523-35.

A patient who wants to take maximally high doses of vitamin C asks to be checked to see if he has a tendency to develop oxalate stones at such high levels—8 grams (8,000 milligrams) a day. Tests reveal he does have this tendency—although he has not yet had any problems. The patient learns eventually he can take this amount in relative safety if he also takes vitamin B_6.

31 High-Dose Vitamin C and Kidney Stones

Michael Williams had been reading extensively about nutrition on his own, and had drawn up a diet and vitamin supplement program to suit his individual needs and preferences. He wasn't ill, but had come in to make sure there were no hidden hazards in his program.

He had one very specific worry. "I've read Irwin Stone's *Healing Factor: "Vitamin C" Against Disease*, Linus Pauling's *Vitamin C and the Common Cold*, and Dr. Klenner's articles about vitamin C, and I'm convinced that to stay healthy I should take an optimum amount of vitamin C every day, not the minimum."

"What do you think is optimum?"

"As much as I can take every day without getting gas or diarrhea."

"That's called the body-tolerance level. I definitely recommend it for those who are interested in optimum health. How much vitamin C are you taking?"

"I can take 8 grams—8,000 milligrams—every day before I

run into gas problems. Of course, I use more if I get sick. And I generally use the time-release form; it's more convenient."

"So far I don't see any problems. The body-tolerance approach is a good one. What's the problem you see?"

"Well, I've read about vitamin C and kidney stones. And there's a history of them in my family. Isn't 8 grams a day risky?"

"I haven't seen anyone develop this problem, but you're right, it's a theoretical risk if you're taking more than 3 to 4 grams daily. It's also not a risk everyone would run. Only a few people out of everyone using body-tolerance amounts of vitamin C might theoretically get kidney stones. The percentages are not definitely known, but they're small."

"OK, but with my family history it might be me. Even if it's only 1 percent risk, or less, if I get a kidney stone, for me it'll be 100 percent."

"That's true. But I don't think you know that there's a method for detecting persons who might be at risk for stone formation induced by vitamin C."

"There is? Good; let's find out. But if I'm one, then I'll have to stop taking vitamin C, won't I? I'd rather not. There seem to be so many potential benefits."

"That is one alternative. However, there are two others. You could cut down the amount of vitamin C to a level that wouldn't cause a stone, or you could counteract this effect of vitamin C with another vitamin. But let's postpone talking about that unless you turn up with a problem."

A very few people who take large quantities of vitamin C start to make abnormally high levels of oxalate, which is then excreted by the kidneys. All of us excrete a small amount of oxalate every day, but when large quantities are excreted, calcium oxalate kidney stones can be formed. In order to test Mr. Williams's potential for this, I asked him to take his 8-gram tolerance level of vitamin C for two to three weeks. During this time he should take no other vitamins. Then, he should collect urine for 24 hours, which we would then send to the laboratory for a 24-hour urinary oxalate excretion test. The vast majority of per-

sons taking such a test show either no elevation of urinary oxalate
or only a minor elevation.

When Mr. Williams returned, he asked about the results of
his test.

"Unfortunately, you are one of the rare oxalate formers," I
told him. "The normal levels of oxalate are 40 milligrams or less
per 24 hours. Yours rose to 383 milligrams, definitely too high."

Mr. Williams looked depressed. "Well, now what?"

"Don't give up yet. I agree that vitamin C at tolerance levels
has many potential advantages. So, let's do more tests. First, let's
see what happens when you take the same amount of vitamin C
and 50 milligrams of vitamin B_6 twice daily."

"Vitamin B_6?"

"Yes. Vitamin B_6 will prevent vitamin C-induced oxalate formation."

Mr. Williams took the same amount, 8 grams, of vitamin C
for another two weeks. But this time, he took vitamin B_6, 50
milligrams twice a day, along with it. His urinary oxalate test
following this was only 57 milligrams.

"Looks like that's the answer," he said. "I'll just make sure to
take my B_6 right along with the C."

"Remember, there's another alternative, too, besides no vitamin C, or maximum vitamin C and vitamin B_6. Why don't you
start with a small amount of vitamin C—say 1 gram a day—and
see how much oxalate you make? Perhaps there's a compromise
level, lower than 8 grams, where you can still take vitamin C, but
not make too much oxalate. After all, it's completely unknown
whether people who are oxalate formers should even take vitamin C, even if vitamin B_6 will counteract the problem."

So, Mr. Williams conducted several further tests. He took
varying levels of vitamin C for two-week intervals, and found that
the most he could take without increasing his oxalate excretion
was 1,500 milligrams. He was very discouraged by this, as from
his reading he had decided he wanted to take more vitamin C for
its potential benefits.

"After all, I didn't start all this until I was 37 years old," he said. "I'm sure I need extra vitamin C."

I agreed that for most people this was probably so. But for him as an individual who tended to make oxalate, I couldn't say.

"Is there any danger in taking my tolerance level of 8 grams, plus the vitamin B₆?" he asked.

"Probably not. You've shown that your oxalate problem is controlled. But all the necessary research hasn't even been done to answer this question, so all I can do is give an educated guess."

"I think I'll take the C and B₆," he said. "I think I'll probably prevent more problems with the vitamin C than I'll cause, as long as I don't forget my B₆."

———

For those readers who wish to take "body-tolerance" levels of vitamin C to prevent disease, or other quantities larger than 2 to 3 grams for a prolonged period of time, the theoretical possibility of calcium oxalate kidney stone formation can be assessed with the 24-hour urinary oxalate test described above. Most readers will need only one test, rather than numerous ones as Mr. Williams did, as most are not potential oxalate formers.

The presently available evidence has convinced me that the body-tolerance approach to ascorbic acid supplementation is likely to produce the most long-term health benefits. Daily body-tolerance doses are full and effective compensation for the metabolic error involved in the genetic disease, scurvy. (See a discussion of this in chapter 29, "A Case of Hepatitis.")

The oxalic acid-kidney stone hazard is at present the only one known in long-term, high-dose, ascorbic acid use. As it's easy enough to test for, it shouldn't be a serious deterrent. As noted above, only a few percent will be found to be oxalate formers.

One other special case of potential hazard in taking high doses of ascorbic acid is during and immediately after pregnancy. If the mother has been taking several grams daily of ascorbic acid, of course the nutritional environment of the fetus is relatively high in this nutrient. After delivery of the baby, if it isn't nursed, but placed on a standard low-ascorbic acid formula, it could potentially develop a relative scurvy.

That is obviously an easily avoidable hazard. The newborn can be given extra ascorbic acid. However, I would hope that if the mother is sufficiently nutrition-and-preventive-medicine oriented to take extra doses of ascorbic acid throughout pregnancy, she also will nurse her infant. If she does, the baby will get plenty of ascorbic acid. It penetrates into the breast milk so well that not infrequently I have to advise new mothers to reduce their own ascorbic acid intake (which they may have raised to fight a cold) because it's giving the baby gas.

What about danger to a fetus from high doses of ascorbic acid? Theoretically, there should be none. But much more important than just theory, Dr. Klenner has reported on over 300 pregnancies during which the mothers took 3 to 10 grams daily. No congenital anomalies were found.

Given my preventive bias, I'm firmly in favor of full treatment of the inborn error of metabolism involved in scurvy, for everyone, whether sick or not. The only present exception is in cases of oxalate formers, since it's not known whether these individuals may simply have an individually very low ascorbic acid requirement, or perhaps some other health problem. I really can't say conclusively whether low ascorbic acid or high ascorbic acid plus pyridoxine is preferable for these individuals; there isn't enough evidence.

The possibilities of disease prevention for each individual with body-tolerance levels of ascorbic acid are impressive. Can you imagine the potential improvement in national health if we all adopted this measure?

FURTHER READING

Anderson, T. W.; Reid, D. B.; and Beaton, G. H. "Vitamin C and the Common Cold: A Double-Blind Trial." *Canadian Medical Association Journal*, vol. 107, September 23, 1972, pp. 503–8.

Klenner, Frederick. "Observations on the Dose and Administration of Ascorbic Acid when Employed Beyond the Range of a Vitamin in Human Pathology." *Journal of Applied Nutrition,* Winter 1971, pp. 61-87.

Pauling, Linus. *Vitamin C and the Common Cold* (San Francisco: W. H. Freeman and Co., 1970).

Stone, Irwin. *The Healing Factor: "Vitamin C" Against Disease* (New York: Grosset & Dunlap, 1972).

A 63-year-old man with all the classic signs of prostate gland enlargement. When examination rules out malignancy, he is asked to take zinc and essential fatty acids as the foundation of therapy. Most of his symptoms vanish after four to five months. . . . One possible reason for his problem is heavy drinking, which causes zinc to be lost from the body.

32 A Case of Prostate Enlargement

"I'm here because my wife asked me to come," Mr. Fife declared. "I told her I'd take her pills, but that wasn't enough. She said there might be something else I could do. So I'm here."

This was the first time I'd met Edwin Fife. He was a slightly heavy man, with graying hair and mustache, apparently in his early sixties.

"As long as you're here, why don't you tell me what your problem's been?"

"I know what that is; I've had it checked already. It's my prostate gland. They told me I'd probably need surgery in a year or two—not a thrilling prospect."

"What symptoms does it cause?"

"It's nothing unusual, just what everybody gets with prostate trouble. I have to get up at night to urinate, sometimes three or four times. I have to wait a long time before I can go, nearly always. It never feels like I've emptied out; sometimes there's dribbling. The stream is kind of weak, too."

"That certainly is a complete set of symptoms."

"It should be. This has been coming on since I was 55. I'm 63 now. I've been through this with three different doctors."

"What happened?"

"I saw two different general doctors when it first started. They told me they couldn't do anything; see a specialist when it got bad. So I saw a urologist eight or nine months ago. He gave me the same blasted examination the other two did, told me my prostate gland was enlarged but no cancer, and I should have surgery."

"Did you receive any other treatment?"

"No," he said, "there wasn't any. My wife asked him about diet or vitamins, but he said I'd just be wasting my money, that surgery was the only thing."

"Have you made any plans for surgery?"

"No! I don't want anyone cutting on me before they absolutely have to!"

"You said you were taking some pills?"

"Yeah, my wife wouldn't listen to the specialist. She just kept looking around to see what she could find out. She got hold of a magazine from a friend; it talked about zinc pills for prostate trouble. I told her that was a laugh."

"Why was that?"

"I've been a metal worker all my life, the last 18 years in sheet metal trades. I told my wife that I was probably full of zinc up to here. But she kept after me. So I figured I might as well try them. I've been taking two a day since. Also, she finally got me to make this appointment."

"How long have you been taking the zinc?"

"Well, it took awhile before I could get in for an appointment. My schedule and yours don't fit very well. So it's been about six weeks."

"Have you noticed any difference?"

"I don't know whether it's my imagination, but I don't seem to have to wait quite as long. And I haven't gotten up as much at night for the last week or two, but that varies."

I made a note of this. "Have you had any other problems with your health?"

"Not that I know of, except a little overweight. But that comes from too much beer, I know." He paused. "You're not going to tell me that that's bad for my prostate, are you? I told my wife I wasn't going to give it up."

"How much beer do you drink?"

"Usually a six-pack or so every night. I've done that for years."

"Zinc is required in the first step of alcohol breakdown in the liver. It works with an enzyme called alcohol dehydrogenase to start the breakdown process. So more alcohol requires more zinc for detoxification."

"Well, I'll just take more zinc to make up for it. Can't teach an old dog new tricks."

"Actually, there are some other things you can do, if your prostate gland isn't too far gone. From what you say has happened already with the zinc, it probably isn't."

"You're going to give me another examination, aren't you?"

"Well, yes. Particularly since this is the first time you've been in."

"I was afraid of that. I told Ethel when I left 'I bet I'll have to have another one of those blasted examinations. That's all those doctors want to do, every time they see me coming.' " Grumbling to himself, Mr. Fife got up and went into the examination room.

Examination of his prostate showed it was definitely enlarged and slightly tender. There were no nodules, which sometimes are indicative of cancer. I told Mr. Fife this.

"I knew that already!" he exclaimed. "Why did it need checking again?"

"I won't be able to tell if it's getting smaller again unless I check to find what size it is to start with. It's also very important to make sure it's not cancerous."

"You mean you're going to check every time I come in here?"

"Probably. But it won't be often."

"Darn right! Now what?"

I gave Mr. Fife a brief note listing the nutrients I especially wanted him to use. It read:

1. Chelated zinc: 50 milligrams, 1 tablet 3 times daily

2. Essential fatty acid capsules: 400 milligrams, 1 capsule 3 times daily
3. Tablets made from whole animal prostate gland: 2, 3 times daily
4. Pollen tablets: 3 a day

Mr. Fife read the note. "I guess there is more stuff than just zinc. I understand about zinc and the prostate tablets, I think, but what about the other two?"

"A report was published in 1941, by Drs. Hart and Cooper, about 19 men with enlarged prostate glands. They found that essential fatty acids, taken orally, reduced the size of the prostate glands in all cases."

"Did you say 1941?"

"Yes, 1941."

"That's long enough for the word to get out. Why didn't the specialist tell me?"

"I don't know. But I do know that most of my colleagues are still of the opinion that only a few rare health problems can be solved with proper nutrition or added vitamins and minerals. So they ignore the whole area."

"And I've had my symptoms for eight years. Well, better late than never. What about the pollen?"

"Many naturopathic doctors, especially European ones, say that pollen is helpful for prostate problems. It seems to work for my patients. So I've put it in to make sure nothing is left out."

"OK. Is that it?"

"Not quite." We went over Mr. Fife's eating habits in some detail. After the usual admonitions about no refined sugar, no white flour, and mostly fresh foods, I asked Mr. Fife to get a good nutrition book.

"What's that for?"

"I want you to look up good food sources of zinc and essential fatty acids. Then make sure to eat lots of those."

"Maybe I'll let my wife do that."

"No, I want you to do it yourself. After all, it's your prostate gland."

Grumbling a little again, Mr. Fife got up to go. "When should I come back?"

"Give it all three to four months. That should be enough time to see how you do. Oh, before you go, let me see your fingernails."

"Fingernails?"

"Yes, fingernails."

"What's that got to do with anything?"

"Look, I'll show you." I showed Mr. Fife the white spots on his nails, a sign of zinc deficiency (as described by Dr. Carl Pfeiffer in his book, *Mental and Elemental Nutrients: A Physician's Guide to Nutrition and Health Care.*)

I'd almost forgotten Mr. Fife, when he came into my office nearly six months later. He'd lost a little weight and was looking considerably more relaxed.

"I was doing so good I just now got around to coming back," he said. "Besides, I got to feeling so frisky, I took Ethel on a second honeymoon. Surprised the heck out of her. Now I'm thinking of early retirement." He laughed. "Is that stuff supposed to do that?"

"I've heard of it before. Dr. Cooper reported that in 1941, too. And don't forget, if you had prostate trouble for eight years, you probably weren't feeling too frisky for all that time."

"Well, no."

"What about your other symptoms?"

"Oh, those. Let me see. There's absolutely no dribbling anymore. I hardly ever have to get up at night to urinate. I can go right away and feel empty now. The stream is even stronger."

"Sounds like nearly a complete recovery—how long did all of that take?"

"Can't really remember, but most of it happened by four or five months."

"Are you still taking all your supplements?"

"Yes, but I cut down to only one of each once a day. I'm eating lots of pumpkin seeds and oysters, though. The book said those were some of the best for fatty acids and zinc, and I like them."

He paused. "I'm still drinking my beer, too! But I've cut down to four cans a day. Now, am I still going to need one of those blasted examinations?"

"I'd prefer to check, to see if the size of your prostate has changed like your symptoms."

"Let's get it over with. I told Ethel I wouldn't get out of it."

Examination showed that Mr. Fife's prostate gland had returned to almost normal. There was only minimal enlargement, and no tenderness at all.

When I told Mr. Fife that, he looked pleased. As usual, though, he grumped: "I could have told you that without the checkup."

He showed me his fingernails. The signs of zinc deficiency were gone.

"I guess that's about all, isn't it?" he asked. "As long as I keep eating my pumpkin seeds and oysters, and take a little bit of the supplements, I should be OK."

I agreed. "I would like you to come back in six months to a year for a recheck, please."

"You doctors are all alike on that. It doesn't matter whether you use vitamins or drugs or cutting, you always want us to come back for a recheck!"

The Nutritional Approach to Prostate

Traditionally, pumpkin seeds have been folk medicine's remedy for prostate gland problems. Likewise, oysters have been mentioned in many folk sources for "rejuvenation" of organs of the reproductive tract.

While folk remedies don't always prove out, pumpkin seeds have been found to be high in zinc and essential fatty acids, the two major components of the remedy noted in Mr. Fife's case; oysters are extremely high in zinc.

Essential fatty acids are chemical substances (essential to life) found in highest concentrations in vegetable oils. Linoleic acid is the best known. It cannot be produced by the body and has been clearly demonstrated to both restore growth when given to animals deficient in it and to prevent dermatitis. For this reason, it is considered essential and must be provided by the diet.

The best sources of essential fatty acids are the seeds and nuts from which vegetable oils are usually derived. Sunflower, safflower, soy, and sesame are only a few. Of course, the oils derived, and even the seeds or nuts themselves can become rancid quite easily by exposure to atmospheric oxygen. This renders the essential fatty acids nearly useless, so the oils must be fresh and protected from air in closed containers.

Recent research by Dr. David Horrobin of Montreal shows that the oil of the evening primrose is probably more effective than anything in current use. It's not generally available yet, though (at least as of this writing).

Besides oysters, nuts and seeds are usually higher in zinc than many other foods; however, the zinc picture is clouded by widespread soil deficiencies. In an article by Pories and Strain, a map is published reproducing findings of a United States Department of Agriculture study done in 1961. At that time, the soil of 32 states was found to be zinc-deficient in at least some areas. The situation is certainly no better this year.

So, even if a food is supposed to be high in zinc, if it's grown in any area where the soils are zinc-depleted, it's not likely to have as much as it should. So the cycle is completed: deficient soil, deficient crops, deficient animals, and deficient people; sometimes, even people who are making every effort to eat a good diet.

Dr. Carl Pfeiffer is a pioneer in zinc research. It's been his observations that have led to the identification of white spots on the nails as signs of need for zinc in a person's system. In my experience, zinc alone, while usually effective in correcting these fingernail spots (and of course treating associated bodily problems) sometimes needs help from pyridoxine (vitamin B_6) and essential fatty acids.

Dr. Pfeiffer has pointed out for years that a certain type of mental health problem is often helped by a combination of zinc and pyridoxine. Very recent research by Dr. Horrobin at the endocrine pathophysiology department, Clinical Research Institute of Montreal, shows that therapy with essential fatty acids and zinc may be very helpful in certain cases of schizophrenia. There's evidence that pyridoxine works on the same enzyme systems that zinc and essential fatty acids do. The "zinc-B_6-essential fatty acid connection" should produce some very exciting research findings over the next few years.

One final note on zinc: some of the original studies on the clinical use of zinc showed that absolute deficiency produced delayed growth as well as delayed sexual maturity. It's been my observation that the age group showing the very highest incidence of white spots on the nails (Dr. Pfeiffer's zinc-insufficiency sign) is from 11 to 18 years of age, when rapid growth and of course sexual maturation are both occurring.

FURTHER READING

Essential Fatty Acids

Hart, James P., and Cooper, William L. "Vitamin F in the Treatment of Prostatic Hypertrophy." Lee Foundation for Nutritional Research, Milwaukee, Wisconsin, Report No. 1, November 1941, pp. 1–10.

Horrobin, D. F. "Schizophrenia as a Prostaglandin Deficiency Disease." *The Lancet*, April 30, 1977, pp. 936–37.

―――. "Prostaglandin Deficiency and Endorphin Excess in Schizophrenia: The Case for Treatment with Penicillin, Zinc and Evening Primrose Oil." *Journal of Orthomolecular Psychiatry*, vol. 8, no. 1, January 1979, pp. 13–19.

Horrobin, D. F. et al. "Prostaglandins and Schizophrenia: Further Discussion of the Evidence." *Psychological Medicine*, vol. 8, January 1978, pp. 43–48.

Mead, James F., and Fulco, Armand J. *The Unsaturated and Polyunsaturated Fatty Acids in Health and Disease* (Springfield, Ill.: Charles C Thomas, 1976).

Pollen

Ohkashi, Masaaki. "Clinical Evaluation of Cernilton in Chronic Prostatitis." *Japanese Journal of Clinical Urology*, vol. 21, no. 1, 1967, p. 73.

Saito, Yutaka. "Diagnosis and Treatment of Chronic Prostatitis." *Clinical & Experimental Medicine*, vol. 44, no. 6, June 1967.

Zinc

Bush, Irving M. et al. "Zinc and the Prostate." Paper presented at the annual meeting of the American Medical Association, Chicago, Illinois, 1974.

Fahim, M. S. et al. "Zinc Treatment for Reduction of Hyperplasia of Prostate." *Federation Proceedings*, vol. 35, no. 3, March 1, 1976, p. 361.

Halsted, James A. et al. "Zinc Deficiency in Man: The Shiraz Experiment." *The American Journal of Medicine*, vol. 53, September 1972, pp. 277-84.

Pfeiffer, Carl C. *Mental and Elemental Nutrients: A Physician's Guide to Nutrition and Health Care* (New Canaan, Conn.: Keats Publishing, 1975).

Pories, Walter J., and Strain, William. "Once Upon a Trace Metal: The Zinc Story." *Medical Opinion*, May 1971, pp. 38-45.

A man who works on his feet all day has large, painful callus formations on his feet. The skin on his legs is rough and red. In addition he has been having repeated sinus infections. All this is suggestive of vitamin A deficiency, but further investigation shows there is a related problem of nutrient absorption. Supplements of the fat-soluble vitamins (A,D,E,) plus digestive enzymes brings about gradual improvement in several health problems.

A Case of Calluses　　33

"I wouldn't have come in at all, but I spend all day on my feet on a cement floor, and they're getting to be more and more of a problem. I've got several years to go before retirement. I don't know if I can put up with my feet this way 'til then."

Lloyd Sykes was a short, muscular, compact man, still dressed in his work overalls. As he finished speaking, he began to take off his shoes and socks.

"Where do you work?"

'I sell auto parts. Busy shop, and I hardly get any time to sit down. I can't find any good help half the time. But it wouldn't be so much bother if it wasn't for these calluses."

He showed me his feet, which had the most impressive set of calluses I'd seen in months. He had thick, hard ridges of callus along both sides of his heels, extending nearly the length of his foot on the outer surfaces, and to his instep on the inner surfaces. The undersurfaces of his heels were hard. Across the underside of his foot, between the front of the arch and the base of his toes, were more thick calluses. Even the outsides of his big and little toes were thickened with callus.

"I see what you mean," I said. "Would you please come into the examination room next door? There are some other areas I'd like to check."

Mr. Sykes picked up his shoes and socks, and went to the next room. I asked him to remove his overalls and work shirt.

His left elbow was a little rough, but his right elbow had a thick callus.

"I forgot about that one," he said. "It's the ones on my feet that bother me."

His skin was a little rough, dry, and flaky overall. Around the hair follicles on his legs, especially on the fronts of his thighs and the outsides of his upper arms, the skin was "built up" and a little red. It looked like lots of tiny pimples, each around a hair.

"How long have those pimples been there?" I asked.

"Years. They don't bother me any."

"Have you had any other problems with your health in the last year or two?"

"Well, nothing new. I've always had a lot of sinus problems, nothing bad though. But this year I've had four or five infections, and had to take antibiotics to get rid of them. Thought the last one would never go away. After that, the wife kept after me to come over here. Must be some reason, she said. Since I've always had a little trouble, I thought it'd pass."

"Anything else that doesn't seem quite right?"

"There's this gas. The wife said to mention that, too. Sometimes it gets so bad it hurts. But I don't see how that could be important; I've had it for years, too."

"Does it happen when you eat?"

"Not right away. Seems like it waits until an hour or two later to act up. Then it just keeps on for awhile."

"Tell me what kind of food you eat."

"Just regular meals."

"Can you be more specific? Go through breakfast, lunch, and dinner."

"Well, breakfast is always oatmeal and coffee. Sometimes I have a slice of toast, whole wheat of course. The wife insists on that. Lunch is two sandwiches, lunch meat, and a Thermos of coffee. Dinner I like meat, potatoes, gravy. Sometimes I have milk."

"Any vegetables?"

"Oh, yeah. Corn, peas, or beans, usually."

"How about green vegetables, or carrots, squash, or sweet potatoes?"

"Maybe once or twice a week."

"Do you take any vitamins?"

"The wife gives me a multiple. That's all I want to take unless I know what it's going to do."

"Do you get constipated?"

"Sometimes."

"How's your eyesight?"

"OK, I guess. A little worse over the past few years, but that's only natural. I don't figure it's going to be as good at 57 as it was when I was younger.

"How about at night? Can you drive at night as well as usual?"

"The lights have been bothering me quite a lot lately. And I'm not seeing as well at night, now that you mention it. I was thinking I needed new glasses, but just hadn't got to the doctor yet. I've been letting the wife drive when we go anywhere at night."

With this final answer, I thought we had enough clues to Mr. Sykes's callus problem. I asked him to get dressed again and come into the consultation room.

When he sat down, he asked "what was that all about? I came in about my feet, and we went from my stomach to my eyes. What's the problem I've got?"

"Don't forget your sinuses," I said. Taking the overall pattern, it looks like you're not getting enough vitamin A for your system, and that it's getting a lot worse lately.

"Vitamin A? There's vitamin A in those multiple vitamins,

10,000 units, I think. I eat butter; there's vitamin A in there, at least that's what my mother said. And I do eat a carrot every once in a while."

"Remember, we all need different amounts of nutrients. I didn't say you didn't get any vitamin A, just not enough for you. Actually, you're not eating an especially high amount of vitamin A. But besides low intake, I think another problem is that you're not absorbing it. Your stomach symptoms suggest a lack or under-production of pancreatic digestive enzymes. If your pancreas isn't making enough of those, you won't absorb the vitamin A you do take in. If that's the case, you're probably not absorbing enough vitamin D or E, either, or essential fatty acids."

"Why don't I show signs of that?"

"You do show signs of insufficient essential fatty acids. I'm sure your dry, flaky skin is due to that as much as to lack of vitamin A. But apparently your system needs vitamin A, especial-ly. Those severe calluses, your night vision problems . . . those are both clear signs of vitamin A problems. Even your sinus problems are somewhat related, although they can be caused by other things, also."

"How's that?"

"Not everyone with sinus problems is necessarily vitamin A-deficient. But if you are, it lowers the resistance to infections inside the sinuses, and you're more likely to have a problem. Haven't your sinus problems gotten worse since your calluses have gotten worse?"

"Well, yes, now that I think of it."

I started to write out a note. "I'd like you to get some pan-creatin at the health food store."

"Aren't you going to take any tests?"

"I don't really think it's necessary. You've got enough signs of vitamin A problems, and your other symptoms fit. We can spend the money if you want to, but in this case, I can't see the need."

I finished writing the note. It read as follows:

1. Pancreatin: 2 or 3 tablets with each meal, as many as

necessary to control gas
2. Vitamin A: 50,000 units, 3 times a day
3. Vitamin E: 800 units daily
4. Safflower oil: 1 tablespoon daily
5. Fat-soluble chlorophyll perles: 1, 3 times a day
6. Vitamin D: 1,000 units, twice a day

Mr. Sykes read over the note. "Isn't that an awful lot of vitamin A?"

"Anyone who takes vitamin A should know what the symptoms of overdose are. If these occur, there's plenty of time to stop taking the vitamin A, and let the symptoms go away. The combination of symptoms of vitamin A excess includes headaches, deep bone pain, very dry skin, and hair loss."

"That should be noticeable enough," Mr. Sykes said.

"I'd think so. Now, in your case, I want you to take a lot of vitamin A because you appear to be quite deficient. As you improve, we'll cut the dose down."

"OK. I understand that. But what are all those other things for?"

"Remember that gas problem, starting an hour or more after you eat? That timing, along with your probable vitamin A deficiency, makes it very likely that you're deficient in pancreatic digestive enzymes. That's what the pancreatin is for. The entire rest of the list contains fat-soluble vitamins that, like vitamin A, are not absorbed if you're deficient in pancreatic enzymes. I'm assuming you probably need them, and in those quantities, they can't hurt."

"What about the safflower oil? I don't know if I can swallow oil."

"Put it on some lettuce. If that doesn't work, you can get it in capsules. It is important, though, as a source of essential fatty acids. Those are as important as vitamins."

"How long do I have to take all this?"

"I can't say exactly, several months. But we'll both know: we'll watch your calluses, and you can't help but notice your vision. Come back in 60 days or so; we'll see how you're doing.

It took nine months for Mr. Sykes's calluses to go away. His night vision improved considerably in six months; his flaky, dry skin was better in just three months. During the nine months it took for his calluses to get better, he had only one sinus infection.

Once his calluses disappeared, he discontinued taking all his vitamin supplements. However, I convinced him to eat more foods containing vitamin A, and other fat-soluble vitamins. He found he couldn't stop taking his pancreatin without his gas returning. Because of this, and the reminder that it was necessary to help assimilate his vitamin A, he has continued to take it with his meals.

Mr. Sykes showed most of the clinical signs and symptoms of vitamin A insufficiency all wrapped up in one person. Frequently, a person will have just one or a few vitamin A-insufficiency symptoms without developing the same overall picture as Mr. Sykes. For example, a slight degree of night blindness or hypercallosity (excess callus formation), treatable with vitamin A, may exist without any of the other problems described.

His vitamin A problem was, of course, complicated by apparent lack of essential fatty acids, and probably the other fat-soluble vitamins. So there were also many interactions between the various insufficiencies of vitamins that probably contributed to his overall picture.

While the most notable features of Mr. Sykes's case were those related to his need for vitamin A, it could equally well be categorized under the heading of poor absorption. True, his vitamin A intake was marginal; but he couldn't efficiently assimilate what he did take in.

In many fields of inquiry, a successful answer to one problem often leads to further questions. Medicine and health problems are a good example of this: in Mr. Sykes's case his symptoms derived from a need for vitamin A and other fat-soluble vitamins. That in turn was largely traceable to a relative lack of absorption, due to a low level of digestive enzyme by his pancreas. What we really need to know is why his pancreas wasn't working. When we have an answer to this question, we'll be further ahead, but then we'll probably have another question to answer.

FURTHER READING

Altschule, Mark D. *"Vitamin A," Nutritional Factors in General Medicine: Effects of Stress and Distorted Diets* (Springfield, Ill.: Charles C Thomas, 1978), pp. 90–95.

A child nearly 4 years old is showing behavioral problems, poor development, and poor appetite. Questioning reveals an environment cause, compounded by deficiency of calcium. Therapy centers chiefly around that mineral plus vitamin C. . . . With a special note on the use of vitamin C as a detoxifying agent.

34   A Case of Lead Toxicity

Kim Jackson would have been a very attractive child, but he didn't appear well. He was towheaded and blue-eyed, but his fair complexion appeared sallow. He had dark circles under his eyes. His behavior was nervous and withdrawn. He stayed close to his mother and kept his thumb in his mouth a good part of the time.

"I don't know what's happened to him," his mother said. "He was such a friendly, outgoing 2-year-old. He didn't suck his thumb nearly as much as he does now. He had such a sunny disposition. I couldn't keep him inside. He wanted to go out and play all the time. Now he just hangs around and mopes a lot of the time. When he does play with other children, he gets into a lot more fights than he used to. He's just not looking well, so we decided to bring him here rather than to a psychiatrist."

"When did you start to notice a change?"

"It's been so gradual, I couldn't give you an exact date. He's 3 years, 10 months now; I guess we noticed the first signs after he turned 3."

"What did you first notice?"

"He just seemed a little more irritable than usual. Nothing major; it's just that when he was 3 I expected his behavior overall to be a little better than when he was 2. That's what everyone told me, anyway. Instead, it's been getting steadily worse."

"What else?"

"He hasn't been eating well for months. Now, I know children eat in streaks; my sister's children are older, and my sister's told me all about that. But he's been just picking at his food for six months or more. He doesn't seem to be growing much, either. He used to be just a little taller than the other 2-year-olds. Now he's definitely shorter than all the children he was taller than a year ago."

"How about those dark circles under his eyes?"

"He's had just faint ones since he was 1. They've gotten much worse this last year. Somebody told me those came from allergies. Do they?"

"Sometimes they're associated with allergies. Has Kim ever shown any other signs of allergies?"

"You mean like skin rashes or congestion?"

"Yes."

"No. As far as we know, there aren't any serious allergies in the family, either. I nursed him for almost a year, too. I read somewhere that might prevent him from getting allergy problems; of course that's not the only reason, it's just better for him. But isn't that right?"

"There is research that indicates that's true. Even so, allergy is still a definite possibility that needs to be checked. It's certainly possible to have no signs of allergy, except behavioral ones. Tell me, did Kim have any big changes in his life when he was about 3? Any family changes? A new baby or anything?"

"No, we're only planning one child. And if you mean between his father and me, no. We have the usual number of fights, but nothing major. We're basically happy with each other. My husband's happy with his job. I work part-time, but I have ever since he stopped nursing."

She thought for a minute. "We moved to a new place just before his third birthday, to be closer to my husband's work. But we live in the same home; it's a big trailer we've had since we were married. We're saving our money to build a house we really want. But if anything, Kim has more friends at this new place than where we were before."

"Are you nearer to a major highway than you were?"

"Yes. It's a large trailer park near a very busy road. But it's fenced so the children can't get on the road, and they have a nice play area."

"How about the last trailer park?"

"Well, we didn't live in one. The trailer was on a piece of property my parents own next to their home. But it was really a far drive to work."

"Was there much traffic?"

"Some. But nothing like now."

"Does Kim eat things from the ground?"

"He still does some. But not as much as when he was younger. Is that a problem?"

"I don't know; occasionally it is. Of course it depends on what's eaten. While we're on that subject, what does Kim eat?"

"He never gets any sugar that I know about. I read up on nutrition and health before I got pregnant, and decided he was going to get the best possible. We don't have any white bread, and we eat lots of fresh, raw foods." She looked a little more depressed and frustrated. "The trouble is, all that good food won't do him any good if he won't eat it. Like I said, he's just been picking at his food for months. I don't want to force him to eat; I know it's not good to make a constant battle out of it. But I don't know what to do. I'm sure he's getting some nutritional deficiencies that way. So I've been giving him extra vitamins and minerals. Luckily, he'll take those most of the time."

I asked her to bring in a list of Kim's vitamins and minerals the next time.

After asking a few other questions about Kim's general health background, all of which was quite normal, I had his mother take him to the examination room. Aside from the dark circles previously noted, and his complexion, there were no other specific abnormalities.

After talking it over with Kim's mother, we decided to have a blood count, urinalysis, hair mineral analysis, and blood test for food allergies (RAST) done. I asked her to make a list of eight or ten foods he ate most frequently. Like most 3-year-olds, Kim didn't appreciate the blood test, and let us know, but it was over quickly.

I asked Kim's mother to return once the test results were back.

Both of Kim's parents came in for the return appointment. Kim's mother gave me a list. "I've been giving Kim a multiple vitamin and mineral formula," she said. "I've written down all the parts of it." It was a fairly typical multiple supplement.

I opened Kim's records to his laboratory tests. "His urinalysis was normal," I said. "His blood count is normal, but just barely so. He's quite close to anemic."

"Could that be his problem?" Mr. Jackson asked.

"A small part of it. But it's probably related to another of his lab tests, his mineral analysis. Before we get to that, though, here's a copy of his allergy test."

I explained the interpretation of the test. "As you can see, he has practically no allergies at all. Only beef appears to be a problem, and at that only a mild one."

"Is that enough to account for Kim's symptoms?" Mrs. Jackson looked disappointed.

"Probably not. But let's have a look at his mineral analysis."

The mineral analysis showed a lead level of 6.3 milligrams percent, or 63 parts per million. His calcium level was low; he was also low in potassium and manganese.

"What's normal?"

"As far as anyone knows, there is no need at all for lead in the human system. There's no known need for it in body chemistry. Unfortunately, lead contamination is so widespread that we all have a small amount in our systems, so some authorities state that below a certain level is 'normal' or 'tolerable.' In fact a level of zero is preferable for optimum health."

"Lead could explain the way Kim's been behaving, couldn't it?" Mr. Jackson observed. "I think I read something about that awhile ago."

"Could it be entirely that?" Mrs. Jackson asked. "Even the dark circles under his eyes?"

"Yes, although you were right before when you thought that usually meant allergies. Also, it probably explains why he's almost anemic. Lead does that, too. Look at his mineral analysis again. His calcium level is low. There's some evidence indicating that a relatively low calcium intake will allow more lead than usual to accumulate."

"Where did all that lead come from?"

"That's probably quite obvious. Remember when you said his symptoms started to become noticeable?"

The Jacksons looked at each other. "It's that trailer park, isn't it?" Mrs. Jackson said.

"Well, not exactly. It's all the lead in the air associated with high-traffic areas. Of course, a crowded trailer park near a busy highway is a high-risk area for lead exposure."

"Why aren't all the other children affected like Kim?"

"I'd guess if you did mineral analyses on all of them you'd find higher lead levels on the average than almost any other area. I can't explain why they don't have symptoms. Maybe Kim's eaten some things from the ground with more lead."

"Kim hardly ever drinks milk," Mrs. Jackson observed. "It gives him gas. He doesn't like cheese either. Will giving him calcium pills help get rid of the lead?"

"That's part of the treatment. Also, look up other foods high in calcium; see if he'll eat those. The main treatment, though, is ascorbic acid, or vitamin C."

"Vitamin C? But Kim gets over 100 milligrams a day now. There's 45 in his multiple vitamin; he drinks at least 8 ounces of orange juice every day; that should have at least 60," Mrs. Jackson said.

"It's a good thing. I'm sure he'd be even worse otherwise. But that's not nearly enough vitamin C. I've treated two cases of much worse lead poisoning than Kim's with 30 to 40 grams (30,000 to 40,000 milligrams) of vitamin C, intravenously with calcium, at frequent intervals. It worked fine, with no toxicity. Of course, Kim won't need it intravenously, and he'll need less, since he's smaller."

"How much?"

"I don't know yet. I want you to start with 1,000 milligrams (1 gram) daily, divided into three or four doses, of course. Each day I want you to increase the total by 500 milligrams, until you find it starts to give him gas or diarrhea. That's a little too much, so at that point decrease just slightly, by 500 milligrams or so, so he doesn't have gas or diarrhea. That's called the body-tolerance level. Then give him that every day.

"Also, for now, give him 600 milligrams of calcium every day, with a little vitamin D, 400 units, to help absorption.

"Last, to protect against the remote possibility of calcium oxalate kidney stones from that much vitamin C, give him 25 to 30 milligrams of vitamin B_6, twice daily. That would probably be best as part of a B complex tablet or liquid."

"How long will this take?"

"Can't be sure, but he actually should start to feel better within just two to three weeks. But most of the lead probably won't be gone for months."

Kim's body-tolerance level for ascorbic acid turned out to be 5,500 milligrams daily. That is definitely unusual for a 3-year-old, but probably had to do with his high lead levels. As he improved, his tolerance lessened, and the dose had to be reduced.

His follow-up hair mineral analysis at four months was distinctly better, at 3.4 milligrams percent (34 ppm). At nine months, it was "normal" at 0.9 milligrams percent (9 ppm), although as mentioned before, lead is really not normal in any amount.

Kim's mother reported that his symptoms were gone by four to six months. His dark circles had nearly vanished; his former sunny disposition had returned. His tense, nervous, irritable behavior was gone. His appetite improved considerably; his blood count improved to a little better than average for his age.

To insure continuing normality, I advised the Jacksons to continue his ascorbic acid at his tolerance point, which settled down to 2,000 milligrams daily, with the calcium and vitamin B_6.

Vitamin C as a Detoxifying Agent

I very definitely do believe in psychiatry and psychology, and refer patients for psychotherapy when I think it would help. I'm also aware that any health-care practitioner uses a certain amount of conscious or unconscious psychology in helping patients.

In this book, as in my practice, I focus particularly on nutritional biochemistry, as that is my particular area of interest. So naturally, the mental health aspects of most cases presented are biochemically related ones. But assuredly, not all mental health problems are nutritional/biochemical.

Having said this, I need to state emphatically that a much larger proportion of so-called psychiatric disease than is generally recognized is nutritional/biochemical in origin.

Kim Jackson's case is one small illustration of this: a factor affecting his entire body chemistry was also affecting his mental chemistry, and therefore his behavior.

Lead poisoning and its effects have been recognized for a long time. In that regard, Kim's case is nothing new. What may not be recognized is that Kim's problem is an "accepted" example of a generally "not accepted" field of study—the relationship of human health to the total environment.

This "health and environment" field goes under the general title of human ecology, and besides numerous individual articles and books, has even produced a textbook, *Clinical Ecology*, edited by Lawrence Dickey (see Corwin in Further Reading).

In medicine, this whole topic has been left to schools of public health. In these institutions, the focus has traditionally been on infectious disease, occupational health hazards, and socioeconomics. As far as I'm aware, no present school of public health is greatly concerned with the various effects on health of heavy metal pollutants; insecticides and pesticides; chlorine and fluoride in the water; electromagnetic field effects such as those caused by high tension wires, electrical substations, microwave ovens and television sets; natural and unnatural atmospheric ionization; fluorescent and incandescent light; synthetic fabrics; petrochemical fumes from automobiles and home furnaces; plastics; supersonic, infra-sonic and "regular" noise. . . . The list could go on, but by now I'm sure the point is made.

If in fact there is a school of public health which is actively involved in all these areas, I will be glad to retract my statement. Being in private medical practice, I may not have kept up with the latest in public health. But if such a school exists, its professors are keeping much more quiet than usual.

Now, back to particular cases. As noted, lead has absolutely no place in normal human metabolism as far as is presently known. In performing routine mineral analysis for patients, it's perfectly obvious that all of us have at least a low level of lead pollution that usually doesn't cause recognized symptoms. But it obviously isn't doing us any good, as demonstrated very clearly by a Swiss physician.

Dr. Walter Blumer made a map of his village and found that the majority of his patients with nonspecific symptoms such as headache, fatigue, digestive upset or nervousness lived within 50 yards of the only major highway passing through town.

Treatment for heavy metal toxicity, designed to remove metals such as lead and cadmium, made a significant reduction in these nonspecific symptoms, as reported in "Cancer Mortality Near Road 9 Times That of Off-Road," in the *Medical Tribune*, September 11, 1974.

Which brings me to my last point—the treatment described in Kim's case. The routine treatment of lead and other heavy metal poisoning uses synthetic drugs such as EDTA and penicillamine. All such synthetic drugs are potentially toxic, particularly if higher doses are used rapidly. Because of this toxicity, they're never used in "minor" cases of heavy metal poisoning which can cause chronic symptoms, even if not disabling or deadly.

Nutritional biochemistry offers a broad-spectrum, almost totally nontoxic detoxifying agent: ascorbic acid, or vitamin C. As demonstrated above, vitamin C will remove lead from the human body. What's hardly known is that ascorbic acid will also remove other heavy metals such as cadmium and nickel. It will also help detoxify many drugs and organic toxins in the human system.

I personally have employed ascorbic acid to detoxify lead, cadmium, and nickel. I've observed the results on before-and-after tests. I've watched an electrocardiogram record the rapid disappearance of digitalis toxicity with intravenous sodium ascorbate (a form of vitamin C). I've used both intravenous and oral vitamin C to detoxify overdoses of drugs such as phenobarbital, Valium, Demerol, and marijuana (in its concentrated form).

Before you conclude that "nothing works that well," I invite you to read *The Healing Factor: "Vitamin C" Against Disease* by Irwin Stone. Containing over 500 scientific references, it presents evidence to back these statements up. (Before it appears I'm claiming the credit, I must say I got many of my ideas from Irwin Stone.)

To physicians reading this, let me say unequivocally that ascorbic acid/sodium ascorbate is extremely effective in both acute and chronic poisonings, with practically no side effects. In emergency room poisoning/overdose situations it's absolutely invaluable and lifesaving. Please write me in care of the publisher for details.

Getting away from emergency situations once more, this nonspecific detoxifying effect of vitamin C is one of its principal uses in preventive therapy as well. Considering air, water, and food pollution, which we all are exposed to and which vitamin C will detoxify, not taking extra vitamin C every day is a definite health hazard.

FURTHER READING

Anonymous. "Cancer Mortality Near Road 9 Times That of Off-Road." *Medical Tribune*, September 11, 1974, p. 14.

Anonymous. "Paint May Not Be Only Source of Lead Poisoning." *Journal of the American Medical Association*, vol. 236, no. 18, November 1, 1976, p. 2035.

Anonymous. "Science." *Chemical & Engineering News*, vol. 54, no. 39, September 20, 1976, p. 22.

Blumer, Max; Blumer, Walter; and Reich, Theodore. "Polycyclic Aromatic Hydrocarbons in Soils of a Mountain Valley: Correlation with Highway Traffic and Cancer Incidence." *Environmental Science & Technology*, vol. 11, no. 12, November 1977, pp. 1082-84.

Corwin, Alsoph H. "Heavy Metals in Air, Water, and Our Habitat." *Clinical Ecology*, edited by Lawrence Dickey (Springfield, Ill.: Charles C Thomas, 1976), pp. 292-303.

Holmes, Harry N.; Campbell, Kathryn; and Amberg, Edward J. "The Effect of Vitamin C on Lead Poisoning." *The Journal of Laboratory and Clinical Medicine*, vol. 24, no. 11, August 1939, pp. 1119-27.

Huisingh, Donald, and Huisingh, Joellen. "Factors Influencing the Toxicity of Heavy Metals in Food." *Ecology of Food and Nutrition*, vol. 3, 1974, pp. 263-72.

Marchmont-Robinson, S. W. "Effect of Vitamin C on Workers Exposed to Lead Dust." *The Journal of Laboratory and Clinical Medicine*, vol. 26, 1941, pp. 1478-81.

Pillemer, L. et al. "Vitamin C in Chronic Lead Poisoning, An Experimental Study." *American Journal of Medical Science*, vol. 200, 1940, pp. 322-27.

Sorell, Michael; Rosen, John F.; and Roginsky, Martin. "Interactions of Lead, Calcium, Vitamin D and Nutrition in Lead-Burdened Children." *Pediatric Research*, vol. 10, no. 4, April 1976, p. 415.

Stone, Irwin. *The Healing Factor: "Vitamin C" Against Disease* (New York: Grosset & Dunlap, 1972).

A young boy has been having recurrent nosebleeds for no apparent reason. When examination rules out other likely causes, a blood coagulation test is run and indicates a probable need for vitamin K. Supplements of fat-soluble chlorophyll which contain natural vitamin K are recommended, along with dark green vegetables. The problem is quickly resolved.

35 A Case of Nosebleeds

Optimum nutrition for good health should always be an overall, integrated plan, including all the known, as well as unknown, factors found in whole, unprocessed, unrefined foods. In addition, there are at all ages certain symptoms or signs that almost always indicate specific nutrient deficiencies or special individual requirements. The next case describes a symptom occurring in children that is most frequently caused by a need for specific nutrients.

———— ◆ ————

"Jimmy's been having a spell of nosebleeds again," Mrs. Robinson said. The Robinsons were relatively new patients; I'd not heard about Jimmy's nosebleeds.

"What do you mean by a spell?"

"Oh, he'll go several months, even a year, without any. Then he'll have one or two a week, six or seven a month, for a few months. Then they go away again."

"Do they last long?"

"Not usually. If he relaxes and squeezes his nose, they usually stop in 10 to 20 minutes. Occasionally one will continue an hour or so."

"You must have taken him to a doctor or hospital."

"When he was younger, he had to have his nose cauterized two or three times. He didn't like that. We also had him checked by a pediatrician, but she couldn't find anything the matter. Another doctor said he'd grow out of them."

"How old was he when they started?"

"Four or five."

As Jimmy was in with his mother, I asked him some questions, also.

"Do you notice anything that makes your nose bleed particularly, Jimmy?"

"Well, not really. It just starts all by itself."

"How about if you're playing baseball or football?"

"Well, maybe sometimes. . . ."

"Do you ever wake up with a nosebleed, Jimmy?"

"Yes, sometimes."

"How old are you now?"

"Eleven."

"Do you get many bruises?"

"I don't know."

I looked at his mother. "He does get his share, but I don't know if he gets any more than any active boy his age. We don't have any other boys."

"Does anyone else in your family have bleeding problems?"

"No, not as far as I know. I even checked all our relatives on both sides, and for years back when the pediatrician asked. But nobody had any hemophilia—is that it?—or any other bleeding problem. Not even nosebleeds."

"If Jimmy cuts himself, does he stop bleeding right away?"

"I can't tell for sure, but I think it takes a little longer than for his father or me. But I don't know for sure."

Although I suspected what the problem might be, I thought it best to check Jimmy briefly first. So I asked him and his mother to go to an examination room.

Jimmy's blood pressure was 92/60, perfectly normal for his

age, and certainly not high enough to make his nose bleed. The inside of his nose looked perfectly normal—no visible polyps, or blood vessels, or other visible abnormality. There wasn't even a trace of blood.

"Did you ever injure your nose seriously, Jimmy?"

"No. I never even got hit in the nose. I got that Danny Turner when he tried to push me around, though. . . ."

By now, I thought I had enough information to ask Jimmy a final question or two.

"How much spinach do you eat, Jimmy?"

The answer was obvious on Jimmy's face before he said a word. "Yuk!"

"How about cabbage, turnip greens, or other green vegetables? Broccoli?"

"I don't like any of that stuff!"

"I haven't been able to get Jimmy to eat green vegetables since he was 3 years old," his mother said. "I keep telling him he should; I didn't know it had anything to do with his nosebleeds. Isn't that unusual?"

Jimmy put it more succinctly: "Weird!" he said.

"It's not really weird at all, once you understand it, Jimmy."

"You mean spinach and broccoli stop nosebleeds?"

"Some nosebleeds, and most probably yours. They don't stop them after they start, though. What I mean is that eating enough green vegetables will probably keep you from having them in the first place. Green vegetables are nearly the only source of vitamin K. When some people don't have enough vitamin K, their noses bleed. It's the most common cause of recurrent nosebleed in children, in my experience."

Turning to Mrs. Robinson, I said, "That's likely what the problem is. We can find out for sure by doing a simple blood test called a prothrombin time (protime for short). In most children with recurrent nosebleeds, it's subnormal. Vitamin K makes it normal again, and of course, takes away the bleeding."

"I know eating green vegetables is the best thing to do, because it's natural. But for now are there vitamin K pills? I'd like to stop this as soon as possible."

"Yes, synthetic vitamin K is available on prescription. I'd rather you got a natural fat-soluble chlorophyll preparation containing vitamin K. That way he'll get other natural factors that go along with it. He should take 6 a day until his test is normal again—assuming, of course, it is abnormal."

Turning to Jimmy, I said, "Unless you want to take pills for the rest of your life, find some green vegetable you can stand. Eating that regularly would be even better than pills. Deep green, leafy vegetables are best."

"You said green vegetables are nearly the only source," Mrs. Robinson observed. "What's another source?"

"The normal bacteria that live in all of our intestines make vitamin K, which is absorbed into our systems. Unfortunately, these bacteria are altered or eliminated, and replaced by other kinds, in people who've taken antibiotics. Even poor diet can eliminate some of these friendly bacteria."

"I read about that. Of course, Jimmy's had penicillin from time to time. I was going to give him those *Lactobacillus acidophilus* bacteria I read about, but just forgot."

"It's hard to say if that's a factor in Jimmy's case. Not eating green vegetables is probably more important. It won't hurt to give him *acidophilus*, though, or homemade yogurt."

Jimmy's protime test came back low, at 57 percent. He took his chlorophyll capsules and learned to eat turnip greens ("of all things," said Mrs. Robinson). His test came up to 100 percent six weeks later. As is usual in cases like his, he's had no nosebleeds since.

Vitamin K: Not Well Understood

Vitamin K is one of the least well known nutrients. Most vitamin K research centers on its role in blood coagulation, where it's involved in the formation of several blood-clotting factors. While there are other roles beginning to be unraveled for vitamin K, research on them is quite sketchy.

Vitamin K, except for one minor form, is fat-soluble. That's why the recommendation above was for fat-soluble chlorophyll capsules, as the water-soluble form is not likely to be very useful.

While there are very numerous reference works on the role of vitamin K in blood coagulation, there are no specific references to the use of vitamin K for spontaneous (not caused by injury) nosebleeds in children. So how do I know it works?

Once again, observation of many cases. The development of this treatment was fairly straight forward. After finding no obvious cause in one child with particularly bothersome nosebleeds, and having had him checked out by an ear, nose, and throat specialist, I decided to have a few blood-clotting tests done, just to be sure. To my surprise, a protime test came back at less than 100 percent of normal. While this frequently indicates liver disease, I didn't think this youngster had that problem, so I decided to ask questions about the various sources of vitamin K in his diet.

It turned out he'd had several prescriptions for antibiotics in the previous few years and had not been given replacement *Lactobacillus acidophilus* to return his bowel bacteria to normal, as should always be done. That deprived him of one source of vitamin K.

Just like Jimmy Robinson, he hated green vegetables. His mother couldn't get him to eat any. Even though there are minor amounts of vitamin K in a few other scattered foods, green, leafy vegetables are the best source.

Just to make sure this was what the problem was, I had him given an injection of pure vitamin K, and nothing else.

The nosebleeds stopped.

So, for about two years afterward, when a green-vegetable-hating child (or even a few others) with otherwise unexplained nosebleeds came in, I'd ask to have a protime run. The majority were returned by the laboratory with values of less than 100 percent. I no longer recommend injection of vitamin K, as I'd rather have the naturally derived form along with its associated cofactors.

Except in children with absorptive problems, it worked. I usually recommend stopping supplements when the protime reaches 100 percent, and relying on green vegetables instead. There's been no toxicity.

Most recently, I've omitted doing the blood test altogether, when the case history indicates a strong possibility of vitamin K deficiency. A trial of natural-source vitamin K usually takes care of the problem.

A 9-year-old girl is in good health except for "growing pains" in her leg muscles. While some people regard these pains as normal, they aren't. A major cause appears to be a lack of vitamin E, and in this case, supplements lead to rapid improvement.

36   A Case of 'Growing Pains'

Amy Parsons' mother had brought her in for a routine checkup. As her mother said, she was generally very healthy. She'd not been back to the hospital since she was born. She was 9 now. She'd only been to see doctors for well-baby checks, immunizations, a case or two of flu and one episode of tonsillitis. She hadn't been ill at all for the last year and a half.

"The main reason I brought her in was because we've been getting interested in nutrition. I wanted to know what kind of vitamins and minerals I should give Amy, if she really needs any," her mother said.

"What does Amy usually eat?" I asked.

"I knew you'd ask that, so I wrote it down," her mother said. "I know it's not as good as it should be, but that's why I'm here."

The piece of paper read:

Breakfast: dry cereal, milk, toast, juice

Lunch: school lunch

Dinner: meat, potatoes, two vegetables, bread, milk, sometimes desserts

Snacks: fruit, milk, cookies

"What kind of cereal?"

"From the supermarket. Usually any kind that's on TV."

"Bread?"

"White, usually. But we're starting to switch to whole-grain."

"Does your school lunch program make a special effort to use nutritious foods? Or is it the usual refined-starch type?"

"I'm afraid so. The PTA is starting to work on that, though."

"At night, what vegetables do you have?"

"I try to use a variety: peas, beans, corn, spinach, broccoli, cauliflower, beets, squash."

"Any raw vegetables?"

"No, I always cook them."

"Does Amy eat vegetables?"

"Oh, yes, she's very good about that."

"I think that's all the questions for now. I'd like you to take her to the examination room for her checkup. Before you do, can you think of any other problems she's had, anything else that has to do with her health?"

"No."

"Mom," Amy said, "my leg aches."

"Those are just 'growing pains,' Amy. I had them myself when I was your age. Lots of children have them."

I'd started to get up, but with this, decided to wait another minute or two. "Please tell me about these 'growing pains,'" I said.

Amy's mother looked puzzled. "Well, she gets pains in her leg muscles on and off. They seem to happen more in the evening and at night, but they can happen anytime. Usually, they're not too bad, but once in a while, one really hurts."

"How often does she get them?"

"Sometimes two or three times a week, sometimes once a month. They do seem more frequent when she has a growth spurt or when she's been running around a lot. But they happen when she's not exercising, too."

"Has she had them long?"

"Since she was 5. But I didn't think to mention it, because I thought 'growing pains' were normal. Aren't they? I had them. Our doctor in Wyoming said lots of children had them, and not to worry because she'd grow out of them."

"It's true lots of children have them, but they're really not normal. It's usually a vitamin lack. But don't worry, it's not a serious illness, and is very correctable. But I'd rather go over this when I give you an overall group of suggestions for Amy. Now, let's go to the exam room."

Amy's height was four-foot-four; her weight, 63½ pounds, quite satisfactory for her age. Her overall examination was also normal, with the exception of slightly dry skin. "She's always had that," her mother said. In particular, there appeared to be nothing the matter with her leg muscles. This was no surprise; children with growing pains don't show physical abnormalities of the muscles.

I asked that Amy get a blood count, a urinalysis, and a mineral analysis using a specimen of hair.

"When do we go over Amy's program?" her mother asked.

"We're collecting data this time," I replied. "Even though her examination and history taking are done, we won't have all the laboratory work back for a week or two.

"Besides, it takes more than a minute or two to go over a program, so please schedule a return appointment with the receptionist."

Amy and her mother returned two weeks later. We sat down in my office to go over her results.

"Amy, I think you should know that a large part of staying healthy depends on the kinds of food you eat. You haven't been really sick for a long time, but you have had leg pains, haven't you?"

"Yes."

"They're not really 'growing pains.' They're pains that usually happen when children don't get enough vitamin E. Have you ever heard of vitamin E?"

"No."

"Vitamin E in food is found particularly in whole grains, like whole wheat bread or other whole grains: rye, oats, barley. There's also a lot of vitamin E in nuts and seeds."

"So if I eat lots of those my growing pains will go away?"

"Yes. Also, it'll be faster if you take some vitamin E capsules or pills, to make up for what you missed. I'm telling you this because it's *your* legs, and *your* pains, so you should start to take care of them yourself."

Amy thought for a minute. "OK."

Turning back to her mother, I said, "She should have 200 units of vitamin E daily until the pains are gone. Usually, there are no improvements for the first two weeks. After that, the pains gradually fade away."

"Does vitamin E always take care of 'growing pains'?"

"Almost always. Occasionally, a mineral or two has to be added. Also, once the pains go, try to cut the vitamin E down to 50 units daily. If they don't return, stay at that level."

"You mean she'll need to keep taking vitamin E? Why's that?"

"Vitamin E is one of the most important nutritional protections against a variety of pollutants and toxins. Since we're all exposed to them, I usually recommend extra."

"What else should she take?"

"Before we talk about that, it's more important to go over the basics of good diet—the everyday food. Since you're here, you're probably aware of most of this, but I want to reemphasize it, and of course, make it suitable for Amy.

"If she likes cereal for breakfast, please make sure it's free of refined sugar. A little honey is OK. Toast should be whole-grain, and juice, unsweetened.

"Until the school changes to a more nutritious lunch program, Amy really should take a lunch. Otherwise, there's hardly any way to get optimum nutrition. At dinner, try to serve as many fresh, raw vegetables as possible. Desserts should be sugar-free. For snacks, give her fruit, nuts, and seeds instead of cookies or crackers. If you do make cookies, find a recipe for whole-grain with honey and seeds or raisins.

"Now, about other supplements. For children, besides vitamin E, I always recommend vitamin C, from 10 to 20 milligrams per pound of body weight. Girls seem to need less than boys, and Amy's been healthy, so let's stick to the lower number. Let's see—that's ten times 63½—635, or to make it easier, 600 milligrams daily. That should be 300 milligrams twice daily."

"Why the extra vitamin C?"

"There are so many good reasons it would take an hour to go over them. However, it's all summarized in an excellent book, *The Healing Factor: "Vitamin C" Against Disease* by Irwin Stone. This is a basic book on good health I recommend to everyone."

"Anything else?"

"Let's look at her mineral analysis."

This showed Amy to be low in selenium, chromium, and manganese. Several others were "low-normal."

"Selenium could be particularly important for Amy as it's very frequently a cofactor with vitamin E." I asked Amy's mother to obtain specific mineral supplements for each of her deficiencies, and to redo the mineral analysis in six months, to see if things were normal.

"What about those low-normal ones?" she asked.

"Remember, the most important thing is an optimum-quality daily diet. Supplements are secondary to this. I expect those low-normals will rise as you make dietary improvements."

Amy's mineral analysis did return to normal by the six-month recheck. Amy's mother had by then changed the entire family to an optimum-nutrition program. Amy had taken her extra vitamin E "almost on her own," her mother said, and her "growing pains" were completely gone, as they are for most children, within a month.

Amy Parsons was actually rather fortunate. Despite a relatively refined and processed diet, she showed no obvious physical signs of poor nutrition. Luckily for her, her mother had become convinced of the desirability of switching her family to a natural-food diet, to help keep everyone healthy.

As can be seen, Amy's diet was relatively low on vitamin E. Since the best sources are whole grains, nuts, seeds, and their oils, she wasn't getting much.

However, this wasn't the source of the clue that vitamin E might help stop "growing pains." Since these pains frequently appear to be nothing more than spasms in the leg muscles, using vitamin E for them is simply a logical extension of the work of Drs. Ayres and Mihan on adult leg cramps. Why vitamin E works isn't at all clear, but it usually does.

In the small minority of failures, I usually suggest calcium, magnesium, or potassium, or rarely, folic acid. By the time we get to the end of that list, there usually isn't a "growing pain" left.

As "growing pains" is really a rather ill-defined, vague term referring to pains occurring in children's legs, with no observable physical abnormalities, there's been no formal study of them, as far as I'm aware.

FURTHER READING

Ayres, Samuel, Jr., and Mihan, Richard. " 'Restless Legs' Syndrome: Response to Vitamin E." *Journal of Applied Nutrition,* vol. 25, no. 3 & 4, Fall 1973, pp. 8-15.

Stone, Irwin. *The Healing Factor: "Vitamin C" Against Disease* (New York: Grosset & Dunlap, 1972).

A chronic low back pain problem, associated with beginning disk degeneration, reaches the critical stage with extremely painful sciatica. Neither drugs nor chiropractic help relieve the pain. The patient is given injections of vitamins B_1 and B_{12} and relief comes quickly. When large doses of vitamin C are added to his program, the underlying back problem also improves.

37   A Case of Sciatica

Herbert Porterfield limped past the reception desk on his way down the hall to my office. As he was obviously in considerable pain, I motioned for him to go into one of the closer examination rooms. Mrs. Porterfield came in with him, and I followed.

"My chiropractor sent me over," Mr. Porterfield said. "He says you might be able to help me with this blasted sciatica. He's given me some help with adjustments for low back pain, but he can't get this to go. I've been off work three weeks now."

As this was the first time I'd met Mr. Porterfield, I thought I'd better get some background.

"Is this the first time you've had this pain?"

"Oh, no," Mrs. Porterfield answered. "Herbert's had it on and off since 1968. He was in a bad auto accident then, and he's had back trouble ever since. This is the worst it's been, though."

"If it's been since 1968, you must have had x-rays and other examinations of your back."

"Oh, yes," Mrs. Porterfield answered again. "He's seen general doctors, and orthopedic and neurologic specialists. A year

ago, the last orthopedic surgeon said he had beginning disk deterioration, and that he could have back surgery when it got bad
enough."

"But that isn't the main problem, Mabel," Mr. Porterfield
said. "Sure, my spine hurts some. But I can stand that. It's this
sciatica. That hurts worse than anything."

"Yes," Mrs. Porterfield resumed. "All the doctors did for
Herbert's sciatica was give him pain pills and muscle relaxers, and
those never did much good. What helped the most seemed to be
just resting. Can you do anything for it?"

"First, I'd like to check Mr. Porterfield to see what the problem is. I know you've been told before it's sciatica, but I'd like to
check myself."

"Of course," Mrs. Porterfield replied. "Herbert. . . ."

"I know," he said. He unfastened his belt and slid down his
slacks.

There was acute tenderness from an area approximately 3
inches to the left of Mr. Porterfield's lower spine, down through
the left buttock and into the back of his thigh. It followed the
course of the sciatic nerve exactly. Mr. Porterfield winced each
time I applied pressure over the nerve. It was fairly typical for
sciatica.

"What is sciatica, anyway?" Mrs. Porterfield asked.

"It just means pain in the sciatic nerve," I replied. "It's probably associated with inflammation of the nerve, but the exact
cause isn't known. It frequently happens after injuries to the area,
as Mr. Porterfield's has; but occasionally it occurs with no known
injury."

"Why does it keep happening this long after my accident?"
Mr. Porterfield asked.

"I really don't know. I don't know if anyone does."

"Can you do anything for it? I've already got pain pills, but I
don't like to take those unless I have to. They make me feel all
doped up."

"There is a treatment which usually will take the pain away.
I don't know why it works; I don't have any research papers
about it. It's a fairly 'traditional' remedy, and usually will settle

sciatica pain right down. It sometimes works on other nerve inflammation, too. But you'll have to learn how to give injections at home, because a shot a day is required to start."

"It's not cortisone, is it?" Mrs. Porterfield asked. "A doctor suggested that for Herbert's back pain once, but he wouldn't take it."

"No, not cortisone. It's a combination of vitamin B_{12} and vitamin B_1: 1,000 micrograms of B_{12}, 50 milligrams of B_1, injected once daily."

"Is there any danger to it?"

"None that I know about. There's a remote possibility of danger from vitamin B_1 intravenously. But this injection goes into the muscle."

"I'm not sure I can learn to give a shot," Mrs. Porterfield said.

"Well, if you can't, I will," her husband replied. "We're not driving all the way over here just for a shot if we don't have to."

"How long does it take to work?"

"Usually after the first or second injection. The pain sometimes doesn't clear up completely for a week or two. And occasionally, it doesn't work at all."

"I hope it works for me. Can I take pain pills with it?"

"Yes. They won't interfere."

"I won't take them unless I have to."

"I'll send the nurse in to show you how to give the injection. Please check back in a week, or sooner if things get worse."

When Mr. Porterfield returned, he still had his limp, but it was considerably less. I had him go to the examination room once again.

"It's not gone, but it's a whole lot better," he said.

"He got about halfway relieved with the first injection," Mrs. Porterfield observed. "It's been a little less with each shot since then."

"She's getting real good with that needle. I think she likes it," Mr. Porterfield grumped. "Can't I stop taking the shots now, and let the rest of it just go away?"

"You could . . . and it might . . . but many times the pain flares up again."

"Don't want that."

I checked Mr. Porterfield's back and leg again. The tenderness was definitely less. "That's a fairly good response. I'd like you to come back in another week. And could you borrow your last set of x-rays from your chiropractor, so I could look at them?"

"Dr. Matthews said he'd be glad to send them over anytime," Mr. Porterfield said. "I'll be sure to bring them along."

The following week, Mr. Porterfield was carrying a large x-ray folder. "These are from Dr. Matthews," he said.

This time, he wasn't limping. "Looks like you're better," I observed.

"Oh, much better," Mrs. Porterfield said. "He's back to his grouchy old self."

"The sciatica pain is completely gone. Now, all I have is my average, everyday, low back pain."

"That must have been quite an accident you were in. Did you break any bones?"

"No, the doctor said I had a really bad back sprain, but no fractures. He said I should use heat, back exercises, and pain pills. I had much worse pain than this in my spine, but I was supposed to learn to live with it. I just put up with it for three years, until I went to Dr. Matthews. He's relieved a lot of the pain, but there's some aching all the time."

I took the x-rays out to look them over. As Mr. Porterfield had reported on his first visit, there was evidence of beginning disk deterioration. I could find no other medical problems.

"Have you tried taking any vitamin C for your back pain?" I asked.

"Vitamin C? For back pain? I thought that was for colds."

"It's for that, too. It also helps in many cases of back pain from slight disk deterioration. Dr. James Greenwood, a neurosurgeon from Houston, Texas, discovered that it helped many of his patients. Your x-ray doesn't look extremely bad. It might work for you."

"But I already take 6 vitamin C pills a day. That doesn't help."

"What dose are they?"

"One hundred milligrams."

"Frequently, the required amount is 2,000 to 3,000 milligrams daily."

"I told you you should take more, Herbert," Mrs. Porterfield remarked.

"I'm not swallowing 30 pills a day," Mr. Porterfield announced.

"You can obtain 500 or 1,000 milligram tablets. You can also get vitamin C in a powder," I pointed out. "If that could be more convenient, why not try it?"

"What does vitamin C do for back pain?" Mrs. Porterfield asked.

"I'm not sure of that, either," I answered. "Vitamin C is a construction material required to mobilize and build collagen—a protein substance responsible for holding the disks together. Perhaps replacing the vitamin C slows down or stops the deterioration; I can't find any further information. I've watched it work enough times to recommend it, though, whatever the reason."

"If it takes away this constant ache, that's enough for me," Mr. Porterfield declared. "I'll try it."

"I've been telling him for years," Mrs. Porterfield complained. "He wouldn't listen to me."

I didn't see Mr. Porterfield again for several months, when he came in with an unrelated problem. I asked him how his back pain was.

"The sciatica never came back," he reported. "That's the first time it's been gone this long since the accident. My lower spine pain doesn't bother me any at all. Two weeks after I started that extra vitamin C, it went away and hasn't been back. Between that, and a little help from Dr. Matthews now and then, I've been pain-free for the first time since 1968."

Mrs. Porterfield, who was with him as usual, couldn't help but observe, "He's been less grouchy than he's been since 1967, too."

———

As in any other professional area, there are many biochemical treatments that "just seem to work," even though the reasons are totally unknown. This case illustrates two such treatments. I have no idea why the combination of vitamin B_{12} and B_1, injected, is frequently so successful in eliminating or at least holding down the pain in cases of sciatica or other peripheral neuritis. But it's certainly not original with me. I learned it from another, more experienced practitioner, who couldn't remember where he'd learned it, either. However, it's a harmless treatment, except for the risk following an injection of anything.

While "degenerating disks" and sciatica are much more common in older age groups, they're not unheard of in younger persons. My recommended treatment would be much the same.

Strengthening exercises are helpful also, once the pain is under control. When a patient has an osteopathic, chiropractic, or orthopedic physician also involved in the treatment, I usually defer to that practitioner for exercise instructions. If not, I usually recommend a gradually increasing exercise series such as the Royal Canadian Air Force program.

At this point, I'd like to take advantage of the role of large doses of vitamin C in helping back problems to briefly discuss natural versus synthetic vitamins.

In almost all circumstances, natural vitamins are preferable to synthetic. Vitamin C is at once the only exception to, and a good (but partial) example of the natural vitamin rule. Let's go over its conformity to that rule before covering the "exception."

Any vitamin, mineral, or other nutritional substance never works all by itself. The B complex vitamins are good examples of this; usually when one B vitamin is needed others are necessary to help it. The connection between essential fatty acids and zinc is another; zinc is necessary to complete a key step in transforming essential fatty acids into one of their active forms in the body.

It shouldn't come as a surprise to anyone familiar with what's known as "nature's economy of design" that if nutrients are found together in the human body, they're usually found together in nature. Thus, the entire B complex is in brewer's yeast or wheat germ; zinc and essential fatty acids are in pumpkin and other seeds.

Now a truly naturally derived preparation of any nutrient is likely to carry along with the "main item" other associated nutritional cofactors. To return to vitamin C as an example, most natural forms of vitamin C include varying amounts of the bioflavonoids, hesperidin being one of the most active. These bioflavonoid factors (jointly named "vitamin P" by their discoverer, Albert Szent-Gyorgyi, Ph.D., M.D.) work together in man and other living systems.

So, whenever possible, naturally derived vitamins are preferable, as they're more likely to contain more of the nutritional package surrounding each nutrient; more of its cofactors.

Having said this, we should proceed to the exceptions, the main one being vitamin C. As you might expect, the principal use for synthetic vitamins is in therapeutics (treatment of illness or its symptoms) where the natural forms are simply not strong enough to do the job in time. Many nutrients are used in "stronger-than-found-in-nature" dosages in nutritional/biochemical medicine. Of course, whenever possible, we try to discontinue these supplements after a period of time.

Vitamin C is the most outstanding example of this, but mostly because of its unique involvement as a "missing product" of our faulty human genetics (see chapter 33, "A Case of Hepatitis"). The important point in therapeutic use of ascorbic acid is that, if our bodies could produce ascorbic acid, they would do so in large quantities under disease stress, but would not produce any rutin, hesperidin, or other members of the bioflavonoid complex, just ascorbic acid itself.

So in the therapeutic uses, particularly involving doses higher than 3 grams (3,000 milligrams), the bioflavonoid factors are not necessary in equivalently excess amounts to help the ascorbic acid work. A small amount is important, and probably vital, but very large amounts are not. The ascorbic acid can be given by itself, and will work fine.

Other single nutrients are frequently used in very large amounts by themselves in nutritional/biochemical therapeutics, but not for the same reasons as ascorbic acid.

FURTHER READING

Greenwood, James, Jr. "Optimum Vitamin C Intake as a

Factor in the Preservation of Disc Integrity." *Medical Annals of the District of Columbia*, vol. 33, no. 6, 1964, pp. 274-76.

————. "On Vitamin C in the Prevention and Treatment of Back Pain." *Executive Health*, vol. 10, no. 12, 1972.

A man in his fifties is suffering from constipation, bleeding hemorrhoids, tiredness, and an extremely powerful body odor. After tests rule out serious physical causes, dietary investigation suggests that a deficiency of magnesium could be at the root of his problems. Eating greens and taking dolomite supplements are chief among the recommendations that bring about great improvement.

38 A Case of Severe Body Odor

It's rare, but occasionally a major source of a person's health problems is instantaneously apparent, even before words are exchanged. This was the case with George Howard. As he entered my office, I became fairly confident of at least one major nutritional problem. But this gets a little ahead of things, so let's go back and follow Mr. Howard's problem through.

Mr. Howard was in his early fifties and worked as a logger. As he said, he'd been "generally pretty healthy" most of his life, but lately had developed some minor problems. He wanted them checked just to make sure nothing major developed.

"The thing that concerns me the most is bleeding with bowel movements," Mr. Howard said. "I've never had that before. It started every once in a while two or three months ago, but for the last two weeks it's been every day. It hurts, too."

"Has the blood been bright red or dark?" I asked.

"Bright red."

"Much?"

"No. At the most, a teaspoon."

"Have you been constipated?"

"Depends on what you mean. I go every day, but it's been very hard."

I asked Mr. Howard about changes in his bowel movements that might indicate more serious problems, such as notable changes in size or shape, or lots of mucus, but none of this had happened. Also, he'd had no recent weight loss.

"It doesn't sound extremely serious," I said. "Of course, the cause should still be found. We'll start to check. But do you have other symptoms, too?"

"Yes. Another thing is, I haven't had the energy I feel I should. Nothing specific, but just overall tired."

"Have you ever been anemic?"

"No."

"Getting enough sleep?"

"Eight to nine hours a night."

"What else have you noticed?"

"Well, it's weird. I've worked in the woods for 30 years, and I always bang myself a little here and there. But in the last six months, I've started to bruise if I even touch myself, practically. The other night, I counted 16 bruises on just my legs. Look!" Rolling up a pants leg, Mr. Howard showed me several bruises in varying sizes and shades of blue, black, and yellow.

He continued, "My wife thought maybe vitamin C would help. So I've taken 3,000 milligrams a day, but it didn't work very well. It only got a little better."

"Anything else?"

"I've been having more muscle cramps than I usually do." He paused for several seconds. "Well, there is one other thing I'd better mention. I'm not sure if you can do anything about it. I've had a terrific case of body odor for months now. I'm a logger, and always work up a good sweat, but it's not just that. Even on weekends I could take six showers a day, and it wouldn't help. Half an hour after a shower, it's back again. I use deodorant soap and underarm deodorant. Nothing helps. My wife says she's never noticed anything like this in the 22 years we've been married. She was even threatening to move to another room, but now she's wondering if she's developing the same problem. I think she is."

Mr. Howard looked a little embarrassed, but relieved at the same time.

"I know that's not a major problem," Mr. Howard said. "But I promised my wife I'd mention it."

"Actually, it may have a lot to do with everything you've mentioned so far," I replied. As Mr. Howard looked surprised, I assured him I'd explain it as we went along.

Of course, this symptom, the "terrific case of body odor," is the "instantaneously apparent" nutritional problem I mentioned at the beginning. It had enough of a characteristic smell that the solution to the problem was apparent right along with the problem itself.

"Can you tell me what you've been eating every day?" I asked.

"Just regular meals," Mr. Howard replied. "Nothing different. I didn't think that could do it, as I haven't made any big changes."

"All the same, go through a typical day's food."

"Well, for breakfast I have eggs and pancakes. My wife always uses whole-grain flour, too, since she's been coming here. Coffee, but not sugar. Just honey, and on my pancakes, too.

"Lunch is two or three sandwiches; lunch meat or tuna fish, and mayonnaise. I drink a thermos of milk and one of coffee. Usually an apple or an orange.

"When I get home, I have two or three beers," Mr. Howard smiled. "My wife gets after me about that, but I tell her it's more nutritional than hard liquor. I never touch that stuff.

"For dinner, I have steak or roast with lots of potatoes and gravy. Sometimes applesauce. No bread. I always have coffee."

"What about vegetables?"

"Oh, yeah. Usually corn or beans."

"No green, leafy vegetables?"

"I can't stand those. Never have been able to. The only ones I usually eat are what Mrs. Howard grows in her garden, and what she puts up for the winter.

"Come to think of it, I haven't had greens at all for nearly a year now, except a few times. You know how wet and rainy it was last summer, just like a regular Washington State winter. Well, the slugs just went wild over at our place, ate our whole garden before it ever got started."

He paused for a minute. "I never thought about that. I guess because I don't like green vegetables, anyway. You think that could have something to do with my problems? Which ones?"

"I hope it's that simple. First let's check that bleeding to see where it's coming from."

Examination showed a problem with internal hemorrhoids, which were irritated and bleeding. No other abnormalities were found.

"I'm sure glad to hear that's all it is," Mr. Howard said. "It had me worried. I'm still a little concerned about cancer, though. Did you check for that?"

"Only in the area of the hemorrhoids. They're definitely bad enough to account for the bleeding. To check further for cancer, you should have x-rays done."

So barium examinations of both the upper and lower gastrointestinal tract were planned. I asked Mr. Howard to return after they were done. A few days later Mr. Howard was back, this time with his wife.

"How were the x-rays?" he asked.

"The radiologist says they were completely normal," I reported. "No sign of any cancer. Remember, though, that's what we expected. The x-rays were just to make sure."

"I told my wife what you said about greens," Mr. Howard said. "But we both want to hear about how it relates to all my symptoms, especially that body odor."

"I'm afraid I'm starting to get that a little, too, doctor," Mrs. Howard said. "We thought maybe we were getting immune to deodorants. We even changed brands several times; it didn't help."

"I'm not surprised," I said. "Most bad odor problems are from inside out, not just surface. But let's start with the hemorrhoids, and go through all Mr. Howard's symptoms one at a time.

"Even though you are eating whole-grain bread, it's obviously not providing enough roughage, so you've gotten constipated. This is one of many things that can lead to hemorrhoids, and even make them bleed.

"Taking vitamin C to stop bruising was a good idea, even though in your case, it didn't work. Unfortunately, a lack of vitamin K can also lead to easy bruising. There's lots of vitamin K in green, leafy vegetables, especially fresh ones.

"Remember you mentioned muscle cramps? A lack of calcium or potassium, or a need for more vitamin E can all lead to this. There's another mineral, though, sometimes associated with muscle cramps: magnesium. Green, leafy vegetables are an important source of magnesium."

"How does that cause muscle cramps?"

"I'm not sure. But it is known that unless there's enough magnesium in a person's system, calcium and potassium aren't properly regulated. I am sure this has something to do with it."

"Is that all?"

"No. The same lack of magnesium is probably the cause of Mr. Howard's problem with body odor."

"That's why I'm getting that problem, too," Mrs. Howard said. "I've been eating some greens from the store, not nearly as many as I usually do, since our garden didn't do well this year."

"It sounds like you both could use some magnesium," I said. "I've found a lack of magnesium to be the first thing to look for when someone's having a problem with body odor.

"Last, Mr. Howard mentioned not having as much energy as he'd like. We'll have to wait to see, but I'm sure this is related to not enough magnesium, too."

"Let me see if I have this straight," Mr. Howard said. "You said my hemorrhoids were because of not enough roughage since I didn't eat green, leafy vegetables. I'm bruising because of not enough vitamin K from green, leafy vegetables. My muscles cramp, I smell bad, and I don't have enough energy because of not enough magnesium from green vegetables. Are you sure?"

"It all fits," I said. "But, of course, you can be tested for it. Let's do blood tests for vitamin K and magnesium, and a hair mineral test for magnesium. OK?"

"Sure," Mr. Howard said. "But it all sounds logical enough. I just want to be certain."

He turned to his wife. "Well, dear, which way to the turnip greens?"

Turning back, he said, "Seriously, won't just eating green, leafy vegetables take a long time to work? It took me a long time to get this way. We'd both like to get over smelling bad as quickly as possible. We haven't been going anywhere because of this."

"Green, leafy vegetables every day are the best," I said. "But other things will help speed you along.

"First, get chlorophyll capsules. These contain the nutrients we're particularly looking for—vitamin K and magnesium—in concentrated but still organically combined form. Of course, they contain other things, too. And the 'bulk' is missing. But they'll still help a lot.

"Second, to stop the bruising more quickly, I've written a prescription for vitamin K. This is synthetic, but it's not known to be harmful. It will stop your bruising quickly until the other form works.

"Also, I'd like you to use dolomite tablets—a naturally balanced form of calcium and magnesium."

"Aren't those inorganic, though?" Mrs. Howard asked. "I've heard that inorganic doesn't work as well."

"They seem to be inorganic, but actually dolomite is composed of the remains of microscopic sea animals that lived ages ago. And they do work well in helping to take away odor more quickly. I've found they do so in nearly all cases."

Mr. Howard took his list of remedies: green, leafy vegetables, chlorophyll capsules, vitamin K, and dolomite. Then he went to have his tests done. I asked him to return in two or three months.

It was 90 days before I saw Mr. Howard again.

"Sorry I didn't come back sooner. It was all working steadily but slowly. So I thought I'd wait until I was cleared up and then come back to let you know."

"It's all gone?"

"All but a last little bit of body odor. It's nothing like it was, at all."

It was certainly true. I could no longer tell what Mr. Howard's problem was, as I could when he'd come into my office for his first visit.

"My bruising went away in ten days. The muscle cramps

took about two weeks. Those hemorrhoids took a whole month. I started to get my energy back in three weeks. My wife says I'm livable again without six showers a day. I guess you were right."

He thought for a few seconds. "I suppose it's a little silly, but I'm still curious. How did those tests turn out?"

"Your blood test was just borderline for low magnesium. Your hair test was definitely low, though. That's not unusual. Blood tests are usually not good indicators of total body mineral content. Your vitamin K test (called 'protime') was only 58 percent of normal. No wonder you were bruising."

Additional Notes on Magnesium Deficiency

Many textbooks claim that magnesium deficiency is very rare. I'll agree it isn't common, but it isn't rare, either. As with many other things, it isn't found unless looked for. I've seen numerous lab slips on my patients reporting below-normal serum magnesium levels. If we include hair tests of magnesium levels, which are to a degree representative of total body magnesium storage, there are more than just a few persons who could use more magnesium. Most of these people are not as symptomatic as Mr. Howard.

Another area where magnesium is clinically important is in cardiovascular disease. Reports from South Africa and Germany indicate that it's useful in treating angina pectoris and lowering cholesterol levels as well as improving blood vessel elasticity. American researchers have found magnesium helpful in treating irregular heartbeat after heart attacks. I've found it helpful in some cases of heartbeat irregularity even if there hasn't been a heart attack.

Another function of magnesium described in all textbooks is a "controlling" action in calcium and potassium metabolism. Frequently, if calcium deficiency or potassium deficiency just won't improve by taking calcium or potassium, even in large quantities, the problem is magnesium deficiency. Once magnesium deficiency is corrected, the calcium or potassium problem normalizes easily.

Returning to Mr. Howard, his neglect of green vegetables

produced signs and symptoms of deficiency in magnesium, vitamin K, and food fiber or "bulk." Other deficiencies that *might* have occurred could include folic acid, vitamin A, or other nutrients. Given biochemical individuality, another individual following Mr. Howard's dietary pattern might have developed an entirely different pattern of nutritional problems, emphasizing the effects of other vitamin/mineral deficiencies.

Magnesium has a very distinct effect on body odors; I'll usually ask a person to try this first, even if the odor isn't "specific." However, another mineral, zinc, is helpful in body odor problems, too. If magnesium doesn't work, or only helps a little, zinc is the next thing to try. Naturally, it's important to look for other signs of zinc lack, too, such as white spots on fingernails, to indicate whether zinc might be helpful.

FURTHER READING

Iseri, Lloyd; Freed, James; and Bures, Alan R. "Magnesium Deficiency and Cardiac Disorders." *The American Journal of Medicine,* vol. 58, June 1975, pp. 837–46.

Malkiel-Shapiro, B. "Further Observations on Parenteral Magnesium Sulphate Therapy in Coronary Heart Disease: A Clinical Appraisal." *South African Medical Journal,* vol. 32, no. 51, December 20, 1958, pp. 1211–15.

Nieper, Hans A. "Capillarographic Criteria on the Effect of Magnesium Orotate, EPL Substances and Clofibrate on the Elasticity of Blood Vessels." *Agressologie,* vol. 15, no. 1, 1974, pp. 73–76.

———. "Mineral Transporters." *New Dynamics of Preventive Medicine,* edited by Leon Pomeroy (Miami: Symposia Specialists, 1974), pp. 43–54.

Parsons, R. S.; Butler, T.; and Sellars, E. P. "The Treatment of Coronary Artery Disease with Parenteral Magnesium Sulphate." *Medical Proceedings,* November 14, 1959, pp. 487–98.

Seelig, Mildred S., and Haddy, Francis J. "Effects of Magnesium Deficiency on Arteries, and on the Retention of Sodium, Potassium, and Calcium." Second International Symposium on Magnesium, University of Montreal, Quebec, Canada, 1976.

The patient, a professor, has very low energy levels, even though he exercises daily and follows a good diet. He has undergone extensive testing to discover the cause of his problem and has read widely on health, all to no avail. Further tests reveal nothing. Finally, the suggestion is made to try B_{12} injections, which the patient believes— along with many doctors—are quite unscientific. Perhaps they are, but the patient is no longer tired. With a special discussion of "Science—Helper or Ruler?"

39 A Case of Unexplained Tiredness

Harvey Constantine was an associate professor at a local university. He came in for his appointment armed with an impressive array of facts, figures, and statistics.

"I've been to the ———— Clinic," he said, naming a major local referral center. "I've had chest x-rays, lower and upper GI x-rays, sigmoidoscopy, blood counts, urinalysis, and everything else they could think of. I saw seven different specialists including a psychiatrist. They all agreed there was nothing wrong with me. I've got all the results right here." He put a small stack of photocopies on my desk.

"You haven't told me what the problem is yet," I said.

"Tired a lot. I don't mean sleepy, just not enough energy. I get enough sleep, I exercise, and I eat right. The doctors at the clinic thought I was a health food nut, but I didn't mind. After all those tests were negative, they thought I was depressed and should see a psychiatrist; at that point, I thought it might be a good idea, so I agreed. But he says I'm not depressed and I'm sure I'm not. After I'd been through all that, someone offered me a prescription for pep pills, but I won't take them. I've read all the studies on side effects."

"Tell me about your diet and exercise programs."

"I run a mile every day. I've read everything on good nutrition. I don't eat sugar, or white flour, or much meat. Most of my vegetables are uncooked. My snacks are sunflower seeds, raisins, and pumpkin seeds. I eat lots of fresh fruit."

"That certainly is a good program."

"I know. I've read all I can on good nutrition." He paused. "I insisted they give me a six-hour glucose tolerance test, but I don't have hypoglycemia. I checked the numbers myself, because I know they don't believe in low blood sugar. But they were normal.

"I'm not anemic. I don't have a weak thyroid. I get outdoors as much as I can. I just can't understand it; I'm still tired. I've got a heavy schedule; I teach sociology and I can't afford to be tired. I've heard you do tests for nutrient absorption. I want those done. I want a hair test, too."

"That sounds reasonable. Let me ask you a few other questions. Do you take any vitamins and minerals?"

"I take them all. A, B, C, D, E, zinc, dolomite, brewer's yeast, multiple minerals, sunflower oil, bone meal, and kelp. I'm still tired."

"How old are you?"

"Forty-four."

"Do you have any digestive symptoms? Gas, constipation, diarrhea?"

"No. And I don't have any other symptoms either."

"As long as you're here, I'd like to check things over."

"My checkup is normal, but you can if you want. I've been thoroughly checked."

"That's so, but it's my policy to check things myself."

However, I could find nothing physically the matter, either. I looked over Mr. Constantine's tests. He was right; they were all normal. As they had been done only two months before, I saw no point in having them done over again.

Since poor absorption of nutrients is frequently a problem

when a person is following a good diet, exercising, sleeping enough, and still not feeling well, I agreed with Mr. Constantine that tests for gastric acidity and pancreatic function should be done, even with a lack of specific symptoms. Since I frequently use hair mineral analysis as a screening test, I agreed this should be done also.

"Sometimes just feeling tired can be a result of chronic low-grade allergy," I said. "Perhaps. . . ."

"Oh, yes, I've read about it. I'm not sure I believe all that, but I did try fasting and pulse testing. I can't say I felt any better or worse. But the ———— Clinic didn't do any allergy tests. I know you have some kind of blood test that's supposed to be good, although I haven't seen as much verification as I'd like. Why don't we check for some of the major allergens, like wheat or milk."

I marked a slip for our usual "screening group." Since neither Mr. Constantine nor I could think of anything more at that point, he left to get his tests done.

Three weeks later he was back about the results.

"I saw on the machine that my radiotelemetry test for gastric acidity was normal," he said. "The nurse said my pancreatic enzyme test was normal, too, and that I didn't show any positive results on the allergy tests. How was my mineral analysis? Let's see," he went on, "I've seen these before. Calcium, magnesium, sodium, potassium. . . ." he mumbled to himself. "All of those are OK; no high levels of toxic minerals. It all looks normal. I've never put much stock in those mineral tests. I've never seen any controlled studies, anyway."

"In the hands of someone who works with them all the time, the mineral analysis can be very useful," I replied. "I find they're invaluable sometimes."

Mr. Constantine didn't answer for a minute. Then he said: "So what do I do now? All the clinic tests are normal. All *your* tests are normal. The psychiatrist says I'm not depressed. *But I'm still tired.*"

He looked almost accusing. "I thought for certain nutrition was the answer."

"No one area of medicine has all the answers. I certainly don't pretend to. There are some people I can't help." I thought for a minute, not sure whether it was worth the argument I anticipated. "Have you thought of trying vitamin B_{12}?"

"I'm disappointed in you, Doctor. Vitamin B_{12} for tiredness? That's just an old country doctor's tale! I thought treatments like that went out with modern scientific nutrition. I've read about that kind of treatment: If you can't find anything the matter, you give them some B_{12} shots, some encouragement, and they feel better. Maybe that was good enough for our grandparents, but today. . . ."

I rarely interrupt patients, but with that it was my turn. "Mr. Constantine, it's been my experience that our grandparents in health care knew many things that modern scientific medicine is just starting to discover. Many of the vitamin and mineral treatments that work extremely well for my patients I learned by studying books and articles written decades ago."

Once I got wound up, I couldn't stop with just that. "Did you realize that the most modern science is in the Dark Ages?" I asked.

"Dark Ages? What do you mean?"

"If you and I are still here, and the world hasn't blown itself up by the year 2050, we could look back at those primitive years of the 1970s as the Dark Ages of medicine. We'd marvel at all the scientific advances since then that have made the best hospitals of those times obsolete. After all, would you want to be admitted to a modern scientific hospital of the 1870s, today?"

"Well. . . ."

"What I'm saying is that we should never think we know it all, in any year. We probably don't come close. . . . And if there's a treatment available that's fairly harmless and has been reported to work by one or more observers, no matter from what year, why not try it? After all, many country doctors are very shrewd judges of health and disease."

"But we might not know if it's safe. . . ."

"That's true. The first rule all medical students are taught is *Primum non nocere*, or, First, do no harm. However, the majority of nutrients are much safer than the majority of drugs. When was the last time you read about a vitamin B_{12} overdose?"

Mr. Constantine admitted he hadn't.

"I've never been able to find a record of one, either." Having unwound my philosophical arguments, and knowing Mr. Constantine's inclinations by now, I went to my filing cabinet.

"Sometimes science does catch up with those grandparents you were talking about," I said. I handed him an article entitled "A Pilot Study of Vitamin B_{12} in the Treatment of Tiredness" by F. R. Ellis and S. Nasser. "We're a little overtime now. Why don't you take a copy of this home, read it, and call the nurse about vitamin B_{12} injections if you'd like?"

I couldn't resist adding, as he left, "I'm sure you'll notice it's a double-blind, cross-over, placebo-controlled study. Very modern science."

I didn't see Mr. Constantine for several months. When he came in, I could see that some things hadn't changed.

"I can't understand it" he said. "I've read as much as I can find on vitamin B_{12} and I still don't know why it worked. I wanted to give it several months to make sure it wasn't just all psychological. But it isn't. As long as I take my vitamin B_{12} shots, I feel fine. If I don't, after two or three weeks I start to run down. It doesn't make any sense."

"What happened?"

"Well, after I read the article, I decided to try it. I decided it couldn't hurt. I took the 3 cubic centimeters—300 micrograms—of vitamin B_{12} 3 times a week for 2 weeks. My tiredness left; I had lots of energy. But after two or three weeks I got tired again. At first I thought I was really crazy, but then I repeated the vitamin B_{12}, felt better, left it off, and got worse again. I finally learned to give my own shots; I'm convinced. But I can't understand why it works; it doesn't make any sense. Why didn't I need it ten years ago?"

"I can't tell you why vitamin B_{12} works that way for some people, even when they have no deficiency. B vitamins function as enzyme helpers in our cells; perhaps some of us have weak enzymes that require more help, especially as we get older. But I really don't know. I do know it won't hurt, so if it helps you out, continue on your own schedule."

"Oh, I will," said Mr. Constantine. "I just feel uncomfortable doing something which I can't explain." He got up to go. "If there were only more research. . . ."

"I'd like to see more research, too," I said. "But by the time all the work that's needed is done, I'm afraid we won't be here for it to help us anymore. So if it doesn't hurt, and it helps, use it, even if it's only an old country doctor's tale!"

Science—Helper or Ruler?

The scientific method—assembling one fact after another, making theories based on observed facts, testing theories, building up a little at a time—is generally held to be responsible for most of the progress in medicine and health care that's occurred in the Western world over the last two to three centuries. Not only progress in medicine, but in most other areas of our lives, is attributed to the discoveries of modern science.

In medicine, perhaps more so than in other scientific disciplines, there is a common tendency to take this helper, the scientific method, and turn it into our *ruler*. What should be treated only as a tool, even though a major one, is instead worshipped as if it were sacred.

Scientifically trained people, especially physicians, repeatedly adopt the attitude that "if it isn't proven according to the methods of science, it isn't so." Mr. Constantine affords an excellent example: even when he experienced the benefits of an "unscientific" treatment, he felt uncomfortable, as they didn't fit his view of a scientifically verified fact. This point of view I call the "scientific ostrich" approach. With head firmly buried in the sand of "scientifically verifiable facts," the "scientific ostrich" not only ignores anything not scientifically proven, but usually also refuses to admit that the possibility might exist.

The "scientific ostrich" description might seem a little extreme or overdrawn. However, having spent several years at various institutions of higher education, I can assure the reader that such institutions, especially medical schools, are full of "scientific ostriches."

There's another approach to health care best represented by one of my favorite medical school professors. To quote from one of his discussions: "I don't care if you do a rain dance around your patient, burning chicken feathers. As long as it doesn't do any harm, and the patient recovers, do it. Your job as a physician is to help all people get well. If you have a scientific explanation for an illness, and a scientific cure, so much the better. If you have no explanation, but can aid recovery through any other means, then do it. You've accomplished your real goal."

Obviously this second approach can be overdone also. If we simply use "whatever works that's handy," to the exclusion of careful scientific study of the whys and wherefores, we'll make very little long-range progress. After all, where were we in health care before the scientific method was brought into use?

The best physicians I know use the scientific approach whenever they can, whenever it has the answers. But when the scientific answers run out, they use anything available that's safe and effective. Their goal is their patients' health, whatever it takes.

Vitamin B_{12} therapy has been in the realm of "unscientific medicine" practically since it was discovered. With the scientific report cited above, its use for tiredness may have "crossed the line" into scientific respectability. It still isn't known why it works; that answer may take decades more.

Vitamin B_{12} therapy also illustrates well the split between academic physicians and practicing physicians. Most medical school staff physicians are inclined towards the purist, "scientific ostrich" approach; the number of professors taking the viewpoint of the professor quoted above is small. Denouncements of vitamin B_{12} and other "unscientific" therapy are common at medical teaching centers.

On the other hand, vitamin B_{12} therapy is in fact used by practicing physicians, who have much more pressure on them from patients every day to help find an answer for their problems, "scientific" or not. Due to embarrassment about being "unscientific," many physicians who use such treatment are reluctant to admit it!

FURTHER READING

Ellis, F. R., and Nasser, S. "A Pilot Study of Vitamin B$_{12}$ in the Treatment of Tiredness." *British Journal of Nutrition,* vol. 30, 1973, pp. 277-83.

Merck & Co., Inc., publisher. *Vitamin B$_{12}$: Merck Service Bulletin* (Rahway, N.J.: Merck & Co., 1958).

Newbold, H. L. "The Use of Vitamin B$_{12}$ in Psychiatric Practice." *Orthomolecular Psychiatry,* vol. 1, no. 1, 1972, pp. 27-36.

We know that changes in light patterns have a profound effect on the germination of plants and the behavior of animals. Is it possible that light can also affect the human reproduction cycle? This case suggests that it is—which would only be one more proof that people are part of, not foreign to, the universe in which we all live.

40 A Deficiency of 'Midnight Moonlight'

There are more things in Heaven and Earth, Horatio, than are dreamt of in your philosophy.
Shakespeare, *Hamlet*, act 1, scene 5

Sarah Worthington appeared very determined. "I know I'm not sick," she said. "I work hard at staying healthy. I eat the right foods, get some exercise . . . and I think my mental health is just fine," she added, a little defensively.

"It's just that my menstrual periods haven't been regular for five years now, and I don't think that's normal. Sometimes when my periods come too early or too close together, I feel more tired or washed out. When they're delayed, I feel more irritable and nervous. The last doctor I saw said I'm just too worried about it, to stop worrying and maybe my periods would get regular again. But I'm sure that's not it; I was under much more stress when I was in college, and my periods were prefectly regular then. I'm sure it's something physical; I even saw a psychiatrist once when my doctor insisted. The psychiatrist talked to me twice, and then sent a letter to my doctor saying there was nothing wrong with me at all mentally; I didn't need to go back."

"Let's go back to the beginning. When did your menstrual periods begin?"

"When I was 13."

"Were they regular then?"

"No. They didn't get regular until I was 16. But all the doctors said not to worry about it then. . . . That's quite usual for young girls just starting."

"That's true. So what happened after you were 16?"

"My periods were regular, no deviation at all, until I was 22, almost 23. Since then, they've been all over the place. At first, I only missed by a few days, but now sometimes I go three months without one; other times I'll have two a month for two months."

"You're how old now?"

"Twenty-eight."

"So this irregularity has been for five, nearly six years?"

"Yes."

"Your physical exams have been normal?"

"Yes, by gynecology specialists."

"Even though you've been through some of this before, I need to get your health background noted and check things over again."

"I know that. That's why I'm here."

Mrs. Worthington was correct: neither her health background nor examination showed any signs of disease. She'd never been in a hospital, had had no surgery, and had no allergies she knew about. She'd never taken the birth-control pill, or any other medication but penicillin for strep throat.

Both her mother and father had some illness, but it didn't seem related. Partly as a result of their illness, her mother had read Adelle Davis and other authors on good nutrition when Sarah was small, and had given her "nothing but good food" while she was growing up. Sarah had been convinced of the value of good diet, and continued after she left home, "even though it was difficult in college."

She'd gotten married two years before, but had no children,

and didn't want to become pregnant for a few years yet. She was working at a branch bank as assistant manager: "almost the youngest in the bank's history." Despite her job, she said the stress was definitely less than in college, where she'd worked hard for "straight A's" so she could get a good job later.

Her job required long hours, but she made sure to go swimming with her husband twice weekly.

After her checkup, which was quite normal, I asked her to have biochemical screening tests, including blood tests, urinalysis, and hair testing for minerals.

Three weeks later, she returned to go over the results.

"Is there anything there that might account for my problem?" she asked.

I looked over her lab results. "You do have two mineral deficiencies, but that's all. It's a much better record than many I've seen. . . . You're not anemic, your Pap smear was normal, the rest of your screening tests were OK, and your physical exam was normal."

"I was afraid you'd say that. I know that doctors have lots of really sick people to take care of, but I just don't feel well when my periods are off. It's not like being sick, but just not as healthy, energetic, alert . . . I don't know how to describe it."

"Please don't be apologetic. Many people think they have to be really ill to go see a doctor, and feel almost guilty if they aren't. Remember, the focus in preventive medicine is on optimum health, not just illness care. Certainly, doctors in the preventive area spend a lot of time helping sick people get better, but that's only a first step. We always have as a goal the optimum in physical and mental health. Even if everyone can't achieve it, we'll do better if it *is* our goal than if we just patch up symptoms as they occur, and wait for the next one.

"Now, back to your own problem . . . you do have two mineral deficiencies, manganese and chromium, but I'm rather doubtful that these are the cause of your irregular menstrual periods. I've seen many women with these mineral deficiencies. Only a few have menstrual irregularities. In those who do, taking chromium or manganese supplementation doesn't seem to help."

Mrs. Worthington looked very disappointed. Then she said "Well, I know everyone's biochemically different. . . . Maybe those minerals would work for me, even though they don't for others."

"That's a good thought, and does apply sometimes. But before you try that, I'd like to ask you some other questions that may be more relevant. Do you get out much at night?"

"Out?"

"Out*doors.*"

"No. I don't have any reason to; besides, where we live, it isn't all that safe for women outdoors at night. We're thinking of moving. . . . We do go out to dinner or movies occasionally, but those are indoor activities.

"You're indoors most of the day, too, aren't you?"

"Can't do much banking outdoors. And on weekends, even though we share the housework, we're generally indoor types."

"Do you go camping?"

"Neither of us can stand it. We know some kind of exercise is important, that's why we go swimming. That's indoors, too, now that I think of it."

"Do you keep your windows shaded at night?"

"Yes . . . always have since I was little. What's all this got to do with my menstrual periods? Is it something about outdoor light?"

"In a way it might be. But until we see if it works or not, applied to you, it's only a theory. But you certainly fit a pattern. However, I'm getting ahead of things; I should explain what I'm talking about.

"Your examination and tests showed physical normality, and, except for minor mineral problems, apparent nutritional normality. You get some exercise and you've checked out the mental health area. There are many other influences on health, however. Scientists are just beginning to find that light, weather, microwave radiation, atmospheric ionization, magnetic fields, synthetic fiber clothing, infrasonic and supersonic sound, color, and many, many other environmental factors have a definite influence on human health. I'm sure many factors haven't even been discovered yet.

"In your particular case, I want to tell you about a discovery attributed to Dr. John Rock, one of the developers of the birth-control pill. Dr. Rock had worked at a fertility clinic, for women who couldn't become pregnant. He had many patients who had very irregular menstrual cycles. Through observation, thinking about the problem, and trial and error, he came to the conclusion that for some women, proper exposure to light would regularize their cycles, with nothing else needed."

"What do you mean, proper exposure?"

"It seems that some civilized lighting patterns are different enough from the natural state that our ancestors were exposed to for millions of years, that it makes a crucial difference for some women. I want to emphasize *some;* like many other influences on health, people have wide degrees of sensitivity.

"But to get back to particulars: Before you try mineral supplementation, I'd like you to get the smallest light bulb you can find—15- or 25-watt is fine—and turn it on in your bedroom overnight on the fourteenth, fifteenth, sixteenth, and seventeenth nights after the first day of your next menstrual period, whenever that is. It needn't be right next to wherever you're sleeping—just somewhere in the room. It doesn't have to shine right in your eyes, either. Do that every month for the next three or four."

"That'll work when I'm asleep, eyes closed?"

"It doesn't work for everyone, but I've asked many women to try it, when no other physical abnormality can be found. It works for 40 to 50 percent, at least in those I've been able to keep track of. It certainly can't hurt."

Mrs. Worthington thought for a minute. "You know, that sounds like simulating moonlight exposure that primitive women got automatically every month."

"Possibly. I don't know for sure, though that's a very logical conclusion. However, we haven't proven a thing until you try it, and then only if it works."

She got ready to go. "You know, my husband's going to think I'm crazy, but I'm willing to try if you say it works sometimes. Oh, should I take any chromium or manganese?"

"Not yet. If you do, we won't know what worked if you do regularize. About your husband . . . most of the women who've tried this system say their husbands think they're nuts, and me too, especially, for suggesting it. But when it works, then we're not so crazy any more."

Sarah Worthington was fortunately in the "good-response" group. Her periods became regular after the very first month, and stayed that way as long as she turned on what her husband called her "midnight moonlight light bulb" every month, on the fourteenth, fifteenth, sixteenth, and seventeenth nights of her cycle. After a few months, she decided to move her bed closer to the window and open the curtain to let the light from a streetlight in, so that it shone on her side of the bed. She found that worked just as well.

This case points up the fact that we human beings are part of, not foreign to, the universe in which we exist. Influences that affect the rest of the universe cannot help but affect us.

The observation that a lack of periodically timed light exposure may be involved in menstrual irregularity shouldn't be a revolutionary idea. Plant scientists have known for years that germination, flowering, and reproductive cycles of plants can be dramatically altered by type and timing of light exposure. Likewise, reproductive behavior in animals is influenced by environmental factors. There's really no reason why humans shouldn't be influenced as well.

Part of the point of this chapter (and several of the other chapters) goes beyond the particular case matter involved. It's intended to act as an eye-opener to encourage you to at least look into "nonstandard" methods of treating illness and promoting health, as well as investigating the usual approaches.

No, I'm not saying that persons with cancer should avoid the usual treatments in favor of the latest unproven natural treatment. Not at all. Just remember that the record of modern medicine in treating cancer, as well as other illnesses, is nowhere close to perfect. Consider standard treatment; consider the alternatives. Pick what seems best for you.

We may not always find the answers, but with open, inquiring, and always critical minds we can usually come closer than we may think. And, if we don't try, we'll get nowhere at all.

FURTHER READING

Dewan, Edmond M. "On the Possibility of a Perfect Rhythm Method of Birth Control by Periodic Light Stimulation." *American Journal of Obstetrics and Gynecology*, vol. 99, no. 7, 1967, pp. 1016-19.

Llaurado, J. G.; Sances, A.; and Battocletti, J. H. *Biologic and Clinical Effects of Low-Frequency Magnetic and Electric Fields* (Springfield, Ill.: Charles C Thomas, 1974).

Ott, John N. *Health and Light: The Effects of Natural and Artificial Light on Man and Other Living Things* (Old Greenwich, Conn.: The Devin-Adair Co., 1973).

Playfair, Guy L., and Hill, Scott. *The Cycles of Heaven: Cosmic Forces and What They Are Doing to You* (New York: St. Martin's Press, 1978).

A woman suffers from persistent headaches associated with stuffy, artificial environments such as her office building and automobile. Questioning establishes the likelihood that she is one of those people who are especially sensitive to changes in the balance of electrically charged particles of oxygen (air ions). Although headaches are her major symptom, respiratory symptoms are often adversely affected by "positive" ions . . . therapeutic alternatives are offered.

A Case of Air Ion Sensitivity

41

"It's these headaches," Kay Jeffers said. "Actually, I haven't been feeling well for a few years, but nothing disabling. But these headaches are starting to get bad. I used to have a real bad one every few months, and mostly little ones in between. But now I have two or three bad ones some weeks, and little ones in between. Of course there are some weeks when I don't have any bad ones at all, but they're getting fewer.

"What's frustrating is I can't really put a finger on what's causing them. They were getting worse when I was going through a divorce two years ago, but that's all over now, and if anything the headaches are worse."

"Can you tell when you're going to get a headache?"

"Sort of. During weeks when they're worse I'm usually more cranky and irritable even when I'm not having one."

"Do they happen at any particular time of day?"

"They don't seem to."

"Any headache when you get up?"

"No."

"Any relationship to meals? Does eating make them better?"

"Not really."

"What happens if you don't eat for several hours? Do you get a headache?"

"No."

"Do you get dizzy spells with them?"

"No."

"Have you ever had high blood pressure?"

"No."

"Do you get pain in your neck, or a stiff neck with the headaches?"

"No, but I know what you mean. I had headaches like that a few years ago, so I went to my chiropractor. He took care of it with a few treatments. These headaches feel different; I get kind of sick with them. But just to make sure, I saw my chiropractor. He says my neck's fine, that something else must be causing them this time."

"What do you mean 'kind of sick' with your headaches?"

"I just don't feel well all over. My sinuses get all stuffy; I have that kind of problem a lot, anyway. I feel tense and anxious with no particular reason. I get a little nauseated. It's like a toxic buildup my body can't get rid of."

"Have you noticed any sensitivity to anything you eat? You said you have sinus problems; do you get allergies?"

"I do get mild hay fever, but I don't think it's that or foods that cause my headaches. I've tried fasting once or twice for three or four days; that's supposed to tell you if you have food allergies, isn't it?"

"Frequently it does. If food allergies are significant, the symptoms caused usually go away on the third or fourth day of a fast."

"That didn't happen. I felt about the same, fasting or not."

"Have you had any other problems with your health?"

"I've got a sinus problem that comes and goes. It does seem to be aggravated by dust in the air. Every time I clean house it's worse. It's also been worse since I went to work in a new office building downtown. They have year-round climate control, heating and air conditioning. We can't even get the windows open. Sometimes I feel so stifled and uptight in there I could scream. I make a point of going outside at lunchtime because it makes me feel better. Some of the other workers there notice the same thing. Maybe I just have claustrophobia and it's all in my head."

"Maybe. But that could also be an important clue. How long have you worked at that office?"

"Two years. I used to live in the country, and work in a small town. But when I got divorced, I decided to try something different and move to the city."

"Haven't your headaches and ill feelings been worse these last two years?"

"Well, yes. Do you think I'm really bothered by that building? I've had this problem longer than two years, you know. It is worse now, but, well, I thought being just divorced and alone and all was just aggravating whatever the basic problem is."

"I won't deny that psychological stress can cause headaches and the other symptoms you have. But in your case it may be more than that. I think you think so too, or you wouldn't be here."

"That's true. I thought of going to a psychiatrist, but there are some things that just don't fit."

"What do you mean?"

"Before I ever got married, I sometimes got headachy and sick spells when the weather was going to change. My grandmother was sensitive that way too; her arthritis always began to ache worse a day before a weather change occurred. She said it was just in the air. My friends used to tell me I should go into forecasting. One doctor said it was just coincidence, but old Doc Cowins—he was our family doctor in the country where I grew up—he said birds and animals were always the first to notice when a storm was coming. He said I was just tuned in to nature. He told me I should only visit the city, never live there."

"Maybe he knew something. How do you feel when you take long trips in a car?"

"Not good. Sometimes I get a headache; when I don't, I feel kind of sick, and more irritable. In the last few years, I've made sure to stop every two or three hours, in the country if possible. If I don't, I get so sleepy, I just don't feel safe."

"What type of heating do you have where you live? Do you have air conditioning?"

"No air conditioning. It's an older apartment building, it has some kind of radiator heat. Now that I think of it, though, I got an electric space heater for one of the rooms where I'm trying to grow a few plants. I really do like growing things. I've noticed when I go in there when the heater's on I don't feel good. I've been thinking of getting rid of it."

"Have you ever been in a sauna?"

"Yes. It made me so sick I never want to try it again!"

"I think there's enough evidence here to form a theory about what your problem is. I'd like you to do two things. First, the next time you don't feel well and get a sick headache on a weekend, I want you to stop whatever you're doing and go to the ocean, even if it's raining. I know you'll have to drive there, but do it anyway. I'd like you to try just sitting as close to the surf as you can get.

"Second, I'd like you to get a book titled *The Ion Effect*, by Fred Soyka and Alan Edmonds. Once you read it, I think you'll understand much better why you're having your symptoms."

"Go to the seashore and sit near the surf? How will that help my headache?"

"It sounds like you're running into a conflict between the way your body is adapted to nature and changes in the natural environment created mostly by civilization and technology.

"Scientists have found that some of the molecules of the air have an electrical charge. Under most circumstances open air in the country has both positively and negatively charged molecules called 'ions.' The natural ratio is approximately five positive ions to four negative ones. Presumably, that is the ratio of air ions in which life on earth has existed and evolved.

"Some people are very sensitive to changes in the atmospheric ion concentrations. One estimate is that 25 percent are sensitive. Research has shown that negative air ions are generally good in their health effects and positive air ions bad. You can find the details in the book. Among other things, an excess of positive air ions causes overproduction of the hormone *serotonin*, which can lead to severe headaches and the other symptoms you've mentioned.

"All of the environments that make you feel ill—sealed office buildings with year-round climate control, automobiles, electrically heated saunas, and your 'plant room' with the electric space heater—all are linked by the artificial overproduction of positive air ions. That's not to condemn modern science and technology; after all, the same science that inadvertently made you ill with positive ions has also developed techniques for finding what the problem is, and means of correcting it.

"Also, in this case 'natural' is not always good or beneficial. Your problems when the weather changes are probably encounters with nature's own high levels of positive air ion production. In fact, there are areas of the world subject to positive-ion winds that recurrently make people ill. Again, you can read about the details.

"Your case seems typical, but some time at the ocean on a bad day is an inexpensive way of testing whether this really is your problem. You see, falling water and crashing surf produce an abundance of negative ions. After an hour or two, you should feel better."

Mrs. Jeffers thought for a minute. "You know, I think you're right. When I'm only feeling a little bit bad, a good shower always makes me feel better. So do walks in the rain. I don't think I need that trip to the ocean; I'm sure you're right, but what do I do about it? I can't afford to quit my job, and I can't take showers while I'm there. From what you say, I'm exposed to many more positive air ions than I used to be, and it's making me more sick."

I went to my file cabinet. "Here are the names of four or five companies that make negative ion generators, machines that produce negative air ions which can counteract the effects of the positive air ions. I can't recommend any one in particular. Write for details. But I do think it's what you need."

Mrs. Jeffers first obtained the least expensive model she

could find. After she found it in fact could help correct her symptoms, she put one on her office desk, one in her car, and one at home. As she said, it was a little expensive, but worth it.

When I last heard, she had eliminated her sick headaches, irritability, tension, and stuffy sinuses. Even her annual mild hay fever didn't come around when it usually did.

The number of people who are sensitive to ionization of the surrounding air isn't known. There are a variety of estimates, but research really isn't far enough along to say. However, from observation in my practice, it appears to me that the proportion is significant, and that air ion sensitivity is not rare or unusual.

In practice, it appears that the group most likely to benefit from negative ions are those who suffer from chronic respiratory tract allergy—hay fever, allergic sinusitis, allergic bronchitis, and asthma.

Besides arousing antibodies, it appears that some allergy-producing substances such as dust and pollens have a positive electrical charge. Negative ions appear to counteract the effects of this on respiratory tissues. Negative ions also have a beneficial effect of their own on respiratory structures (see Llaurado and Soyka).

The response among my patients has been variable, but generally favorable. Only a few have had no help for their respiratory allergies. Most have reported considerable relief, with a few clearing up entirely. The majority have been able to cut down on other treatment, nutritional/biochemical or drug, that they were taking.

Research on the effects of atmospheric ionization on human health is still relatively sparse and in the preliminary stages. There are a few indications, however, that a lot more than allergies and headaches may be helped by manipulation of the ions of the air around us.

This is an appropriate place to reemphasize briefly another point: all that is natural is not good for health; and everything unnatural or technological is not necessarily bad. This case is an excellent example.

Positive air ions, which at present appear to be uniformly bad for humans, have been around much longer than science, technology, or civilization. Nature produces them quite nicely without any help from man, right along with negative ions. For millions of years, man and positive ions have interacted unfavorably. As detailed in one of the books below, folk knowledge has attributed evil effects to certain seasonal winds, which science has identified to be highly charged with positive winds.

Certainly, civilization and technology can aggravate this problem, but did not originate it.

Likewise, it's been a technological innovation, the negative ion generator, which has provided the most practical remedy for most persons bothered by positive ions. Certainly, nature had been making negative ions long before man made generators, but most of us can't just quit our jobs and leave for regions higher in negative ions, even if it is good for the health.

Even though it seems obvious that as natural beings, humans will stay healthier by observing natural laws and, whenever possible, applying natural remedies, faith in this principle should never be blind. People also become ill and even die prematurely from entirely natural causes, as well as by violating natural principles.

In matters of health, take nature as your guiding principle, but always try to illuminate your path with the light of reason.

FURTHER READING

Llaurado, J. G.; Sances, A. Jr.; and Battocletti, J. H. *Biologic and Clinical Effects of Low-Frequency Magnetic and Electric Fields* (Springfield, Ill.: Charles C Thomas, 1974).

Rosen, Stephen. *Weathering: How the Atmosphere Conditions Your Body, Your Mind, Your Mood—and Your Health* (New York: M. Evans, 1979).

Soyka, Fred, and Edmonds, Alan. *The Ion Effect* (New York: Bantam, 1977).

Part II

Your Personal Health Improvement Program

The preventive, natural approach to health emphasizes the fact that our body engineering is designed to cope with—and thrive on—a lifestyle and diet followed for millions of years. Just in the last century or so, that lifestyle has all but disappeared from industrialized societies. By modifying some of our habits to accommodate the needs of our heritage, we can greatly increase the ability of our body to maintain health and optimize the natural healing process.

42 The Seven Principles of Good Health

Unlike conventional medicine, nutritional therapy is not merely a collection of individual stratagems designed to suppress illness or its symptoms. It is much more "of a whole piece," a kind of unified system, the basis of which is to accommodate the true needs of the body. So I'd like to begin by discussing the general principles I ask my patients—well or ill—to follow.

If well, following them will help to maintain health. If ill, other special treatments are necessary, of course, but only as fitted into the overall background of general principles of good health.

As you'll see, what this does for an ill person is to remove all impediments to the healing forces of nature. Until harmony with nature is restored, true, full health is not possible.

To start, we should look at what it *is* we are trying to keep healthy.

Your body, your mind, all that is uniquely "you," is probably no older than 90 years. If you are much older than that, you're truly exceptional. Some people might consider you *ancient*.

But compared to the basic metabolic processes churning away within you, you are practically a flash in the pan. For the design of those internal processes, your "engineering," so to speak, is literally *millions* of years old. The way your stomach digests food is probably the same way that human stomachs have digested food for countless generations. The way each of your cells makes and uses energy; the way your cells store starch and fat or build proteins; the way the living chemicals of your skin and eyes respond to light—all of these processes, with very minor variations, take place in your body in exactly the same way as they have for millions of years.

Millions? Yes, almost certainly. The earliest specimens of *Homo sapiens*—our own species—that we know about date back 40 to 50 thousand years. But the earliest specimens of what we often call "early man"—a being probably remarkably similar to us except in some external details—go back, as far as can be told, some 3 to 4 million years.

What difference does all this ancient history make to your health?

More, I believe, than most of us realize.

According to anthropologists, the only reason you and I are here today is that our species has, over this vast long haul of time, managed to survive by *adapting* to our environment. Our bodies are the gloves, so to speak, that we as a species developed to fit the hand of nature. Everything that goes on inside our bodies can be interpreted as an adaptive response—you might even call it an "intelligent" response—to the challenge of the environment. We can't always understand what the adaptive purpose is to any given process in our body, but it's safe to say that precious little happens by accident.

Now let's look at the nutritional environment of humans over the past millions of years. During all that time—with practically no exceptions—the food eaten was whole, natural, and unrefined. Our ancestors ate no white bread, refined sugar, or steam-blasted canned foods impregnated with chemicals to keep them looking fresh. They drank no sugar-drenched chemical concoctions called soft drinks. They ate no foods designed by some chemist for the sole purpose of looking cute and amusing the taste buds. Our ancestors ate only what they could hunt, gather, dig up, or (in the last ten thousand years) grow.

One reply is: "So what? Our ancestors lived in caves, huts, or tents. They were little better off than animals. And they had no books or TV or airplanes. Why should we try to copy them when we have everything that modern technology can give us?"

I'd agree that modern technology does have many advantages. But despite the changes we've created with our technology, our biochemical systems (our body cells) have changed scarcely at all since the discovery of fire, and probably since long before that.

Your body's cells are adapted to the same foods humans have eaten for three or four million years. We might theorize that if the human race continues to eat modern convenience foods for *another* three or four million years (and survives it!) our descendants might be well adapted to them and we'll stay healthy on such a diet. Maybe.

Unfortunately, that won't help you or me at all. We need to stay healthy *now*. So, our first principle for good health should be: *All of our food should be whole, unrefined, and cooked as little as possible.*

Don't let anyone confuse you by labeling such a diet "faddism." It is the consumption of highly processed convenience foods which is faddism, a reckless chemical experiment with the natural course of human evolution.

There are two other basic principles for good health which involve diet. To appreciate them, we must also go back in time.

Butylated hydroxytoluene. Propylene glycol. Tartrazine. Nordihydroguaiaretic acid. All of these synthetic or partially synthetic chemicals, and thousands more, have been added to our food supply at some point in very recent history. They derive from test tubes and not from nature. Almost none of them are more than 150 years old.

None of these has been absolutely proven to have killed any individuals outright. Furthermore, according to apologists for the very large and profitable food chemical industry, they've been used for many decades now, so they must be safe.

That is nonsense. First, we know for a fact that even a common additive like monosodium glutamate (MSG) can cause susceptible people to be seized with terrible headaches and other alarming circulatory disorders. And it is almost certain that susceptible children can become hyperactive as a result of eating artificial colors and probably other additives.

But more convincing than these recently discovered specifics is our understanding that our bodies simply have not had time to adapt to these chemical invaders. After all, what is 150 years compared to 2 million?

That applies not only to intentional food additives, but to synthetics such as insecticides, weed killers, and other agricultural chemicals which find their way into our systems. What the long-term effects of consuming these chemicals may be has given rise to some nightmare speculation. But rather than worry, it's best to try to avoid all synthetics in our diets unless they are absolutely necessary or somehow proven utterly harmless.

Our second principle for good health, then, should be: *Avoid all synthetics in your diet.*

These first two principles apply in the same way to all of us. The third diet-related principle, though, varies from individual to individual.

According to the best presently available evidence, hunting for game or gathering wild vegetables and roots has been the human way of life for all but the last 10 to 15 thousand years of the total three-to-four-million-year human history. The earliest evidence of farming and animal domestication comes from the Middle East and Southeast Asia and dates from about 8000 to 15,000 B.C.

Now ten thousand years seems like a terribly long time to you and me. But in perspective, it's only about ½ percent of the total time of human existence. Stated another way: for 99½ percent of the history of humans on earth, hunting and gathering has been the source of all food.

So it shouldn't be much of a surprise that foods only recently introduced into the human diet as a result of farming and animal domestication should frequently be the source of symptoms or diseases. Wheat, corn, eggs, milk; these and many other natural and wholesome foods are perfectly capable of causing illness in persons whose body chemistry isn't suited to them.

Similarly, the vast improvements in transportation of both people and foodstuffs which have occurred in the past few centuries have brought people into contact with foods their ancestors never knew existed. Considering this, a reaction of a descendant of Scandinavians to pineapple, or a reaction of a black person to Scandinavian cheese might be perfectly understandable.

Unfortunately, reactions of this sort, *particularly minor ones*, can go overlooked for years. Frequently, it takes careful investigation by a physician trained in nutritional medicine to ferret out such a source of what may be puzzling and obscure symptoms.

Your third principle for good health should be: *Beware of possible adverse reactions to even wholesome, natural food.*

Our last health principle dealing with diet is: *Diet supplementation is always necessary for good health.*

Some may call this principle highly controversial, citing pronouncements by the Food and Drug Administration that practically no one needs diet supplementation. Few health professionals who have really studied nutrition, however, believe that reckless and potentially dangerous assertion.

If there are any exceptions to the rule of general supplementation, it might be someone who lived in the middle of a wilderness, a thousand miles from all sources of air and water pollution. These pollutants increase our need for detoxifying nutrients such as vitamin E and vitamin C. And if that same person grew all his or her own food from fertile, undepleted soil, always eating it fresh, the need for diet supplementation would be even less. And if he spent most of his time outdoors and worked hard physically, it would be still less.

Actually, because not every area of the world has an abundance of all vitamins at all times, even primitive peoples frequently resort to diet supplementation by eating unusual foods such as raw animal glands, insects, or special herbs or roots which tradition has taught them are rich in vital nutrients. So the idea of making dietary supplementation part of your daily life is not only necessary, but quite natural.

Now, briefly, I would like to give my present recommendations for such supplementation. You should understand that these apply if you are healthy. They need alteration in case of illness. Further, they are based on presently available evidence and may well be changed in the future. Given these cautions, the list is as follows:

1. A high-quality multiple vitamin and mineral supplement, including all known useful nutrients
2. Additional ascorbic acid (vitamin C)
3. Additional vitamin E

These are general recommendations. I am not opposed to using other vitamins and minerals, as well as whole natural substances, as dietary supplements. However, this must be done on an individual basis, after careful consideration. Preferably, it should be done under the supervision of a physician experienced in nutritional medicine.

Now let's go over some nondietary but entirely naturally derived principles.

Airplanes, cars, washing machines, mixers, vacuum cleaners—most of us wouldn't be without these and other examples of our civilization's machinery. Unfortunately, while taking advantage of all these machines, most of us neglect nature's *original* work-accomplishing devices—our muscles!

Can you spend most of your day digging a field by hand? Can you run a mile (even at a moderate pace) in pursuit of game, and not fall on your face? Can you do any type of rugged work all day and not wake up in the morning sore and aching all over? If you can, you are an exception to the rule.

Yet, this is the kind of activity which our muscles were designed to accomplish, and to which our body structure and chemistry are adapted.

Let's be realistic and admit that for some of us it would be difficult to get more than an hour or two of exercise every day. But even this much is an enormous improvement over nothing.

And age should be no excuse or barrier. The peoples of Hunza, Peru, and the Caucasus who often live well past 100, all remain extremely active in the fields after a century of work.

Putting off exercise until tomorrow because there just isn't time today is all too easy. If you want to stay healthy for as long as possible, do it today! What's more, try to do it outdoors, so you enjoy the benefit of natural sunlight.

Your fifth principle for good health must be: *Get enough exercise, regularly, to stay fit.*

Enough has been written on the effects of stress on health that I'm sure you're well aware of them. And stress is nothing new. Our early ancestor constantly glancing over his shoulder to see if a saber-toothed tiger was sneaking up on him had his full share of stress. And surely family fights and problems with in-laws are even older than civilization.

I'm not going to elaborate further except to agree with those who say that the rapid changes of the past few generations have probably worsened the stresses we must all face.

Obviously, each of us has to deal with stress in his own way. Some prefer meditation; others find solace in traditional religious activities. Many go off to the hills for a day or two, while still others obtain help from psychiatrists or other professionals in learning new ways of coping with or eliminating stress. However you do it, the important thing is to realize that dealing positively and creatively with stress is important to each of us in staying healthy.

So your sixth principle should be: *Recognize stresses in your life; don't ignore them. Find a way to adjust, or eliminate them.*

These six principles all involve what you can do to keep yourself healthy. Of course, there are certain preventive and health-maintaining measures that only a physician can help you with. I'll make a list of the procedures I currently recommend, but remember, if you were to ask three or four different doctors, you would probably get the same number of different lists. And that is as it should be. All good physicians I know have highly individual ways of helping their patients, as individual as each of their patients.

My present recommendations are:

• A thorough physical examination every three to four years, more frequently with advancing age. For example, once every two years in your sixties and annually in your seventies.

• An annual blood pressure check.

• An annual Pap smear and breast check for women.

• An eye pressure check for glaucoma with every physical, if you're past 40.

• Completed immunizations in most cases (although I know there is debate on this).

• A treadmill or "stress" EKG (electrocardiogram) if there is even a remote suspicion of heart disease. This is the most reliable method we currently have of assessing the likelihood of having a heart attack.

• With every physical examination, these basic laboratory procedures: blood count to determine if you are anemic; urinalysis to look for such things as diabetes or kidney damage; cholesterol and triglyceride readings to determine blood fat levels; a blood sugar and/or glycohemoglobin (Hgb Al_c) determination to check the carbohydrate metabolism, and a hair test to analyze for minerals and check for possible imbalances or toxic levels of minerals or trace elements.

If you're wondering why I haven't mentioned smoking, drinking alcohol, or coffee and drug abuse, that is because I consider these practices to be drug usage rather than ordinary lifestyle habits. But drug usage is another topic.

As a final note, let me point out that these principles for health owe as much to a study of human adaptation and evolution as they do to a study of medicine. I believe this is the most helpful perspective with which to look at something as important as health.

Which brings me to a close with a quick review of our basic principles for good health.

1. All your food should be whole, unrefined, and processed and cooked as little as possible.

2. Avoid all synthetics in your diet.
3. Be aware of possible reactions to wholesome, natural foods.
4. Diet supplementation is necessary for good health.
5. Get enough exercise, regularly, to stay fit.
6. Recognize stresses in your life; don't ignore them. Find a way to adjust or eliminate them.
7. See a doctor, at whatever intervals he or she recommends, for health-care measures you can't take on your own.

FURTHER READING

Allergy and Environment

Breneman, J. C. *Basics of Food Allergy* (Springfield, Ill.: Charles C Thomas, 1978).

Dickey, Lawrence D., ed. *Clinical Ecology* (Springfield, Ill.: Charles C Thomas, 1976).

Randolph, Theron G. *Human Ecology and Susceptibility to the Chemical Environment* (Springfield, Ill.: Charles C Thomas, 1978).

Man and Prehistory

Cohen, Mark Nathan. *The Food Crisis in Prehistory: Overpopulation and the Origins of Agriculture* (New Haven, Conn.: Yale University Press, 1977).

Fagan, Brian M. *People of the Earth: An Introduction to World Prehistory* (Boston: Little, Brown and Co., 1977).

Refined Carbohydrates

Cleave, T. L. *The Saccharine Disease* (New Canaan, Conn.: Keats Publishing, 1975).

Refining and Nutrient Loss

Christensen, James J.; Hearty, Patrick A.; and Izatt, Reed M. "Determination of Chromium in Several Proposed Standard Samples and of Zinc and Chromium in Wheat Milling and Beet Sugar Refining Samples." *Journal of Agricultural and Food Chemistry*, vol. 24, no. 4, 1976, pp. 811–15.

Ferretti, Renato J., and Levander, Orville A. "Effect of Milling and Processing on the Selenium Content of Grains and Cereal Products." *Journal of Agricultural and Food Chemistry*, vol. 22, no. 6, 1974, pp. 1049–51.

Schroeder, Henry A. "The Role of Chromium in Mammalian Nutrition." *The American Journal of Clinical Nutrition*, vol. 21, no. 3, March 1968, pp. 230–44.

———. "Losses of Vitamins and Trace Minerals Resulting from Food Processing and Preservation of Foods." *The American Journal of Clinical Nutrition*, vol. 24, May 1971, pp. 562–73.

———. *The Trace Elements and Man: Some Positive and Negative Aspects* (Old Greenwich, Conn.: The Devin-Adair Co., 1973).

Many commonly prescribed drugs cause nutritional side effects, some of which can be quite serious. Among these drugs are antibiotics, diuretics ("water pills"), anti-inflammatories, cortisone, oral contraceptives, digitalis, antacids, laxatives, and anticonvulsants. Protective measures are outlined. . . . Also, a special section on the ecological approach to controlling recurrent yeast infections, through the *Lactobacillus acidophilus* - yogurt treatment.

43 Surviving Drug Therapy

The best way of combating disease is to prevent it in the first place. However, despite our best efforts, ill health will still occur sometimes, and accidental injury can't always be foreseen.

So there are times when turning to health-care professionals is unavoidable, and in fact, modern medicine does have a lot to offer in the way of crisis care. Unfortunately, it is frequently difficult, in fact often impossible, to locate a physician with anything but a sketchy knowledge of nutrition and the effects of drug treatment on both nutritional substances and normal body ecology. Even though this is only another way of saying "applied biochemistry and human ecology," the vast majority of physicians are woefully undertrained in this very basic area.

It's the intention of this chapter to bring together information about nutritional and ecological side effects of some of the more common drug therapies, and what to do about them. I have not included an exhaustive list, and of course recommend only those measures which can be taken with safety by a nonprofessional. I hope that readers will find this useful, and set it aside for the next time a visit to the doctor is necessary.

Antibiotics

Aside from allergic reactions, antibiotics cause other disturbances of body ecology that may go unrecognized, sometimes for years. In addition to killing off the "bad" (or at least, unwanted) germs, antibiotics also eliminate numerous good or "friendly" germs at the same time. These good germs don't always return on their own, and since each has a definite place in body ecology, problems may arise.

Let's start with one of the most common, often-recurring problems seen in a general doctor's office, vaginal infection, particularly yeast infection. Women frequently arrive for the first time at our offices saying, "I've had this yeast infection for three years," or "This is the sixth time I've had this!" The problem is frequently traceable to a long-forgotten antibiotic treatment, which may have helped whatever the problem was, but also killed the normal germs of the vaginal area. Once these are gone, yeast or other germs will invade, and sooner or later cause a full-scale infection.

Women frequently are given the first step in treatment of such an infection, an anti-yeast medicine. But the crucial second step (described at the end of this chapter), replacement of friendly germs which will keep the yeast out, is usually omitted. So the yeast infection keeps returning.

Antibiotics also alter the normal intestinal bacteria. This is easily recognized in children who get diarrhea from antibiotics, but also happens in adults, with no symptoms. The friendly germs are often replaced by antibiotic-resistant organisms. Problems that can occur because of this are decreased bacterial synthesis of vitamin K, and decreased intestinal utilization of a variety of nutrients, including calcium, magnesium, folic acid, and vitamin B_{12}. Almost all of this can be avoided with the help of *Lactobacillus acidophilus*. As a general rule, persons taking antibiotics for a few days or long-term should take either *Lactobacillus acidophilus* tablets or eat home-made yogurt every day they're taking the antibiotic.

Diuretics

Also known as "water pills," these medications are frequently given for fluid retention and high blood pressure. They cause a variety of nutrient losses, the most important of which are potassium, magnesium, and water-soluble vitamins (B and C).

Before discussing what to do for these nutrient losses, an equally important question is: are "water pills" always necessary? As you could guess from the question, the answer is definitely *no!*

"Chronic fluid retention" with "no known cause" is a frequent problem, especially in women. Diuretics are frequently prescribed as the answer. However, most often increasing the dietary protein and foods rich in B vitamins is the real solution. This takes time to work. In the meantime, there is another nearly 100 percent effective and natural remedy for women in their menstrual years: vitamin B_6, also called pyridoxine. I've recommended pyridoxine amounts from 50 to 600 milligrams daily (in several doses) to nearly 1,000 women with fluid retention, and it's worked on all but one or two. That it's really getting at the cause of the problem is shown by its frequent side effects of calming the nerves, improving the complexion, and helping a variety of problems not related by the patient to either fluid retention or vitamin lack.

For others, the cause of chronic fluid retention is frequently an unsuspected food allergy, or eating too much sugar and refined carbohydrates. Simply eliminating these problems can lead to an elimination of retained fluid.

But back to diuretics. Sometimes, as in cases of high blood pressure, there seems to be no alternative and the doctor orders them. In this case, foods rich in potassium (raw vegetables, fruits, nuts), magnesium (nuts, whole grains, greens), B-complex vitamins (wheat germ, liver, beans), and vitamin C (fruits, melons, peppers) should be eaten daily. It's usually advisable to take at least a low- to medium-potency supplement of these nutrients also, for as long as the need for diuretics exists.

Anti-Inflammatories

This is another group of frequently prescribed medications, including aspirin, Butazolidin and Indocin. (These last two often go under other trade names or generic names, so always ask your pharmacist what sort of medication you're getting.) They're frequently prescribed for a variety of arthritis-, bursitis-, tendonitis-, and rheumatism-type of complaints.

All of these medications greatly increase the body's requirement for vitamin C. A gram or two a day of vitamin C, some taken at each meal, is a minimum requirement when taking these medications. Since these medications all put stresses on the body, the other "antistress" vitamins (B complex) should be added if any medications in this group are used for prolonged periods of time.

Cortisone

Cortisone and other cortisonelike medications are frequently given, despite their well-known side effects, including gastrointestinal ulceration, delayed wound-healing, hypertension, and suppression of natural immunity. (In extreme cases, suppression is the desired effect, and the reader is advised to inquire about the exact purpose of a cortisone prescription before taking any nutritional-preventive measures to counteract these side effects.)

Vitamin A is probably the most important supplemental nutrient for a person on cortisone therapy. It has been shown to counteract the ulcer-causing tendencies of cortisone, and to restimulate the suppressed production of white blood cells. Fifty thousand units daily is probably adequate and should be accompanied by 100 to 200 units of vitamin E, which helps protect the vitamin A from oxidation.

Zinc is another nutrient that should be supplemented by persons on cortisone therapy. Fifty to 100 milligrams (preferably of a chelated form) is probably adequate. Zinc has been found to stimulate enzymes involved in wound healing which might be suppressed by cortisone.

Long-term therapy with cortisone is a major stress on the body; regular supplementation of the antistress B and C vitamins is also necessary in these cases. Last, long-term cortisone therapy can produce osteoporosis, often signaled by persistent pain in the mid-back. Calcium supplementation in the range of 800 to 1,200 milligrams a day, plus vitamin D to utilize it, would be indicated.

Oral Contraceptives

The list of nutrient problems caused by oral contraceptives is a long one. The list of symptoms caused by these nutrient problems is also long, including mood swings, depression, sleeplessness, irritability, complexion problems, dry or flaky skin, fluid retention, hair loss, "lifeless" hair, and many others. Fortunately, most of these effects can be corrected with appropriate nutrient supplementation.

Probably the most-researched nutritional deficiency caused by oral contraceptives is vitamin B_6. Recognized experts in this area of research advise that 25 to 30 milligrams of vitamin B_6 be taken daily by any woman on oral contraceptives.

However, this is not the only B complex vitamin that oral contraceptives can affect. Riboflavin, vitamin B_{12}, and folic acid have all been found variably deficient in women taking oral contraceptives.

Mineral abnormalities have also been detected. Depressed levels of zinc and elevated levels of its some-time "mineral antagonist," copper, have been found. Other trace minerals are also affected.

I usually ask any woman for whom I prescribe oral contraceptives to make sure she's eating foods rich in B complex vitamins and minerals. Also, taking a medium- to high-potency B complex supplement (with at least 30 milligrams of B_6) and a multiple mineral supplement is a must. These supplements will not interfere with the desired actions of oral contraceptives.

Digitalis

The standard remedy for "heart failure," digitalis, is an invaluable drug remedy. (Interestingly, this remedy is found in the natural form in the foxglove plant, and was prescribed as "digitalis leaf" into the early years of this century. As might be anticipated, it was considered an "old wives' tale" for many years after its discovery.)

The most important nutrient to be aware of if you're taking digitalis in any form is potassium. If body levels of potassium drop too low, digitalis can cause abnormal electrical rhythm in the heart. Bananas, orange juice and other fruit juices, and fresh greens should be eaten every day. Also, to be sure, I recommend potassium supplements to all of my patients on digitalis.

This supplementation is even more important for persons taking a very common combination of digitalis and a diuretic. As noted above, diuretics cause potassium loss. A potassium supplement is absolutely mandatory for anyone taking this combination.

Some of the potential toxic side effects of digitalis can be prevented by vitamin C, in my opinion. I recommend 1,000-milligram doses, taken 2 or 3 times a day, to all my patients who must take digitalis.

Antacids

Most antacids have potential for interfering with vitamin and mineral absorption. Over two to three days, this probably isn't important, but if taken for any prolonged period of time, it can be. The vitamin most affected is B_1, or thiamine. Thiamine-rich foods and a 10- to 20-milligram supplemental dosage should be taken by anyone on prolonged antacid therapy. New work has shown that calcium, phosphorus, and probably other minerals are blocked from absorption when aluminum hydroxide gel is taken over a long period of months or years. Either generous amounts of milk or a calcium-phosphorus supplement should be taken—not at the same time antacids are taken.

Mineral Oil and Laxatives

The most important thing about mineral oil is not taking it. It causes serious impairment of absorption of vitamins A, D, E, and K. Over a period of time, that can seriously affect health.

The same thing can be said about laxatives. There are enough natural alternatives to them that there should never be any reason to swallow one. A commonly available and effective bowel regulator is bran.

Anticonvulsants

Anticonvulsants have been found to impair absorption of vitamin B_{12} and folic acid. The most widely prescribed one of these is Dilantin. A caution here, though: although vitamin B_{12} can be taken with safety, there's definite question about whether folic acid supplements will interfere with the antiseizure effect of Dilantin. At the present time, it's wisest to limit supplementation to vitamin B_{12}.

In Conclusion

As I mentioned at the beginning, this is not a complete discussion of natural treatment of drug-caused nutritional problems, but only a brief survey of the more common ones, and what to do about them. Except as noted above, all of these things can (and should, for good health) be done by a nonprofessional person on his or her own. In this way, one can get the maximum benefit from needed drug therapy with a minimum of problems.

Of course, preventive medicine is always the best. But when and if these measures fail, I hope the above discussion will be of help in surviving drug therapy.

A Special Note about the Ecological Approach to Recurrent Yeast Infections

It would be advisable at first to check with your physician about whether or not you do have a yeast problem. If you are in some doubt about the diagnosis, it never hurts to gain a second opinion. That is perfectly acceptable to most physicians. Once you have ascertained the cause of the problem to your satisfaction, carry on.

1. *Killing off the yeast as much as possible.* This is quite necessary as a first step in getting rid of the yeast infection. The bacteria replacement outlined below frequently doesn't have a chance if there is too much yeast around. Therefore, any of the commonly prescribed anti-yeast medications should be used for the recommended length of time, which is frequently one to two weeks. This recommendation should be checked with your own doctor or pharmacist.

2. *Replacing the normal bacteria.* The reason yeast infections often return is that while the yeast is killed, the normal bacteria are not replaced. That leaves an opportunity for the yeast to return. Unfortunately, the normal bacteria are not usually transmitted from person to person. Therefore, they must be deliberately replaced.

   A good analogy for this is the lawn or flower bed. If you first pull up all the weeds (as in killing off all the yeast), but then do not plant either your grass seed or the flowers in the flower bed, the weeds will soon return. No matter how often the weeds are pulled up, they will return once more unless something else is planted.

   The normal vaginal bacteria is Döderlein's bacillus. This is not generally available commercially. Therefore, a good substitute is the *Lactobacillus acidophilus* commonly available in health food stores and frequently in drug stores under the trade name *Lactinex*. Instructions for its use are as follows:

   A. Obtain half a cup of plain yogurt. It does not matter

whether it is pasteurized or not, just so it is plain. Second, obtain the above-mentioned *L. acidophilus.* This can be purchased as noted in either health food stores or drug stores. It should be obtained in either tablet form which can be crushed to a powder, or in capsules containing powder. It is available in a liquid suspension, but this does not make as neat a mixture and should be avoided if possible. However, it probably will work if nothing else is available.

B. To the half-cup of yogurt, add approximately 2 tablespoons of *L. acidophilus* powder. Mix very, very well. This mixture is for both bacterial replacement and to provide a suitable growth material for these bacteria. The mixture should be put in the refrigerator and may be used each night.

C. The mixture should be inserted into the vagina. The applicator may be either a medicine applicator, tampon applicator, a syringe with the end cut off, or any other suitable device for introducing the mixture into the vagina. Approximately 2 teaspoons will suffice. If the applicator is not big enough for this, a little less will probably work. It should be put into the vagina for five nights in a row, beginning on the night of the day when you have completed using your anti-yeast medication for the prescribed period of time. It should not be repeated in the morning (see below); once at bedtime is sufficient.

D. In the morning, a douche with water and approximately 2 tablespoons of vinegar should be used. The usual quantity of water is just fine. This is to inhibit the growth of yeast and to promote the growth of the bacteria (and also for the sake of neatness). After the period of five nights, this treatment should be stopped as the bacteria should be well established.

3. *Other details.* The anti-yeast medication and the bacteria replacement should be done on consecutive days. If a menstrual period intervenes, it might not work out. So

wait until there is time for both the medicine and the bacteria replacement. This is not absolutely foolproof; it usually works. However, if there are other complications besides the yeast infection, or if it is not a yeast infection, it very well might not work. Also, the next time you have to take an antibiotic or other medication, including hormones, which might affect the vaginal bacteria, it may return anyway. If so, the whole routine should be followed again. However, we have found that the recurrence rate for yeast infections drops off drastically when following this routine.

FURTHER READING

Ahmed, Faizy; Bamji, Mahtab; and Iyengar, Leela. "Effect of Oral Contraceptive Agents on Vitamin Nutrition Status." *The American Journal of Clinical Nutrition*, vol. 28, no. 6, June 1975, pp. 606–15.

Basu, T. K. "Interaction of Drugs and Nutrition." *Journal of Human Nutrition*, vol. 31, no. 6, December 1977, pp. 449–58.

Clark, F. "Drugs and Vitamin Deficiency." *Journal of Human Nutrition*, vol. 30, pp. 333–37.

Hunt, Thomas K. et al. "Effect of Vitamin A on Reversing the Inhibitory Effect of Cortisone on Healing of Open Wounds in Animals and Man." *Annals of Surgery*, October 1969, pp. 633–41.

Palmer, A. "Vaginitis." *The Practitioner*, vol. 214, May 1975, pp. 666–72.

Prasad, Ananda et al. "Effect of Oral Contraceptive Agents on Nutrients: I. Minerals." *The American Journal of Clinical Nutrition*, vol. 28, April 1975, pp. 377–84.

Roe, Daphne A. *Drug-Induced Nutritional Deficiencies* (Westport, Conn.: Avi Publishing, 1976).

Schneider, Howard A.; Anderson, Carl E.; and Coursin, David B. *Nutritional Support of Medical Practice* (New York: Harper & Row, 1977).

Wynn, Victor. "Vitamins and Oral Contraceptive Use." *The Lancet*, vol. 1, no. 7,906, March 8, 1975, pp. 561–64.

Some of the side effects that can be caused by antibiotic therapy are illustrated in the case of a woman who had persistent vaginal and fungal infections, cramps, and other problems. . . . Why antibiotics should be considered "pesticides for human use."

44 How Antibiotics Can Disrupt Body Ecology

Like most physicians in family practice and other specialties who give ongoing health care for women, I urge annual Pap smears as one of the more important preventive precautions. Frequently, women will save up several "minor problems" until the time of their annual exams, and in fact, this is what Susan Bing had done.

"I have several other problems today, too," she said. "Could we take care of these?" I said I didn't know if we could fit everything in, as well as her Pap smear, but we could at least make a start. So, she listed the following:

1. A persistent vaginal infection. She said she'd had this on and off for nearly a year. It tended to get much worse before menstrual periods. She'd seen doctors about it, and was always told it was a "yeast infection." Despite several anti-yeast medications, it always returned. She was becoming more and more uncomfortable. But "even worse, it's putting a strain on my married life. If nothing else, I'd like to get rid of this."

2. Sores inside her nose. She reported that there were almost always yellow brown crusted scabs that hurt. Sometimes her nose would bleed a little. She'd been using Vaseline, but it hadn't helped.

3. A little fungus between her toes on both feet. "This," she said, "wasn't bad," but itched and was a nuisance. But "lots of people have fungus, and if I can't get rid of it, it's OK."

4. Intestinal cramps which came and went. The cramps didn't seem to relate to food, or anything she did. But she didn't have diarrhea or constipation, so she figured this might be normal.

5. "A funny kind of numbness" in her fingertips and toes. This symptom also came and went. It had only been present for two months.

Mrs. Bing said, "I'd been ignoring all the rest, as a lot of people have those problems. But when my fingers and toes started acting up, I felt like I was falling apart all over. Also, I've been feeling more and more tired and run-down. So I thought I'd better at least ask about it, anyway."

As she'd proceeded with her list of "minor problems," I'd become increasingly suspicious that something was interfering with her normal overall body ecology—in this case, the many types of normal bacteria that live in and on us all. But, as one of my medical school professors liked to point out, "jumping to obvious conclusions is a dangerous sport, even when you're right!" So I thought I'd best inquire further.

Starting with the last symptom, the numbness in her fingers and toes, I asked if she'd ever been suspected of having diabetes mellitus. Even though she was only 31, this is of course a rather frequent diabetic early warning signal. But she said no, and that there was none in her family either. Further, she had no numbness, tingling, or interference with sensation or movement anywhere else, so, for the present, I thought neurologic disease unlikely.

Going to the problem of intestinal cramps, I asked if she'd had any other symptoms such as nausea, vomiting, fever, blood in bowel movements, mucus, or abrupt change in bowel habits. She said no, and that she also had looked for a pattern to it and found none. She'd tried to relate it to what she ate, but this didn't seem to have anything to do with it either.

I then asked about the fungus infection on her feet, the yellow brown crusted sores in her nose, and the vaginal yeast infection. Since the "immediate cause" of these problems, infectious germs of several types, was fairly obvious, what I wanted to know was when they had started. She repeated that the yeast infection had begun about a year before, the nasal sores about six months ago, and the fungus about six months ago, also.

At this point she looked quite puzzled, "You don't think this is all the same problem, do you," she asked. "I talked to my other doctor about some of this, and he didn't think so. Is it serious?"

I thought by now I'd looked around enough before leaping, and the mention of her other physician seemed a final clue. So I asked her if she'd been taking any medicine she hadn't mentioned. (I should have noted that this was the first time Mrs. Bing had come to the office for herself. She'd brought her children in before, but I'd no records yet for her.)

"Why, yes," she replied. "But I thought it wasn't important because my other doctor, who's a urology specialist, has been taking care of it. He's had me taking penicillin for a year for a kidney infection." She paused and looked up. "Could that have anything to do with it?"

I told her it probably did. However, of course, I wanted to examine her first.

Her pelvic exam was normal except for the presence of a yeast infection. (Microscopic examination confirmed this.)

The skin between her toes was cracked and red. There was a slight yellowish cast to the adjacent skin. This appeared to be, as she had said, fungal.

The sores inside her nose, as previously described, were yellow brown crusted, cracked, and inflamed. The appearance was typical for infection with staphylococcal bacteria. That wasn't a surprise. Likewise, her fingers and toes (aside from the fungus) showed nothing visible to account for the numbness and tingling.

So we concluded the examination, and went back to my office from the examination room.

Mrs. Bing immediately asked, once more, if I thought the penicillin might be causing the trouble. When I said yes, she appeared skeptical: "I never heard of a penicillin reaction like that." So I asked if she was aware of "normal body bacteria." She said she was. So I pointed out that this was not a direct penicillin reaction, but an indirect series of associated results from the penicillin. Symptom-by-symptom, it worked this way:

1. *The recurrent yeast infection.* The main thing that prevents women from having yeast infections *all* the time is a healthy vaginal area. A key part of this normal health is the presence of normal bacteria in the vagina. Penicillin kills these in many women, and they usually don't return on their own. So unless the bacteria are replaced, yeast just keeps coming back.

2. *The staph infection in her nose.* Most normal intranasal bacteria don't cause infections. However, penicillin kills many of them off, and then "abnormal" bacteria, such as staphylococci, will get a foothold. As it is penicillin-resistant, it will continue to grow despite continued penicillin.

3. *The toe fungus.* Once more, the absence of normal bacteria will cause increased susceptibility to fungus.

4. *Intestinal cramps.* Naturally, there are normal bacteria present in the intestine, particularly the colon. When the normal bacteria are killed by penicillin and replaced to varying degrees by penicillin-resistant germs, a variety of unusual symptoms may happen. In small children, diarrhea frequently occurs. In adults often there are no symptoms. In her case, though, it was likely the cause of the cramps.

5. *Variable numbness in the fingers and toes.* Here, I didn't think the problem was due to absent bacteria on the fingers and toes. It sounded more like a problem with B vitamin metabolism. Although I couldn't be positive, I suspected it was due to lack of production of small but crucial amounts of vitamins by the missing normal intesti-

nal bacteria, or to interference with normal B vitamin absorption by penicillin. This is known to happen with vitamin B_{12} and folic acid, and suspected with other vitamins. Either way, something could be done about it.

"Well," Mrs. Bing said thoughtfully, "that certainly seems logical. But what am I to do about it all? Should I stop taking the penicillin? What will my urologist say? What about my kidney infection? I just don't know."

As we'd already run overtime, and there were others waiting, I told Mrs. Bing it would be best if we made another appointment time to go over all this. Also, I said I would call her urologist in the meantime and discuss the situation with him. She said that it seemed reasonable, and promised to return.

During the time before she returned, I telephoned her urologist. As I expected, he told me that what I explained couldn't be true. He'd never heard of penicillin causing any such thing. He even sounded as if he was angry with Mrs. Bing for bringing up the matter of her treatment. "But," said Dr. ———, "if it hasn't helped her kidney infection in a year, it's probably not going to, so she might as well stop it anyway." I thought that this had probably been the case ten months ago, but didn't mention it as the conversation wasn't all that friendly anyway.

At her next visit, Mrs. Bing seemed a bit more cheerful. She'd called her urologist also, and his nurse had advised that she stop the penicillin. So she'd already done so. As her back pains—attributed to the kidney infection—seemed unchanged, she'd decided the penicillin really made no difference. Besides, she was anxious to get rid of the rest of her symptoms.

I advised her that since the staph infection and toe fungus had taken firm hold, it would be necessary for her to use ointment-type medications to get rid of them. Logically enough, she asked if that wouldn't interfere with normal body germs too. I agreed it would, but only temporarily. As soon as these specific germs were gone, the medications should be stopped. Normal skin bacteria would return on their own, either from other areas of her body, or by simple contact transmission, as they pass from one person to another easily.

However, the bacteria in the colon and vaginal areas would

actually need replacement. When I mentioned this, Mrs. Bing seemed very surprised. "You mean you want me to eat germs on purpose?" she said. "That doesn't sound too good!"

So I asked if she hadn't ever had buttermilk or yogurt. "Oh, yes . . . I guess those are made with germs, aren't they?" Mrs. Bing replied. "So do I just get those?"

I reminded her that most commercial dairy products are pasteurized and that this kills the bacteria. What were needed were live bacteria. She could get these at a health food store, usually under the name *Lactobacillus acidophilus.* Two or three tablespoons of this for a week to ten days should be just enough. Or, she could get them at the drugstore as Lactinex tablets. Three or four tablets with each meal for the same length of time should also replace the normal intestinal bacteria sufficiently.

"Will this take care of the yeast infection, too?" she wondered. I reminded her that the problem here had two parts: First, getting rid of the yeast, and then replacing the normal bacteria.

(As mentioned before, the bacteria usually considered to be normal for the vaginal area, called Döderlein's bacillus, is not commercially available. However, *Lactobacillus acidophilus,* the bacteria mentioned above, is a good substitute and is widely available.)

First, she would have to use another anti-yeast medication for ten days. "Oh dear," Mrs. Bing looked disappointed. "I'd hoped I was done with those." I replied that this would probably be her last one for a long, long time if all went as usual.

After finishing with the anti-yeast medication, she would need to mix approximately ½ cup of plain yogurt and 2 tablespoons of *Lactobacillus acidophilus* powder. A part of this mixture should then be used for each treatment. It should be kept in the refrigerator. I told her she should use about 2 teaspoons of this mixture inserted just like the medicine for 5 nights in a row. In the morning, it would be best to use a water and vinegar douche.

Of course, Mrs. Bing had lots of questions. "What's the yogurt for? How do I get the mixture in? Do I have to use the douche? What if my menstrual period arrives? And what will my husband think?"

I answered that it was best to use the medication first, and then the yogurt and bacteria together without interruption. So, if her menstrual period was due soon, it would be best to wait.

The douche was partly because the treatment was messy. But just as important, the vinegar's slight acidity inhibits yeast growth, and promotes the growth of the *Lactobacillus acidophilus*.

The yogurt is a good bacterial growth material. It helps make the mixture a little more sticky so the bacteria would stay in place long enough to grow in the vagina. Also, by itself, it's soothing.

Inserting the mixture could be done with the medication applicator or a tampon applicator. Perhaps a syringe with the end cut off would do. This problem could always be overcome.

As for the last question, I replied: "I don't know what your husband will think. But tell him to wait until after the yeast infection is finally gone, and then decide."

"Well," Mrs. Bing answered. "I guess all that will keep me busy for a while!" Gathering up her prescriptions and direction notes, she left the office. But 30 seconds later, she was back. "We forgot! What about my numbness? And my kidney infection?"

I answered that I thought the numbness would clear up on its own after the normal intestinal bacteria were replaced. As for the kidney infection, if her back pain didn't change much, then I wanted her to check back in a few weeks to look into this further.

Nearly six weeks later, Mrs. Bing returned. Her back pains were no worse, but as they'd not improved, she thought she'd try again to find out what the problem was.

Of course, I asked how many of her "minor problems" remained. "You know, I couldn't believe it," she said. "Every single one of those other problems is gone. I never thought the answer was as simple as that!"

Body Ecology and How We Unwittingly Damage It

Even though we don't spend much time thinking about it, all of us spend our entire lives in close contact with a wide variety of invisible-to-the-eye microorganisms, known to all of us since childhood as "germs." Both bacterial and viral, they live on our surfaces, in our insides, and sometimes right in our tissues.

Before this becomes too nauseating a thought, and we all start to reach for our cans of germ killer, we need to remember what our elementary school science teachers told us: the vast majority of these little beasties are beneficial, doing us no harm and in fact much good.

For example, the most-studied friendly bacteria, those that reside in the intestine, help to break down certain sugars and produce small quantities of vitamins. Without these little helpers, we'd all be in big trouble.

That kind of cooperation, of course, isn't unique to humans, but is just part of the overall natural scheme. All larger living things have working relationships with a variety of microorganisms. And the microorganisms have many interrelationships with each other.

Naturally, there are a very few of these germs that cause us a lot of trouble. Some names, like "staph" and "strep" are so frequently associated with disease that they've become household words. (Please note, I said "associated with" disease, not necessarily "causative of." More about that later.)

Antibiotics, killers of some of these bothersome germs, have become some of the most widely used drugs of the past four decades. Hailed as one of modern medical science's most spectacular advances, the use of antibiotics has been said to be the major contributor to modern medicine's conquest of disease.

Anyone who's had a grandmother saved from dying of pneumonia, or a child rescued from serious infection with antibiotics, has reason to be grateful. Most hospitals couldn't exist without them. Along with my advocacy of nutritional/biochemical means, I employ antibiotics when necessary.

In another, more important way, antibiotic therapy and its success has been detrimental to real progress in medicine. Antibiotics should really be used much like fire extinguishers, to put out acute emergencies. The need for them should be rare; most of our effort should be going into "fire prevention"—preventing the infections from happening in the first place.

Medicine's present use of antibiotics is exactly analogous to a fireman dashing from fire to fire, an extinguisher in each hand, stopping at one after another, and foolishly ignoring most of the factors involved in preventing the outbreaks. Yet any modern fire department emphasizes that preventing fires is more efficient and productive of less damage than dousing them.

In my office, any person who comes in with more than a very occasional infection is invited to discuss what the underlying problem might be. In my internship-residency days I saw many children come in repeatedly, all winter, with "another earache, another bronchitis." Or adults who "just kept catching things." The routine was to prescribe another antibiotic and hope for the best.

Except in very unusual circumstances, that just doesn't happen in nutritional/biochemical practice. Recurrent infections can be stopped.

But back to antibiotics. In a way, antibiotic overuse is exactly analogous to the overuse of pesticides and herbicides in agriculture. The very same sorts of problems can be produced. We're slowly learning that drenching our crops with poisonous chemicals kills not only the unwanted pests, but quite a lot of valuable insect and bird life right along with them. In some areas, honeybees, so valuable to the pollination of crops, are in dangerously short supply.

In some human beings, antibiotics have killed off so many of their beneficial bacteria that important functions aren't taking place, or are working only marginally. In many ways, antibiotics are "pesticides for human use." While they're cleared for safety by the various drug authorities, this is only short-term safety, making sure that they're not directly poisonous or toxic. The ecological implications aren't considered. Truly, an "environmental impact statement" for any antibiotic would be disastrous.

Mrs. Bing's case was an excellent example of a typical "environmental impact" of penicillin. I won't go back into the details; suffice it to say that even if you don't take penicillin or any other antibiotic for a year, all of these effects still happen, albeit briefly. Before this case is dismissed as untypical, remind yourself of another very widespread example of long-term antibiotic use: treatment for acne. I don't know how many teenagers and young adults I've had to take off antibiotics they were given for acne as the ecological disruption started to appear.

Now, let's take a look at another controversy for a moment: do germs really cause disease?

Of course they do, you say. My doctor says they do; I've had strep throat, or "Hong-Kong" flu virus. If that wasn't a germ, what was it?

Then why is it that a room full of people can be exposed to an infectious germ, but not all of them get it?

Sometimes everyone in a family gets a cold, but not always. Why doesn't everyone who's exposed become ill?

Just luck, you say? More likely, you'd say the exposed-but-not-ill person has more "resistance."

There's the key to the problem. What's this *resistance* that some have, and some lack? Obviously, all the factors in resistance aren't known, or they'd (hopefully) be more widely applied. But it's the opinion of many experts in preventive medicine and nutritional biochemistry that factors of both heredity and environment are important.

It's my opinion that a major factor is the dietary environment. From clinical experience, it's perfectly clear to me that food allergy, particularly in children (as well as inhalant allergies), is a major factor. So is improper diet, including refined sugar, refined carbohydrates, and various vitamin and mineral insufficiencies.

If germs were the sole cause of infectious disease, then altering the above factors, eliminating allergy, cleaning up and supplementing the diet would make no difference. The same germs still would be out there waiting to leap onto the same individual, and infect him or her just as much as before.

With proper attention to nutrition and biochemistry, it usually doesn't happen.

Certainly proliferation of harmful germs is *associated* with infectious disease. But they're only the last or most noticeable manifestation of an underlying biochemical problem. A seed will only grow well in the right soil; likewise infection will only spread under the right circumstances for its growth.

Modern medical science has been lulled for too long by the apparent success of antibiotic therapy. The time is long overdue to get back to the fundamentals of infection prevention, which can only be done through overall health improvement.

Severely impaired ability to absorb nutrients is rare, but a slight to moderate impairment of absorption is more common than most people realize. As we grow older, the chances of developing such an impairment increase significantly. It's possible that nearly half of all senior citizens have this problem, which, if undetected, can negate much of the effect of dietary improvement. . . . Causes, diagnosis, therapy—and cautions—are discussed.

Poor Absorption 45

"I took zinc for my skin condition, but it didn't do any good at all."

"I've been eating a good healthy diet for ten years, and I still don't feel good."

"My doctor says my osteoporosis is getting worse. I don't understand it, because I've been taking calcium, bone meal, and dolomite for six years."

These statements, and others like them, are unfortunately frequent among those who have tried to better their health by dietary improvement and supplementation. You not only have to eat a good diet, vitamins, and minerals, but you also have to *absorb* them to get their full advantage.

Every day at the office, I see people whose health problems trace mostly back to faulty digestion and absorption of nutrients, particularly minerals, but often other nutrients as well. Occasionally, the number will go as high as seven or eight persons a day. Of course, my viewpoint about the frequency of "poor absorption" problems may be distorted by my occupation; people whose nutrient absorption is good (and who are eating good foods) are much less likely to need to visit a doctor's office. Even so, health problems tracing back to this cause are among the most frequently seen in nutritional medicine.

Faulty absorption of nutrients is described in standard medical textbooks under the general heading of "malabsorption syndrome." That diagnosis is considered to be a relatively rare one; symptoms usually have to be severe for the diagnosis to be made.

The "textbook" type of malabsorption syndrome is not the same as the common forms of nutrient malabsorption described below. These are much more common, milder versions with chronic, insidious effects and many fewer symptoms. In some cases, there are no specific symptoms at all. Because of this, many digestive-absorptive problems are not recognized by those who have them. So they can continue for years, with possibly serious results which are never related to the unrecognized absorptive problem.

If you are on a good diet, taking what appear to be the right supplements for you, and you're still not doing well, absorption may be the problem.

Chronic, excessive intestinal gas is probably the most frequent symptom of absorptive problems. Many are troubled with chronic constipation; fewer have a low-grade diarrhea. If you don't feel like it's digesting when you eat quantities of meat, you probably have a problem. The frequent appearance of a variety of undigested foods in bowel movements is of course an excellent clue. Many persons "bloat" after meals.

As we all get older, the chance of poor digestion-absorption increases. Particularly after age 60, it's extremely common. Some estimates have gone as high as 40 to 50 percent of all those past that age.

I should note, though, that youth is no guarantee of good digestion and absorption. I have records of over 50 children under the age of 3 who definitely have problems with nutrient absorption. As mentioned, some people have no symptoms of absorptive difficulties, particularly in the early stages. How can these be found?

One way is with mineral analysis of a specimen of hair. Hair analyses are available without seeing a doctor (even though for proper interpretation, this isn't always a good idea).

Most mineral analysis companies include roughly the same group of minerals, including the following: calcium, magnesium, iron, copper, manganese, zinc, chromium, and selenium. If five of this group are low, I suspect poor nutrient absorption. If six or more are low, then it's highly probable.

By far the most frequent cause of poor absorption is a lack of sufficient stomach acid production. A total lack of stomach acid (achlorhydria) is very rare, but an insufficient quantity—a relative lack—of stomach acid (hypochlorhydria) is quite common (see Goodman and Gilman). Apparently, having enough stomach acid is important to the absorption of all minerals except sodium, potassium, and lithium. For example, I've seen any number of older persons show no improvement or only marginal improvement of hair tests for calcium, iron, or magnesium, despite taking relatively large quantities, until it was discovered they suffered from hypochlorhydria. Upon correction of this problem, their minerals were much better absorbed. The same applies to other minerals.

The most useful tool for accurate diagnosis of hypochlorhydria at present appears to be radiotelemetry. This test uses a small plastic-enclosed, battery-operated, pH-sensitive radio transmitter, which is swallowed. Once in the stomach, it radios out to a recorder the pH (degree of acidity or alkalinity) of the surrounding fluids. Using a variety of challenge and stimulation tests, it is possible to diagnose hypochlorhydria with a much higher degree of accuracy.

Another frequent cause of poor nutrient absorption is a lack of pancreatic digestive enzymes. If you have less than optimal digestion, it's easy to guess if this is the cause. There are many digestive enzyme preparations sold without prescription. As there are no known hazards in taking them, except allergy, they can safely be tried. If the symptoms are corrected, this is quite likely the problem. However, deficiency of pancreatic enzymes often is related to lack of stomach acid. So taking enzymes and correctly interpreting what happens is not always as simple as it first appears.

A third cause of poor nutrient absorption is chronic, undetected food allergy. There are ways of detecting this on your own—fasting and pulse testing being two—but this is frequently a sufficiently involved problem to require professional guidance.

If you have a lack of sufficient stomach acid, heavy protein meals may not digest properly. Most minerals are suboptimally absorbed. The consequences of this are incredibly variable. They depend on which minerals are most poorly absorbed and the long-term consequences of a lack of that mineral. Also, the need of each individual for each mineral varies. That's why it's nearly impossible to predict exactly what else will go wrong with the health of a person with hypochlorhydria, if the condition persists. The only thing definitely predictable is that anyone with hypochlorhydria will have health problems of some kind long before he or she would have had if absorbing nutrients properly.

Pancreatic enzymes are concerned with the digestion of carbohydrates, fats, and proteins, as well as fat-soluble vitamins A, D, E, and K. With this wide range of digestive functions, it's once again impossible to say exactly what will go wrong if the enzyme deficiency persists.

This is where preventive rather than curative medicine is definitely important. Instead of waiting to find out what the disease will be, subsequent to poor digestion and absorption, it's best to stop whatever it may be before it happens.

It is not known how safely and reliably to induce a stomach to produce more acid on its own. The solution to this problem at present is taking hydrochloric acid supplements. If you have a symptom such as excess gas or indigestion that is correctable with acid supplementation, it is usually safe to take enough to correct the symptom, and no more.

I usually recommend taking betaine hydrochloride or glutamic acid hydrochloride tablets, available from most health food stores. On three consecutive mornings take 1, then 2, then 3 on an empty stomach. If you have no bad reactions, then take 1 or 2 before each meal for a week, and see how your digestion feels. If it's better, we can safely assume that your stomach hasn't been producing enough acid for proper digestion.

A bad reaction is anything that feels bad. Heartburn, worse gas, pain in the stomach—anything. If it hurts, don't take any more. Neutralize the reaction with milk or baking soda in water. Remember too, that aspirin or aspirin-containing compounds, or "anti-inflammatory" drugs such as Indocin, Butazolidin, or cortisone should never be taken when hydrochloric acid is being taken (or vice versa). The risk of ulcer becomes much greater.

Several years' experience with hundreds of patients with hypochlorhydria has shown me that the dose of betaine hydrochloride or glutamic acid hydrochloride needed for gastric acid replacement is highly variable. A few persons require as little as 5 to 10 grains; others need 50 to 60 grains. The right dose can be estimated, but has to be finally adjusted by trial and error.

The necessary dose cannot be found just by relief of digestive symptoms such as gas, constipation, bloating, or just not digesting. Frequently these symptoms are alleviated by less of a dose than it takes to substantially improve generally low mineral levels. Therefore, I follow mineral analyses at roughly six-month intervals until "normalization" is achieved.

I consider the correct dose to be that which improves nutrient absorption significantly, not the symptom-relief dose. As mentioned earlier, there are a few who have no physical symptoms but in whom testing reveals hypochlorhydria or occasionally achlorhydria. I have no explanation for this.

The combination of mineral analysis and radiotelemetric testing is invaluable in the management of hypochlorhydria.

More than half the time, persons who have digestion-absorption problems, from whatever cause, cannot absorb vitamin B_{12} from food or from supplemental tablets. Even if the problem is corrected by acid or enzyme supplementation, or removal of allergenic foods, a series of vitamin B_{12} injections usually helps to improve symptoms. That is particularly applicable to "nonspecific" nervous system symptoms, such as tiredness, anxiety, or depression. Folic acid should be taken at the same time.

It should be noted that this procedure is helpful at times

even when blood tests for vitamin B_{12} are reported as normal.

I'd like to digress for a moment to say a few words about clinical testing of nutritional therapies. In large population group studies, nutritional therapies frequently give disappointing or highly varying results. I've very rarely read in such studies that the digestive and absorptive capabilities of the persons tested have been verified as optimum or at least good—especially in older persons, where poor absorption is frequent. This is very important. If a supplement is not absorbed, it won't work. As far as I'm concerned, any clinical test of nutritional therapy that ignores this factor is just not accurate and might as well not be done.

Suboptimal nutrient absorption is a much more frequent problem than is generally realized; its frequency increases with age. It is also likely (although there is no proof) that with increasing consumption of unnatural foods, the condition—much like cardiovascular diseases, diabetes, cancer, and other "diseases of civilization"—will become increasingly prevalent.

FURTHER READING

Bray, George W. "The Hypochlorhydria of Asthma in Childhood." *Quarterly Journal of Medicine*, January 1931, pp. 181–97.

Goodman, Louis S., and Gilman, Alfred. "Digestants; Hydrochloric Acid." *The Pharmacological Basis of Therapeutics*, 5th ed. (New York: Macmillan, 1975), pp. 970–71.

Montgomery, R. D. et al. "The Aging Gut: A Study of Intestinal Absorption in Relation to Nutrition in the Elderly." *Quarterly Journal of Medicine*, vol. 47, no. 186, April 1978, pp. 197–211.

A general discussion of the role of food allergy in health problems. Specifically discussed are self-testing methods, medical testing methods, adverse reactions to food which are not allergic in nature, and a note on food chemicals. Six books for further reading are listed.

A Look at Food Allergy 46

You don't eat junk food. It's been years since you had any refined sugar or white flours; instead it's honey and whole grains.

You're reasonably sure your food is being digested and absorbed properly. You don't get gas or stomach upset when you eat; there's no chronic diarrhea or constipation. You've never seen any evidence of undigested food.

So, now you can relax, eat good food, apply other self-care measures such as exercise and mental attitude techniques, and stay healthy, right?

Obviously if you've come this far, you must suspect there may be another health hazard in nutrition lurking about somewhere, and you're right.

As stated in a recent textbook, *Basics of Food Allergy* by J. C. Breneman, "food allergy can do anything to any part of the body." This is just another way of saying that practically any symptom ever experienced could be caused by food allergy. Of course a disclaimer should be entered at once: not all symptoms of all diseases are allergy caused. Instead, it's simply necessary to keep alert to the possibility that food allergy may be involved in just about any disease.

This same textbook contains a brief outline of "common manifestations of food allergies." These include the familiar itching, asthma, hives, and eczema that most of us associate with allergy. But the list also includes arthritis, bursitis, low back pain, fainting, bronchiolitis, sinusitis, bladder infections, kidney failure (nephrosis), canker sores, ulcers, hypoglycemia, colitis, gallbladder disease (including stones), malabsorption, diabetes, epilepsy, headaches, schizophrenia, tension-fatigue syndrome, and learning disabilities!

Remember this is a list of health problems commonly associated with food allergy. As I mentioned, the list of symptoms that can be caused by food allergy, even if uncommon, is practically endless.

Self-Testing Methods

There is a long list of methods for determination of food allergies. Most of them require professional help, particularly in finding exactly which foods are "trouble." There are self-diagnosis methods, though, so let's start with those.

First, it is necessary to find out whether food allergy in general is causing symptoms before trying to identify particular allergens. The simplest way to find out whether food is a culprit is, of course, not eating, or fasting.

A word of caution: fasting is not for everyone. Some of us just cannot stand the stress. For example, persons with severe hypoglycemia, or who are underweight, or those with chronic illness should not fast. As these health problems might be caused by allergy, allergy testing could still be worthwhile, but probably should be done by some other means. If you have any question about being able to go on a fast, you should check with your physician.

Most physicians who work with fasting as a means of food allergy diagnosis have observed that symptoms frequently get worse during the first, second, and even into the third day of fasting. Usually, if the symptoms are due to food allergy, they'll be gone by the fourth and fifth days.

If you're careful, and lucky, by carefully reintroducing foods into your diet one at a time, at intervals of several hours, you may be able to identify which foods are causing which problems. Unfortunately, some foods don't react right away; wheat is notorious for delayed reactions of two to three days. Pork is another example; joint pains caused by pork allergy can take five days to appear, according to Dr. Breneman.

So, for identifying food allergy in general as a problem, fasting on your own can be very helpful. For specific food identification, professional help is probably wise.

Two other points about fasting: of course drinking water should be continued. I usually recommend distilled water, as a small percentage of us react to the various additives in tap water. Second, some have greater success with single-food fasting, whether for physical or psychological reasons. This is done by just eating one food for the test period. Hopefully, the food chosen isn't an allergic one, or nothing will be learned. Don't pick your favorite food; experience has shown this is frequently the worst allergy offender.

Another self-testing system for diagnosis of food allergy that works extremely well for some is pulse testing. Simply stated, allergic foods may cause an increased pulse. If this was the case with everyone, it would put a lot of allergists out of work, but it doesn't apply that uniformly.

The pulse-testing system was worked out by Arthur F. Coca, M.D., a prominent allergist/immunologist. In his book *The Pulse Test: The Secret of Building Your Health,* Dr. Coca describes his finding that many allergic individuals have a pulse elevation after eating foods to which they are allergic. He outlines a method of self-testing for these food allergies. The major drawback is that it takes considerable time and effort, as does fasting.

Other Testing Methods

Traditionally, skin tests have been used by some clinicians

for allergy diagnosis. While skin tests are very helpful for inhalant allergies (pollen, dust, etc.), they are useless for the diagnosis of food allergy. As I am an "allergist by necessity" and not by professional specialty training, I'll quote Dr. Breneman, whose credentials are impeccable (and of course, whose opinion I share): ". . . skin tests for the diagnosis of food allergy are so unreliable that most clinicians use them very little."

Presently, I make considerable use of a blood test for food allergies. While it is relatively new, I've found that the clinical results are excellent. Technically entitled the "radioallergosorbent" method or RAST, it involves the detection of antibodies to specific foods in the serum fraction of the blood.

If you're allergic to something, your system usually produces antibodies to help fight off the offending allergen. Even after the allergen is gone, antibodies circulate in your blood for months.

The RAST test concept is simple: the test blood serum is exposed to specific food antigens. If the serum does not contain antibodies to that food antigen, no reaction will take place. If a reaction does occur, its relative strength can be measured. That way the test can determine which foods you're allergic to, and how badly.

Like most other tests, there is a caution with this one: There are certain types of allergic reaction that it won't detect; it can't be considered foolproof.

Some physicians use cytotoxic testing. In this test, white blood cells are exposed to food antigen solutions, and disintegrate more readily if there is allergy. When done by well-trained individuals, this test may be very helpful.

Another relatively new system, applied by some chiropractors and a few D.O.'s and M.D.'s, uses kinesiology. While kinesiology is at present not generally accepted, I have seen a few remarkable results with its use.

Obviously, there are many testing systems. None is so universally superior as to recommend it for everyone under all circumstances. Allergy determination is an area where frequently the ability and judgment of the person doing the testing is just as important as the type of test employed.

What to Do

If you find that you are allergic to a specific food or foods, the most effective treatment is not to eat it. That is far and away preferable to any other treatment system. Despite the considerable life disturbance that this can cause, once alternative foods are found, the symptom relief is usually worth it. Disruption caused by changing eating patterns is usually temporary.

For those with an overwhelming number of food allergies, allergy desensitization is worth trying. Although this sometimes works well, other times it doesn't work at all. There isn't any way to tell in advance about the chances of success. (A useful book in the care of overwhelming allergy problems is *Management of Complex Allergies* by Natalie Golos.)

Persons who haven't done so already frequently find that "cleaning up" the diet—getting rid of junk food, especially refined sugar, artificial flavors, colors, and preservatives, and adding in vitamin/mineral supplements—frequently cuts down on allergy symptoms. Vitamin C and the B complex are especially helpful. However, since we're discussing food allergy here, I should say once again that avoidance of the food(s) involved is the best solution.

Nonallergic Food Reactions

Some bad reactions to food aren't allergy. A good example would be poisonous mushrooms: this isn't allergy, but toxicity. The difference is that poisons or toxins usually function by interfering with chemical processes within each body cell. If the interference is bad enough the cell dies.

Unfortunately some toxically reacting foods are insidious, taking literally years to produce their bad effects. The result is frequently not death, but chronic disability.

The most recently identified and spectacular discovery in this area is that of nightshade-caused arthritis. The foods involved here are tomato, potato, pepper, eggplant, and the nonfood, tobacco. According to Professor Norman Childers of Rutgers University, for some people these are "slow poisons." Before we all stop eating tomatoes, it should be emphasized that just as with food allergy, nightshade sensitivity is an individual matter. A few of us are sensitive; most are not. This underlines the old principle that nutrition is a highly individual matter.

As nutrition research accelerates, most likely other toxic reactions to some foods for some people will be found.

Food Chemicals

Obviously, I'm in favor of the total elimination of artificial flavors, colors, and preservatives as rapidly as possible. The more they're investigated, the more they're found to be potentially toxic.

What isn't generally recognized is that the above substances, and also a whole host of other food chemicals—insecticide sprays, antibiotic feed additives, antifungal seed treatments, to name only a few—can be the source of both toxic and allergic reactions that are extremely difficult to detect. (For further discussion, see *Human Ecology and Susceptibility to the Chemical Environment* by Theron G. Randolph, M.D.)

In Conclusion

Even the best health food diet isn't good and safe for everyone. If you're on such a diet and still not well, allergy might be the cause. Food allergy is the cause of an incredible diversity of symptoms; it must be considered as part of the evaluation of any health problem of unknown origin.

FURTHER READING

Breneman, J. C. *Basics of Food Allergy* (Springfield, Ill.: Charles C Thomas, 1978).

Childers, Norman Franklin, and Russo, Gerard M. *The Nightshades and Health* (Somerville, N.J.: Horticultural Publications, Somerset Press, 1977).

Coca, Arthur F. *The Pulse Test: The Secret of Building Your Health* (New York: Lyle Stuart, 1967).

Dickey, Lawrence D., ed. *Clinical Ecology* (Springfield, Ill.: Charles C Thomas, 1976).

Golos, Natalie. *Management of Complex Allergies.* HEAL, Suite 6506, 505 North Lake Shore Drive, Chicago, IL 60611.

Randolph, Theron G. *Human Ecology and Susceptibility to the Chemical Environment* (Springfield, Ill.: Charles C Thomas, 1962).

47 You Can Keep Yourself Healthy

The most important person involved in keeping yourself healthy is you. Only you have the capability of knowing how you feel, 24 hours a day. You're the first to know when something is going wrong; you're first to know when you're feeling well.

Staying healthy involves some work. Certainly, many people wait for illness to arrive before paying any attention to health, noticing health only when it's absent; as our grandparents would say, locking the barn door once the horse is gone.

Taking care of your health is really not as hard as it might seem. If you're not actively involved in staying healthy already, it probably will take considerable effort to get organized. Like any other new enterprise, getting started can be a chore. But once you've invested the initial time and effort, the job of keeping yourself healthy should run smoothly, requiring only a little extra effort from time to time.

Is it worth it? Ask anyone whose health isn't good. Despite all the marvelous advances of modern scientific medicine, organ transplants, wonder drugs, antibiotics, and vastly improved diagnostic techniques, avoiding all of these through the help of preventive measures is still preferable.

There's more to keeping good health than good nutrition. Picking healthy ancestors is a help. So is exercise, enough sleep, sunshine, a proper balance of work and relaxation, a healthy mental attitude. Don't wait for someone to tell you what to do about these things: investigate on your own. But since this is obviously a book concerned with nutrition, I'll leave advice on those topics to more qualified experts, and try to help you with the nutritional aspects of staying healthy.

Excellent nutrition is extremely important to staying healthy. After all, the raw material of which your physical body is made is obtained entirely from what you eat and drink. When you're building a home, you want the highest quality materials you can afford. Why should you build and maintain your body with anything less? Would you purposefully erect your home with junk?

Good Health Requires Good Water

I've not said much in this book about water. But your body contains from 50 to 75 percent water, so let's spend a little time considering this important body component.

If you're like most people, you don't really know what's in the water you're drinking. (If you do, skip this section!) Actually, most of us have had no particular reason to spend much time thinking about it. Just turn on the faucet and there it is. Quick, easy, effortless. What could be more harmless?

Now, let's picture early man for a moment. In whatever environment, forest, desert, grassland, mountain, or jungle, he didn't just step around the nearest tree and open a spigot. His sources were rain or various forms of groundwater. Most of the time, a few traces of minerals such as calcium or magnesium might have been present, or a few "organic" contaminants. Except in isolated instances, man over thousands of generations has been well adapted to these naturally occurring, accidental additives. In fact, much of the time, they're beneficial. There's considerable evidence, for example, that "hard" (mineral-containing) waters are associated with less death from cardiovascular disease.

But as humans increased in numbers and congregated in cities, just wandering down to the river for a drink, using a common well or pump, or even a common piping system became more and more hazardous. From time to time, mysterious epidemics of diseases such as cholera would break out. Early public health authorities traced some epidemics directly back to contaminated public water supplies. Unfortunately, along with the growth of cities came problems with disposal of human wastes, which most frequently were the source of contamination.

As knowledge of the association between microorganisms and certain diseases grew, particularly in the latter nineteenth and early twentieth centuries, public health authorities began to add chlorine to public water supplies, as a germ-killing disinfectant.

Public water chlorination for prevention of infectious illness has been extremely successful. The number of acute infectious disease cases and deaths from waterborne sources has been drastically reduced.

Unfortunately, the long-term effects of chronic exposure to chlorine in the water supply have scarcely been investigated. Reasoning from principles of natural adaptation, it can be predicted that there might be adverse metabolic effects from even the small amounts of chlorine present in public water. The explanation for this prediction is simple. First, the chlorine in water combines very easily with various living organic substances, including bacteria. This is, of course, the basis for chlorine's germ-killing action. During such combinations new organic compounds are formed, including chloroform. (The chlorine added to water is chemically different from chloride found in sodium chloride or salt.)

Second, human beings have not been exposed to even the supposedly "nontoxic" levels of chlorine found in public water supplies for even one hundred years. Water for millions of years has been chlorine-free.

So going back to the basic premise that any chemical molecule that humans have not adapted to for millions of years is more likely than not to be harmful if introduced into the body, and combining this with relatively modern knowledge of chlorine's high degree of reactivity, it could be harmful.

There is a very small amount of animal research indicating that in fact this is so. But this research is not conclusive; much more work needs to be done.

It's been argued that chlorine in water is in such small amounts it "couldn't possibly" be harmful. True, it's not acutely toxic, but chlorine is in fact poisonous in larger quantities. There's at least the possibility that sublethal quantities over a long time could be metabolically toxic.

No, I'm not saying there shouldn't be chlorine in public water; I'm just as bothered as any public health authority by the possibility of waterborne disease epidemics. Ideally, though, I'd like to see chlorination replaced by safer disinfecting methods such as filtration, exposure to ultraviolet light, or other less potentially toxic means (with of course, consideration of potential long-term problems from these means, also).

In the meantime, chlorination is a necessary evil in public water. But that doesn't mean it has to be in you. For good health, for the reasons cited above, it shouldn't be.

Chlorine isn't the only potentially harmful substance in water. As environmental studies have become more prevalent, reports have been released showing a variety of synthetic chemicals and other substances of industrial origin in varying amounts in different areas of the country. Asbestos has been found in some; potentially cancer-causing chemicals in others. Of course, some water supplies have been relatively clean.

Last, there's the hotly debated topic of fluoridation of public water. I'll confine my remarks here to the same observations I made about chlorine: Fluoride is a highly reactive chemical (in fact, in the same family as chlorine), and there needs to be more study of potential risk.

What of fluoride and tooth decay? There are better ways of preventing tooth decay. In a long-neglected study, Dr. Weston A. Price, a dentist, demonstrated that certain primitive people kept tooth decay at zero or close to it without one speck of added fluoride. Close study showed this to be due to good diet. *(Nutri-*

tion and Physical Degeneration: A Comparison of Primitive and Modern Diets and Their Effects.°)

Now, back to taking care of your health. For the reasons noted above, I don't think it's wise to expose yourself to the unnecessary risk of chlorine, fluoride, and other miscellaneous chemicals in your water supply. On balance, the risks, even if small, outweigh the possible benefits from the good minerals found in some public water. (These minerals, principally calcium and magnesium, have been in groundwater drunk by humans for millions of years. Only in very isolated instances have naturally occurring waterborne minerals been found to be toxic.)

If you have your own well water, you can have it tested to see if it's reasonably safe. If not, the only presently practical means of obtaining reasonably pure water are using bottled water of known composition, distilled water, or distilling tap water at your own home. Obviously, only water that you or your family consume needs to be distilled or otherwise free of chemicals; for other uses it doesn't matter. Of course, when not at home, an occasional glass of impure water is to be expected.

Two other water problems: some historians think that the ancient Romans were poisoned by lead from water pipes and other water containers. Many modern preventive and nutritional physicians point to extremely high levels of copper found on mineral analysis of a small percentage of individuals. Most often, the source of this copper is water piping. It's not known why most persons tolerate waterborne copper well, while a few accumulate large excesses.

Copper is an essential mineral, but at high levels it can be toxic. Among my patients, high levels of copper are most frequently found in hyperactive children, very moody or emotional teenage girls, and in women with relatively severe premenstrual mental/emotional problems. Dr. Carl Pfeiffer has linked high levels of copper with certain types of schizophrenia. Bottled water or distilled water will eliminate this potential problem.

The remaining water question is, of course: What about the

° Books mentioned in this chapter will be found under the appropriate headings in chapter 49, "A Resource Guide to Nutritional and Natural Therapy."

beneficial minerals? Some bottled waters contain them, but distilled water is mineral-free.

The best-known beneficial minerals are calcium and magnesium. As for the more minor trace minerals, other natural sources such as kelp or alfalfa will take care of whatever might be found in water.

Is water really that important? Does it really make sense to go to the expense and trouble of buying bottled or distilled water, or distilling your own? Can't you get by with chlorinated, fluoridated, possibly chemically contaminated water? Of course you can. And there will be those who say that it's just silly, fanatical, health-food-nuttiness to do otherwise.

But I'm talking about keeping yourself healthy in an optimum way, not just getting by. Remember also that your individual biochemical system is like that of tens of thousands of generations of humans, which have not been exposed to, or had any chance to become adapted to anything in water other than a few naturally occurring minerals.

It's your health. My present recommendation is unchlorinated, unfluoridated, unchemicalized water, with a little mineral supplementation. The decision, as always, is up to you.

Choosing Food that Builds Health

Some readers have already gone ahead and adopted many of the recommendations I'll be making. A few very nutritionally aware readers may have progressed even further, years ago. I apologize in advance to those who've already gone through this process. I hope the rest of the book has been both useful and enjoyable.

Before going into specifics, I'll note a mental test you can use when trying to decide whether or not a particular food fits into a keeping-yourself-healthy diet plan. Ask yourself if it's a food that primitive man ate, or could have eaten, somewhere in the world, a million years ago. This "primitive man test" immediately divides foods into acceptable and not acceptable categories, with only a few gray areas.

Of course, this test isn't foolproof: primitive man could be killed by poisonous mushrooms just as we can, for example. But it's a good starting place. Also, some foods available to primitive man have been altered by modern agricultural practices. Primitive man didn't pasteurize or homogenize milk, if he drank it; the eggs he might have eaten weren't produced by caged chickens in egg factories. Any fruit he ate wasn't sprayed with insecticide.

Which brings us to the next point: if you have it available to you, it is best to obtain foods grown or produced in a natural manner (sometimes called "organic"). Vegetables should be relatively free of pesticides and herbicides and fertilized with natural wastes and natural sources of trace minerals, rather than with chemical fertilizers. Animal proteins should have no synthetic hormones or antibiotics, and should be raised in natural conditions, rather than force-fed in feedlots. Eggs from chickens allowed to live somewhat freely and scratch around a hen yard are preferable. Choose whole-grain breads without chemical additives.

I think the overall point is clear. If you can raise most of your own food, you have a substantial head start. If you can't, try to find as many foods that fit into the entirely natural category as money and time will allow.

Enough said about ideal circumstances. If you can attain an entirely natural food diet, please do. You'll be much healthier for it. The more the rest of us keep searching for the ideal, and demand it from our usual food suppliers, the more likely it is we'll get it. But in the meantime, what? What if you're an average suburbanite or city dweller, dependent on the shopping center or corner supermarket? Is a good diet unattainable? Of course not! I'd definitely recommend you use more vitamin and mineral supplements than your organic country cousins, both to detoxify chemicalized foods, and to make up for what's missing. But a relatively natural diet is still within reach.

At this point, a general review of good, whole foods available at most supermarkets, along with discussion of the not-recommended-for-good-health items would be very helpful. *The Supermarket Handbook: Access to Whole Foods* by Nikki and David Goldbeck is an excellent guide, enabling the aware shopper to find worthwhile nutrition in the junk food jungle. If you haven't been able to sort the good from the worthless at your supermarket with certainty, this book will make your job much easier.

Even though it's impossible to give diet and supplementation specifically for you in a general book, discussion of nutritional needs of various *groups* can at least come closer than everybody-should-do-this advice. Let's start with a very basic division: women and men.

The Special Dietary Needs of Women

Nearly everyone with a television has seen, at one time or another, a commercial featuring a smiling, attractive woman holding a bottle of iron tablets and proclaiming that she keeps her husband happy, her children cared for, and her house spotless all with the aid of brand X. Of course, there's some truth to this: women do require more iron than men to stay healthy, throughout the menstrual years.

As always, food sources should be the number-one choice. Liver is absolutely the best source of food iron. Other relatively high iron foods include other organ meats, meat in general, fish, beans and other legumes (lentils, peas, chick-peas), potatoes, dried fruits, blackstrap molasses, and wheat germ.

It's been found that iron is better absorbed from animal sources than from plant sources. However, accompanying iron-containing foods with vitamin C can double the absorption of iron.

How can you tell for certain whether you're getting enough iron from your food? Unfortunately, it's impossible to tell for certain on your own. Of course, an absolute shortage of iron leads to anemia, with its usual telltale symptom of fatigue. But not everyone gets this symptom; also, it's possible to have a minor shortage of iron and not feel it. The only surefire way of telling is to have a blood count done; more about how to help yourself with your doctor's help, too, later.

If food sources of iron just aren't enough, then of course supplemental iron should be taken. In practice, 30 to 50 milligrams from a chelated or ferrous gluconate source is right for most women. (I realize that's more than the so-called Recommended Dietary Allowance [RDA], but I've given my opinion of the RDA already.)

In case you hadn't read it elsewhere, it's always advisable to separate supplemental iron tablets from supplemental vitamin E by at least three to four hours. While you're at it, it's just as well to separate iron tablets from supplemental vitamin A or concentrated sources of essential fatty acids (vegetable oils), too. As noted, iron goes with vitamin C.

Next on the agenda of nutrients for women to be especially careful of is calcium. Once again, due to persistent advertising, nearly everyone is aware that milk, cheeses, and other dairy products are extremely good sources of calcium. There's no question about that.

However, there's considerable suspicion among practitioners of nutritional medicine that cow's milk is a two-edged sword, both harmful and helpful. Looked at strictly from the point of view of the plan of nature, cow's milk is for calves and not for humans. Human babies should have human milk; human adults, none at all.

In fact, around the world the majority of humans are actually intolerant of cow's milk. The Caucasian (or "white") race is an exception, with only a minority unable to digest milk. Incidentally, symptoms of milk intolerance are headed by excess intestinal gas, then constipation or sometimes a little diarrhea. Even among those who can digest milk, it's sometimes implicated as one of the contributing causes of sinus symptoms and degenerative arthritis.

So what are alternative sources of calcium? Deep green, leafy vegetables, especially beet tops, dandelion greens, Swiss chard, kale, parsley, turnip greens, and watercress are all good sources. So are soybean products, salmon, and sardines.

All this doesn't mean I don't think you should use milk. Not at all. Just try to be especially aware of whether milk is causing you any symptoms of any kind. If not, go ahead. It might be wise to test your system's ability to make use of milk and dairy products in the same way self-testing is done for allergy. Abstain from milk and dairy products for at least five days; as long as you're eating other foods, a week or two is better. Then eat and drink a lot for a day or two, and see how you feel. Remember, anything with milk in it has to be omitted for the test period, too.

Despite the best calcium-containing diet, it's wise to use some supplementation as menopause approaches, and, of course, throughout the postmenopausal years. Entirely too many women develop osteoporosis and osteomalacia (bone pain), interfering with what could otherwise be productive and enjoyable years.

There's an accumulating body of evidence showing that diets high in animal protein may predispose women to the development of osteoporosis. These foods produce more acidity which is thought to correlate with calcium loss; also they're relatively high in phosphorus, which can promote calcium loss, also. Diets higher in foods from plant sources have neither of these drawbacks.

Many women use bone meal, dolomite, or just calcium supplements. All of these are good calcium sources, but due to problems of mineral balance, not everyone should use each or all of them.

Remember, diets high in animal source foods are high in phosphorus. This is part of the reason for the often quoted statement that "the average American diet is high in phosphorus." In practice, I've observed many women following a relatively high phosphorus diet trying to obtain extra calcium from bone meal, and getting nowhere. Of course, bone meal is relatively high in phosphorus, too (as is another common supplement, lecithin), so the total phosphorus intake overwhelms the extra calcium intake, defeating the purpose of taking it.

That doesn't mean you shouldn't consider bone meal as a calcium source, but how can you tell if it's right for you or not? Probably the best way is by mineral testing on both hair and blood specimens; again more about this later.

Short of medical testing, consider the rest of your diet. If it's low in animal protein, containing no processed foods (also high in phosphorus), then bone meal is probably best for you. If not, more consideration should be given to alternative sources of supplemental calcium: dolomite, calcium from oystershell, chelated calcium and calcium lactate (for those without milk intolerance), and calcium gluconate.

Without specific testing for mineral balance and advice from a nutritionally oriented physician, my own general recommendation is for a combination of plain calcium and dolomite, giving a calcium-to-magnesium ratio of from 4:1 to 10:1, and approximately 1 gram of total calcium daily.

Moving on from calcium, the next group of especially-for-women nutrients are the B vitamins. Any woman who suffers from premenstrual "anything" should always try B complex vitamins, with special emphasis on vitamin B_6 or pyridoxine. Nervousness or depression frequently respond to B vitamin supplementation.

Once again, food sources of B vitamins deserve emphasis. Whole grains, nuts, seeds, beans, lentils, liver, and other organ meats are all good sources. Wheat germ and brewer's yeast are two especially good supplemental food sources.

If you're eating an entirely whole food diet, which is of course best, a supplemental food source of B vitamins such as brewer's yeast may well be enough. However, under conditions of stress, if you find yourself especially nervous, or if your diet isn't all it should be yet, sometimes a B complex supplement is advisable.

How much is enough? Ordinarily, any quantity of B complex vitamins between 10 and 100 milligrams daily is sufficient (since there are so many different formulations of B vitamins, for now I'm just assuming roughly 10 to 100 milligrams of each individual B vitamin in a single tablet).

With the exception of B_3, or niacin, in high doses, usually 1,000 milligrams or more daily, there is practically no chance of toxicity from the vitamins of the B group. Therefore, it is fairly safe to experiment until you find an amount that helps you feel better.

Also, remember that if you have a particularly hormone-related problem, pyridoxine is often the most important B vitamin and needs to be taken in excess of the other B vitamins.

This brings us to another question. Sometimes the statement is made that B vitamins should always be taken in a "balanced" formulation. The only problem is that no one has been able to define exactly a balanced formulation. It's true that in nature where one B vitamin is found, the rest of the B complex is always close by. However, the proportions are variable. Usually, the amounts of niacin are highest, with B_1, pantothenic acid, and B_6 next, but not always in that order, and other B vitamins in lesser amounts.

So, if nature varies in B vitamin balance, no vitamin supplement manufacturer can possibly achieve a "perfect balance" in a pill. Obviously, the best thing to do is to use various natural sources whenever possible.

One last point: not only are refined sugars and refined foods in general missing the B vitamins (not to mention minerals) that originally accompanied them in nature, but they also "use up" more B vitamins in the process of being metabolized. So any refined food, especially sugar, creates an extra B vitamin demand.

Just for a little change, there's one nutrient not to take, at least by itself, without specific professional advice. That's copper. Nutritionally oriented physicians have observed that in general, estrogen promotes the accumulation of copper in women's tissues. If a multiple vitamin and mineral formula happens to have a very small amount of copper in it, it's not likely to hurt. But all by itself, for some women, it will accumulate in excess. Even without taking a specific copper supplement, some women take up too much from water and food sources.

How can you tell if you've got too much copper? Without a mineral analysis of hair, it's generally impossible.

To summarize, if you're female, it's wise in general to use supplemental iron, calcium, B vitamins, and not to take copper.

What about vitamins C and E? I usually recommend these for women, too; almost everyone should supplement these. Just for the record, though, 400 units of a natural-source vitamin E (remember, not with iron) and one or two grams of vitamin C daily are advisable.

Eating for a Healthy Pregnancy

This section wouldn't be complete if we ignored women's special—but temporary—state of pregnancy (although more than one woman has told me that temporary seemed like forever, especially in the last two to three months).

Now, in this chapter, I'm generally trying to accentuate the positive, going over what to do, and only touching on what not to do from time to time. But being entirely responsible for the raw physical materials of which your baby's body is made is such an important job that here I'm going to go through the don'ts, first. Please bear with this; it really is important.

Eating for two doesn't start when you get pregnant. If you were going to grow a garden, you wouldn't just walk over to a patch of ground, poke in the seeds, and walk away, would you? Not if you wanted the best results. You'd dig up or till the ground, removing any unwanted weeds or stones. You'd fertilize the soil (hopefully with an organic-source fertilizer). You might even add small quantities of trace minerals. After this careful preparation, you'd plant the seeds. Of course, you'd continue to tend the plants as they grew, but much of your work would be done beforehand.

Doesn't a new human life deserve the same attention? Don't wait until you're pregnant. Start preparing yourself ahead of time, months ahead if possible.

Nearly all physicians, not just nutritionally oriented ones, want you to be especially careful of your baby's growing body. You've certainly heard "If you're pregnant, don't take any drugs, not even an aspirin, without asking your doctor." I agree with this 100 percent, and think you should go farther.

Months before you become pregnant, if you're still eating junk food or chemicals, you should get all of this out of your diet. The more that's learned about synthetic chemicals, even "generally recognized as safe" chemicals, the more it's being discovered that they have unrealized potential for damaging human cells, especially rapidly growing ones, even if in subtle or minor ways.

Leaving aside specific evidence of harmfulness, we can go back to the history of tens of thousands of generations. Except during the last one hundred to two hundred years, human fetuses have simply not been exposed to synthetic chemicals. Remember, if it hasn't been around for as long as humans have, or longer, it's quite likely we haven't fully adapted to it. On balance, a new chemical introduced into the human system is more likely to cause harm than good, especially when whole organ systems and tissues are just being formed; the wrong chemical in the wrong place at the wrong time can literally cause a lifetime of trouble.

Unless a synthetic chemical has been proven harmless beyond a doubt, don't take it without a compelling medical need. This applies especially during the first three months of pregnancy, but is just as important for months before, too, as some chemicals "hang around" in the tissues for indefinite periods of time.

The routine use of food with artificial flavor, color, or preservative is not good at any time. Especially before and during pregnancy, such food chemicals should be avoided completely.

Is this just "fanatical health-food nuttery"? I'm sure some will say so. It's your baby; the decision is up to you.

For the same reasons, avoid all refined sugar and refined foods. You know they're not good for your health: why feed your growing baby junk?

Having put yourself on as healthy a general diet as possible, what items require special attention? Let's start with protein. If you've read chapter 16, "A Case of Preeclampsia," you can see why enough protein is important when you're pregnant. Not only does your growing baby need protein, but many nutritionally oriented physicians believe that adequate protein is essential to prevention of toxemia of pregnancy.

The best sources of protein are eggs, muscle and organ meats, cheeses, nuts, seeds, beans, lentils, and fish. If you're not a vegetarian, getting enough high-quality protein shouldn't be difficult. If you are, then some care with protein combining is important. How much is enough protein? Recommendations vary, but I'd prefer to see from 70 to 100 grams of well-balanced protein daily during pregnancy.

Remember, a gram of any particular protein source is not equivalent to a gram of balanced or "complete" protein. Even egg protein, the most complete of any, is not perfectly balanced.

For an excellent brief review and explanation of complete and incomplete protein sources, how to figure various equivalents and protein combining, I'd suggest you see *Diet for a Small Planet* by Frances Moore Lappé.

Other special-attention nutrients are our familiar especially-for-women nutrients, calcium and iron. During pregnancy, there's even more need for these two. Particularly during the latter half of pregnancy, supplemental calcium intake should be 1½ to 2 grams, and chelated iron in the range of 50 to 100 milligrams; the higher amount if the blood count is low.

In the past decade, much more attention has been given to adequate folic acid intake during pregnancy. Nearly every prenatal vitamin preparation presently available contains 1 milligram of folic acid. While supplementation is a wise idea, also strive to get folic acid from food, especially deep, green leafy vegetables, lima beans, salmon, and brewer's yeast.

There are a few special-situation nutrients, also. The most frequently used is vitamin B_6 (pyridoxine).

According to the American Medical Association, pyridoxine has no value in the treatment of nausea and vomiting of pregnancy. I don't know where the person who wrote that opinion got the information, but it obviously wasn't from my pregnant, previously nauseated patients. I'm not an obstetrician, but I've had occasion to recommend pyridoxine to over one hundred women suffering from nausea and/or vomiting with pregnancy. In all but a few cases, adequate pyridoxine has controlled the problem.

That should come as no surprise to anyone knowledgeable in the biochemistry of the interactions between estrogen and B vitamins, especially pyridoxine. That should also be of no surprise to anyone familiar with pyridoxine's ability to counteract most of the side effects of birth-control pills and other externally administered forms of estrogen.

Perhaps a key word here is "adequate." The amounts of pyridoxine required are sometimes as little as 25 milligrams daily, but can range as high as 200 milligrams, 3 times a day. Rarely, injected pyridoxine will work when it's not effective orally. It should be emphasized that there's never been a case recorded of pyridoxine toxicity, even in 600-milligram-a-day doses, for either mother or baby. For further reading on this, I'd suggest the work of Dr. John Ellis, described in his book *Vitamin B₆: The Doctor's Report.*

As I've mentioned before, even reports of effective natural therapies are frequently buried. Only recently, I came across a report printed in a respectable medical journal about the use of vitamin K in the nausea and vomiting of pregnancy (*The Practitioner,* November 1952, p. 573). So far, I've only had occasion to recommend it a few times; it works fine, as reported.

Although it's not mentioned in the report, there exists the theoretical possibility that the natural form of vitamin K found in plants, called "phylloquinone," may work better than the synthetic form. Both types are available commercially. Your pharmacist can tell you which is which.

Besides pyridoxine and vitamin K, magnesium has an occasional place as a special-situation supplement. If you've had a history of preeclampsia with pregnancy, or if it's in your family, it's probably wise to use a little magnesium along with pyridoxine and a high protein diet as preventive measures. For further details, see chapter 16, "A Case of Preeclampsia."

A good multiple vitamin and mineral supplement is always wise during pregnancy. However, since all nutrients important to health aren't known, it's also wise to regularly use supplemental food sources of a wide range of nutrients, such as brewer's yeast, alfalfa, kelp, rice, bran, and that old standby, liver.

After the baby's born, I hope you'll be nursing as long as possible. In this case, make sure to maintain a high-quality protein diet, and even more calcium: 2 grams a day are probably wise.

Many cases of postpartum blues and depression have been helped with B vitamins. But if you're nursing, watch out for too much vitamin B_6. Two excellent studies have shown that pyridoxine is even more effective than estrogen in shutting off normal lactation. The amounts of pyridoxine used were high, 200 milligrams, 3 times daily. But some women are more sensitive to this action of pyridoxine than others. At present I recommend a postpartum intake of no more than 10 milligrams of pyridoxine daily if you intend to continue nursing. (*The Journal of Obstetrics and Gynecology of the British Commonwealth,* August 1973; *South African Medical Journal,* December 1975.)

Special Diet Recommendations for Men

There are fewer special recommendations for men at present than for women; as more is learned about nutrition that may change. Let's cover the few recommendations there are.

Men don't seem to use vitamin C as efficiently as women. The reasons for this aren't known, but it's been observed clinically. My usual minimum recommendation for vitamin C for men is 1 gram twice daily as opposed to 1 gram daily for women. (For those who want to make optimum use of vitamin C for good health, I recommend the body-tolerance level for both sexes. For discussion of this concept, see chapter 31, "High-Dose Vitamin C and Kidney Stones."

It's well known that men are more prone to heart attacks, at a much younger age than women. Particularly if you have a family history of heart attack, it's wise to take precautionary diet and supplement measures.

The rate of heart attacks is definitely lower among vegetarians than among animal protein eaters. No, this doesn't mean I think everyone who's concerned about heart attack prevention should become a vegetarian immediately, but some thought should be given to a compromise that's comfortable for you. More fish and poultry can be substituted for beef and pork; the overall quantity of animal products can be cut down.

What about eggs, butter, cheese, and the whole idea of low-cholesterol diets? For a variety of reasons, I think some of this type of effort is misguided, especially when eggs are excluded. For a review of this topic, see chapter 12, "A Case of Heart Disease."

Even if you don't care for them, there's good reason to include onions and garlic fairly regularly in an anti-heart attack diet. If you do like them, so much the better. If all else fails, supplemental garlic capsules are available for daily use.

Although it's quite controversial, evidence developed by Dr. Kurt A. Oster indicates that the homogenization of milk may contribute to heart attacks. I concur with Dr. Oster's opinion, and likewise recommend that homogenized milk be avoided especially if you have a family history of heart attacks.

Other supplements I'd recommend would include lecithin (1 tablespoon daily), vitamin E (400 units), essential fatty acids contained in 1 tablespoon of safflower or sunflower oil daily, along with vitamin C. If you must drink homogenized milk, include several milligrams of folic acid daily. There are a large number of other supplements that are useful and could be recommended, but for going much further it'd be wise to check with a knowledgeable expert if at all possible.

For obvious reasons, only men develop prostate gland problems. While this appears to be a problem of age, appearance is deceiving. It takes years for an enlarged prostate to become symptomatic. It's not too soon to start working on prevention.

It appears that zinc and essential fatty acids are two very important nutrients in the maintenance of the health of the prostate. In one of nature's happy coincidences, nuts and seeds, especially pumpkin seeds and sunflower seeds, are good sources of both nutrients. Seafoods are excellent sources of zinc; so are liver and mushrooms.

In addition to safflower and sunflower oils, others rich in essential fatty acids include linseed (flaxseed), wheat germ, and corn oils.

If you haven't gotten a head start on prevention of prostate symptoms, it's probably wise to use a supplemental source of zinc. Twenty to 30 milligrams of a chelated source is probably adequate.

Two cautions: if zinc is taken for years in a supplemental form, there's a small possibility of producing copper deficiency. It's wise to have a mineral analysis from time to time to check mineral balance. Second, as has been previously noted, always take vitamin E when using supplemental sources of essential fatty acids.

Diet for a Small Person

In infancy and very early childhood, there's absolutely no question about the best food available: mother's milk. It seems absurd to me that anyone would feel a need for biochemical and biological studies to prove this point, as the plan of nature is perfectly obvious. However, when such studies are done, they invariably prove that nature is right.

How long should you nurse? As long as you can. One of the ironies of modern civilization is that women who try to nurse for more than just a few months are looked upon as "unnatural." Anthropological studies show that in primitive communities, much closer to nature, the average age of weaning is about 30 months. This doesn't mean the children aren't eating other foods (as well as anything else they can get their hands on). They are. This age is when nursing is stopped entirely. Once again, this isn't weird or strange. It's nature's way.

If you haven't heard of it already, the La Leche League is an excellent source of information about nursing, as well as general support. Usually doctor's offices know who the local representatives are. If not, write to the address given in chapter 54, "A Resource Guide to Nutritional and Natural Therapy."

Small children are frequently picky eaters. When I ask mothers "What do you feed your 3-year-old?" I often get the reply, "Whatever I can get down!" For this reason, it's extremely important that all food presented a child provides excellent quality nutrition.

Vitamins A and D are usually recommended until your child will eat his or her vegetables and liver reliably. Ten thousand units of A and 400 units of D daily are usually adequate.

Multiple vitamins and minerals are also wise. To insure adequate quantities, it's probably wisest to get separate multiple vitamin and mineral tablets. Tablets that combine both vitamins and minerals are frequently inadequate.

What about vitamin C? Recommendations can be quite variable. In my own practice, I ask parents to give a minimum of 10 milligrams per pound, and more when ill. For those interested in optimum rather than minimum, I encourage the body-tolerance approach.

No, I've never seen a kidney stone develop in child or adult on body-tolerance vitamin C and neither has Dr. Klenner, a physician with extremely wide experience in the use of optimal vitamin C therapy.

However, it is a theoretical possibility. Especially if you have kidney stones in the family, there are several choices: don't give your child so much vitamin C; run a 24-hour urine test for oxalate; or give additional vitamin B_6 (see chapter 31, "High-Dose Vitamin C and Kidney Stones").

But back to supplements for children. As with adults, a vitamin E supplement is advisable. However, no more than 50 units for smaller children, and up to 200 units for older ones is wise.

Last, I'd like to invite you to make a tour of any junior or senior high school and inspect everyone's fingernails. No, not for dirt, for white spots. Identified as a sign of a need for additional zinc by Dr. Carl C. Pfeiffer, "white spotting" is at its highest level in the most rapidly growing and maturing age groups. When supplemental zinc is given to children with white-spotted nails, the spots disappear over 90 percent of the time, within a few months. (*Mental and Elemental Nutrients: A Physician's Guide to Nutrition and Health Care* by Carl C. Pfeiffer.)

No one ever died of white-spotted nails. However, I'm convinced that the white-spotted fingernails of our junior and senior high-school-age children are evidence of widespread subclinical zinc deficiency.

Zinc is extremely important for full growth and sexual maturation. In fact, the first reported cases of human zinc deficiency were sexually immature, physically stunted individuals. Children in the maturing years use up a lot of zinc.

Zinc is processed out of many foods. It's also lost from the body under the onslaught of sugar and junk foods. Hopefully, your children are well trained enough in nutrition to avoid such foods. But not all teenagers are.

In the 1960s, the United States Department of Agriculture released a report showing that the soils of 32 states were zinc depleted in at least some areas. That situation hasn't improved since. If the zinc isn't in the soil, it won't get into the plants, animals, and people.

So, we have children in high zinc-need years, and also in the years with the most free access to junk foods, often sold by the schools themselves. In addition, soil deficiency of zinc is common. It's no surprise that so many show signs of need for additional zinc.

If high-zinc foods don't take care of the problem, 30 to 50 milligrams of chelated zinc daily is a good starting place. Some teenagers, especially those with acne, may require more. To be on the safe side, it's wisest to stop when the white spots disappear.

In sum, we have extra vitamins A and D (for the younger children), a multiple vitamin, a multiple mineral, vitamins C and E as general rules, and zinc for those who show a need. Except with specific guidance, it's probably wisest not to go further.

Except for calcium. If your child's nursing, you take the calcium. If he or she is drinking lots of milk, eating lots of cheese, and showing no ill effects, probably whatever is in the multiple mineral will do. However, if not, then a total of approximately 500 milligrams of supplemental calcium is best.

The Special Dietary Needs of Older People

At the other end of the age spectrum, nutritional supplementation can be even more important in the effort to stay healthy. I suppose I should define the age group I have in mind; in Western society, the line between middle age and old age is usually crossed somewhere between 60 and 70 years of age.

Which is really too soon. With good self-care, it should be possible to postpone so-called old age into much later in life. Those readers who started conscientiously following a good diet and other health practices years ago hopefully will discover just how true this is for themselves.

As you've seen, an all-too-frequent problem with advancing age is proper digestion and absorption of nutrients. Before paying attention to specific nutrients, it's wise to make sure they'll be used. See chapter 45, "Poor Absorption," for further details.

Speaking of memory and mental function in general, it's not necessary to let your mind just slip away. At the top of the list for mind-preserving supplements are the B vitamins, especially niacin, B_{12}, folic acid, and choline.

Food sources of B vitamins have been covered above. As usual, food should be relied on first. However, I always recommend extra B complex for older age groups, beginning with a B complex tablet—usually, a 50-milligram supplement, twice a day. If you're not feeling alert enough with that, extra niacin might be the answer. As an added bonus, it can aid in the control of pain from osteoarthritis. Most prefer niacinamide, as it doesn't give the vascular flush that niacin can give in doses of 100 milligrams or more. Vitamin B_3 in large quantities can have definite side effects (see chapter 31, "A Case of Degenerative Arthritis").

Usually, there's enough choline in a B complex tablet. However, choline has shown promise as an antisenility vitamin; some may prefer to take extra as insurance. Remember that lecithin is a good source of choline. An extra tablespoon of lecithin should be enough for all but those with definite problems.

I've been told frequently by some other physicians that giving vitamin B_{12} injections to older people is only justified for pernicious anemia. To do so otherwise is a "rip-off."

Nonsense. And worse than nonsense: to withhold vitamin B_{12} injections is sometimes to sentence older persons to chronic tiredness and less mental alertness than they could otherwise have.

It's a known fact that as we age, we absorb nutrients less

efficiently. (For example, see chapter 24, "A Case of B Vitamin Deficiency in a Healthy 90-Year-Old.") Vitamin B_{12} is usually the first to go. Blood levels of vitamin B_{12} are also completely useless as guidelines for using or not using injectable B_{12}. (What's probably needed is to find a blood test measuring some crucial function completely dependent on vitamin B_{12}. Then we'd probably find that different individuals need different amounts of B_{12} to make that function work.)

Last, no one ever died of an overdose on vitamin B_{12}. So there's no harm done trying. The placebo argument has been shot down in at least one study (see chapter 39, "A Case of Unexplained Tiredness"). As for "rip-off": there's no reason you can't learn to give B_{12} injections yourself; all my patients do. That way it is less expensive.

I don't mean to imply that everyone in the older age group needs vitamin B_{12} or other vitamins by injection. Many do just fine taking it orally. But it is a relatively frequent problem, increasing with age. If despite your best efforts you're still tired, try injectable B_{12}. If you can just get a prescription. . . .

Folic acid is our last special-need B vitamin. Folic acid absorption also falls off with age; however, it doesn't need to be injected nearly as often as vitamin B_{12}. Usually, from 2 to 4 milligrams extra by mouth are enough. There are no known side effects.

I've mentioned body-tolerance levels of vitamin C for optimum health so many times I'm sure you're getting bored with it. But old age is a good time to start this, if you haven't already. Vitamin C may help retard deterioration of disks, joints, and other aging tissues. It won't stop the process; just slow it some. Fifty milligrams daily (the RDA) won't do an optimum job.

While on the subject of antiaging vitamins, extra vitamin E should be mentioned. One of the many theories of aging is the free radical theory, which holds that destructive molecules get loose in the tissues, causing aging changes. Vitamin E (as well as vitamin C) acts as a trap or scavenger for free radicals.

Eight hundred units is a good starting point for vitamin E supplementation if you're in an older age group, unless you have hypertension or rheumatic heart disease. In either case, it's wisest not to go over 200 units without some sort of medical attention. (For further details, see *Dr. Wilfred E. Shute's Complete Updated Vitamin E Book.*)

Specific supplementation for osteoporosis and prostate problem prevention has been covered above. As these are frequent aging problems, don't overlook them.

In general, it's wisest to use a little bit more of everything if you're in the older age group. Not only is absorption less efficient, but it just takes more of everything to keep older cells going.

Most emphatically, this does not mean obtaining a bottle of every type of vitamin or mineral pill made. What I have in mind is concentrating on vitamin- and mineral-rich foods, and adding in several supplemental foods known to be rich in numerous nutrients.

Most of these have been mentioned before, but let's go over them again. Alfalfa and kelp are excellent sources of minerals (watch the salt content in kelp if you have hypertension). Brewer's yeast is an excellent source of B vitamins and other nutrients. Wheat germ, desiccated liver, and rice polishings are also good concentrated nutrient sources.

One final note: before going and getting your glasses changed again, try 50,000 units of vitamin A and 50 milligrams of zinc for three or four months first. You may be pleasantly surprised.

Know Your Family History—and Eat Accordingly

It's well known that certain diseases tend to run in families. Part of any good health evaluation should be a family health history. Just because Aunt Tillie had a particular ailment doesn't mean you'll get it for sure; it's just that your odds are a little higher. Another way of trying to keep yourself healthy is to be aware of any diseases that may be in your family and to take dietary measures to keep them from occurring in you.

I've already noted some general recommendations you might

follow if your family suffers from heart attacks. Let's add in the somewhat related problems of hypertension (high blood pressure) and stroke. It's widely accepted even by non-nutritionally oriented physicians that cutting down as much as possible on sources of salt is important. Eliminating bacon, ham, cottage cheese, most other cheeses, lunch meats, olives, pickles, sausage, and most important, the contents of the saltshaker from your diet may help prevent hypertension.

It may be just as important to concentrate on foods high in potassium to help control blood pressure. Keeping sodium low is important; changing the sodium-potassium ratio in favor of potassium is important, too. Instead of the negative "throw the sodium out" approach being the only theme, add in the positive with as many high-potassium sources as possible.

The best sources of potassium are fresh fruits, vegetables, and fruit juices. It's probable that putting fresh vegetables through a thorough juicing will release even more potassium by disrupting somewhat hard-to-digest plant cell walls. Good supplemental food sources include brewer's yeast, wheat germ, blackstrap molasses, and sunflower seeds.

One other consideration: sodium is present in softened water. If you have a water softener, don't use this water for drinking. As mentioned before, at the present time distilled water is probably best.

In addition to controlling the sodium-potassium ratio in your diet, the overall animal source food-vegetable source food relationship is important to hypertension. Generally speaking, the more vegetable source food, the better, as long as it's not high in salt.

If your family suffers from diabetes, it's especially important not to include in your diet refined sugars and processed foods in general. Medical science can't say exactly what causes diabetes, or even whether there's just one cause or many. But over and over again, medical anthropologists have shown that a switch from a natural food diet to a highly refined and sugared fare is accompanied by a rise in the incidence of diabetes. This has happened in such diverse groups as North Canadian Eskimos, New Zealand Maori, South African blacks, and Yemenite Jews.

Whether recognized by modern medical science or not, this has happened to black, white, red, and Oriental Americans, too. It's so common and all around us that it seems hard to recognize. (I should mention that diet-related diabetes is called "maturity-onset diabetes" and usually comes on after age 50. It's thought that juvenile diabetes has another, as yet undiscovered, major contributing cause.)

Other than overall attention to diet, it is known that in some cases the trace element chromium may be extremely important. This is sufficiently old news that I'm sure many have read it often before, so I'll just mention that good supplemental food sources of chromium are brewer's yeast and liver.

At present writing, one government regulator or another has limited the size of supplemental chromium tablets to 200 micrograms or smaller. I haven't been able to discover why. It's been my observation that at least 1,000 micrograms (1 milligram) of supplemental chromium daily are necessary to bring up subnormal levels.

If there's a history of kidney stones in your family, particular attention to magnesium, pyridoxine, and vitamin A is all-important. These factors are much more important than the traditional low-calcium diet, which wasn't too helpful anyway.

Magnesium is found particularly in nuts, seeds, and whole grains. Pyridoxine is, of course, found in foods high in all the B vitamins, especially liver, seeds, nuts, beans, and lentils. Again, brewer's yeast and wheat germ are good supplemental food sources. Last, all deep green and yellow vegetables are good sources of vitamin A.

For extra insurance, 10 milligrams of pyridoxine (as part of the B complex), 50 milligrams of magnesium, and 20,000 IU of vitamin A might be advisable.

Does your family background contain cases of cancer? Make sure to include plenty of nuts in your diet (remember, peanuts are not a nut, but a legume). Millet, berries, and fruit are other good dietary items. Although it's controversial, 3 or 4 peach or apricot kernels daily for an adult (don't take more) can't hurt, and are probably beneficial. Make sure to include also lentils, chick-peas, and beans.

A high-fiber diet is associated in some areas of the world with a decreased prevalence of cancer. American dietary surveys show likewise that there's a lower rate of cancer generally among vegetarians.

Even the Food and Drug Administration admits that vitamin C is capable of blocking some of the carcinogenic effects of certain food chemicals called nitrites. Most nutritionally oriented practitioners would go further, pointing to numerous animal studies showing the relationship of vitamin C to the detoxification of carcinogens. If your family history shows several cases of cancer, extra vitamin C, 1 to 3 grams daily, or more, shouldn't be omitted.

It's also advisable to include vitamin E, 400 to 800 units daily. I'd recommend small quantities of B complex vitamins, 10 to 20 milligrams daily. Vitamin A also has antitumor activity; 20,000 units daily would be advisable.

I don't mean to imply that the above dietary supplementation is capable of curing cancer. Rather, there are indications it may help prevent it. The subject of dietary and other natural treatment of cancer is so controversial that it could and has filled many books.

This time, I've left the "don'ts" till last. They're a familiar list: leave out all synthetic chemicals, flavors, colors, and preservatives from your diet. This doesn't mean there aren't any natural cancer-inducing substances; there are. But why add to the load and multiply the risk many times over?

If you have a family history of degenerative arthritis, there are several things to watch for. (The type of arthritis meant is said to come with age or from wear and tear, not rheumatoid arthritis, or arthritis from gout.)

Avoidance of the nightshade family—tomatoes, potatoes, peppers, eggplant, and tobacco—may be very important (see chapter 26, "The 'Nightshade' Elimination Diet for Arthritis").

Unfortunately, at present there's no predictive test for this, so what to do if you just love tomatoes (or one of the other nightshades)? Prudence would advise simply a lessening of nightshade intake, or, if arthritis has just appeared, an immediate no-nightshade trial could be started.

Food allergy also appears to be very involved in some cases of arthritic pain. If your family has a history of both arthritis and allergies, it would be wise to determine if you have any food allergies before they cause trouble. Several methods of allergy detection are available (see chapter 46, "A Look at Food Allergy"). Before you have any problems from allergy-related arthritis, why not try to prevent them?

Two B vitamins seem especially related to arthritis. Thanks to Dr. William Kaufman, the link between niacin and arthritis is firmly established. Likewise, Dr. John Ellis has demonstrated the importance of pyridoxine in another type of degenerative arthritis.

Food sources of B vitamins, as well as supplemental foods high in B vitamins have already been noted. I'll add only that as the arthritis years approach, it's wise to add extra B vitamins in the form of supplemental tablets, 20 to 50 milligrams.

Vitamin C is important here also. A minimum of 1 to 3 grams is probably advisable. Good sources of minerals, especially for calcium and magnesium, would also be helpful.

What if your family has allergies? The best thing you can do about a food you're allergic to is not eat it. Even if the number of food allergies is very large, so that some intake of allergenic food is unavoidable, then a dietary rotation including each allergenic food no more often than every four to five days is a good idea.

Just because you don't have any typical allergy symptoms, don't assume you're allergy-free, especially if there are allergies in your family. Remember, just about any symptom might be allergy-related. If there are allergies in your family, and you're not feeling healthy, check yourself.

Vitamin C is always first on the list of antiallergy supplements. I usually recommend body-tolerance doses of vitamin C, especially in moderate to severe cases. (As noted before it should be accompanied by extra amounts of pyridoxine, approximately 50 milligrams, to avoid the remote but theoretically potential hazard of kidney stones.)

Many find pantothenic acid (also called pantothenate) to be very helpful against allergy symptoms, in general. It's another nontoxic B vitamin and can be used in amounts from ½ gram to several grams daily. The best food source is green, leafy vegetables. Other B vitamins are very helpful also; usually 50 to 200 milligrams of B vitamins, or more in a few cases, are helpful against allergy.

Last, a word about allergy prevention. It's not known what exactly causes allergies to form in some people, and not others, but there are clues. Work with small children indicates that the longer a child is nursed the lower the incidence of allergy. From this point of view, there's nothing we can do about me and you, but we can try to help our children.

Selecting the Optimum Diet

By now, I'm sure you've noted a recurrent theme in many of the foregoing brief discussions. There does seem to be a dietary pattern associated with a lower incidence of a variety of diseases. That pattern has often been called an "optimum diet," and certainly isn't original with me. However, in concluding this chapter, I think it should be repeated.

Not everyone can immediately adopt an optimum diet. Some won't even want to. Certainly, not all of my patients do, even though it would be better for their health, and I often wish more would.

If you look up food items highest in a wide variety of nutrients, nuts, seeds, beans, and whole grains are at the top of the list. Modern scientific means have determined many of the exact values, but common sense could have predicted the result of such analysis before it was ever done. After all, a nut, seed, bean, or whole grain is the embryo from which the whole plant grows. Every nutrient needed for the plant's initial growth has to be in the seed. It only makes sense that nuts, seeds, beans, and whole grains are continually referred to as sources of fiber, niacin, magnesium, pyridoxine, pantothenic acid, zinc, thiamine, riboflavin, manganese, calcium, essential fatty acids, copper . . . I think the point is clear. Just about any nutrient needed for cell growth and development is packed into a nut or seed as part of nature's plan. Why not take advantage of this yourself?

Next on the optimum diet list are fresh, raw vegetables. Various sprouts, carrots, turnips, kale, endive, Swiss chard, cabbage, spinach, watercress, beet tops, dandelion greens, onions, garlic, parsley, peppers, radishes, tomatoes, and many more you can think of. But as wide a variety of fresh, raw vegetables as possible should form another major portion of an optimum diet.

Apples, oranges, bananas, melons, cherries, peaches, figs, nectarines, blackberries, raspberries, cranberries . . . the whole list of fruits and berries is on any optimum-diet-for-good-health list. In our present century, though, we must be extremely careful to remove as many traces of pesticides, insecticides, and other chemicals from fruits and vegetables as possible. Food grown without chemicals is, of course, preferable.

Nuts, seeds, beans, whole grains, raw vegetables, a few cooked vegetables, fruits and fruit juices, berries, pure water . . . these items complete the absolutely optimum diet list, for the best health results. Accompanying such a diet is a reduction in a long list of diseases: less cancer, heart attacks, high blood pressure, strokes, diabetes, gallbladder disease, osteoporosis, diverticulitis . . . and this list probably isn't complete.

Now back from the optimum to the practical. Few persons are going to be able to adopt an optimum program; many won't want to. There are some who've tried, and find they just don't feel good without more traditional foods. Then there are the obvious questions: What about protein? What about iron? Vitamin B_{12}? Won't most people develop dietary deficiencies from such a program?

Protein is entirely adequate on such a diet, particularly if attention is paid to "complimentary amino acid" matching. (The book *Diet for a Small Planet* by Frances Moore Lappé covers this.) Overlooked by generations of dietitians in this country is the fact that thousands of generations of humans have gotten enough protein from the above type of diet, when the quantity of food was adequate.

Iron nutrition can also be adequate on a nut-seed-bean-whole grain-vegetable-fruit-and-berry plan, as long as enough attention is paid to iron-rich foods. As noted before, beet greens, kale, dandelion greens, dried fruits, molasses, and wheat germ are all good sources.

Vitamin B_{12} adequacy is probably the trickiest question. For the Western scientist, there's not really enough data to make an absolute statement. Unanswered questions abound, such as: How much B_{12} is needed in the metabolism of a diet high in animal source foods compared to one high in vegetable source foods? How much B_{12} is produced by the intestinal bacteria, particularly if the bacteria of carnivores and vegetarians are compared? What's the incidence of pernicious anemia (produced by absolute lack of B_{12}) among strict vegetarians, as compared to meat-eaters? Are there further plant sources of vitamin B_{12}?

Until all these questions are answered, no absolute statements can be trusted (although many are made). I suspect that when all the answers are in, if they ever are, that it will be found unnecessary to include animal source food to obtain enough B_{12}. But since all the answers are far from being in, it's probably wisest to include vitamin B_{12} supplementation even with an optimum diet. (The supplements are derived from a plant source—bacterial synthesis.)

Descending from the optimum diet, there certainly are other good foods to include in your nine-to-five, hurried, urban or suburban existence (even rural sometimes), or in your busy-busy clean the house-cook the meals-watch the children world. In fact, there are so many other good foods that there's absolutely no excuse other than bad habit for resorting to dietary junk.

Seafood and eggs are at the top of the next list. Admittedly, our oceans are increasingly polluted, and most eggs are produced by factory chickens. But that's the best many of us have available, so we'll just have to use dietary supplementation and countermeasures to make up for these problems.

A wide variety of fish should be next on the list of foods for good health. Cod, herring, salmon, haddock, perch, pike, sardines, tuna . . . the list goes on. Shellfish should be at the bottom of the seafood list.

Eggs also deserve inclusion in an optimum-diet-for-good-health list. Yes, eggs are high in cholesterol, but I've observed that when fish and eggs are the main sources of animal protein, high cholesterol is rarely a problem.

Eggs are the most complete protein food in nature. They're high in many other important nutrients; again, this is only to be expected. Although they're not usually thought of in this way, eggs are simply the animal form of one of nature's basic concepts, the seed. The completeness and range of nutrients are characteristic of any seed.

Further down our list of acceptable foods are chicken, turkey, other poultry, and rabbit. As a matter of practicality, many families rely on these foods as protein sources. Just keep in mind that the more animal source foods, the more the statistical association with a wide range of ailments.

What about milk, pork, and beef? These are still within the acceptable group, but definitely at the end. Before getting too upset about this categorization, remember they're not on the don't-use-at-all list.

Many persons, especially mothers, may still be upset about the end-of-the-list position of milk, so let's go over the reasons for it.

Remember nature's plan? Human mother's milk is absolutely the best thing for human babies; cow's milk is the best for calves. But after infancy, the continuation of milk as a principal component of the diet is actually, in the long course of human history, an unnatural dietary practice.

Yes, cow's milk has been around in all of our stores since any of us can remember. It's heavily promoted as a source of calcium and protein. But over the tens of thousands of generations of people, dietary liquids have been mother's milk, and then water and fruit juices (excluding for the moment the long human history of alcoholic beverage consumption). Until the domestication of cows and goats, which appears to have taken place at a relatively recent point in the course of human history, there was nary a glass of milk in sight.

That doesn't mean I'm totally against cow's milk consumption. In persons who detect no symptoms, some milk from time to time is probably innocuous. But there are other sources of both dietary protein and calcium, and it's not true at all that no one can stay healthy without milk.

Keep in mind that the cow's milk most of us get is both pasteurized and homogenized; that's not the way it came from the cow, and that qualifies it as a processed food. I've already mentioned Dr. Kurt Oster's highly suggestive evidence that homogenized milk is a possible cause of atherosclerosis. If there are heart and blood vessel diseases in your family, I'd advise against much homogenized milk in the diet at all.

Last, beef and pork. I usually recommend to my patients that they avoid much consumption of these animal proteins. The correlations between heavy consumption of fatty animal proteins and all the diseases noted are simply too strong to be ignored. Once again, many people don't want to, or can't, eliminate these items entirely. That's understandable, and for some people, they won't necessarily cause health trouble. It's a statistical correlation, and statistics don't necessarily apply to any one individual. In going over evidence for a generalized optimum diet, beef and pork at present have to be placed on the acceptable list, but at the bottom.

Now, for the list of definitely health-damaging foods. I'll make it brief, as you've seen it in this book before. At the top of the list are all sorts of synthetic food chemicals, artificial flavors, colors, and preservatives. Not far behind are refined sugars, white flour, and other highly processed foods. Hopefully in the future we will all have learned enough to relegate this sort of nonfood to the junk pile of human history.

Don't be discouraged or give up if you can't obtain a 100 percent optimum diet. Yes, that's the ideal, and I'd recommend you work toward it. Realistically, though, how many of us got 100 percent every time when we were in school? Come as close as you can, as often as you can. You'll be healthier for it. It's your life and your health.

48 Keeping Yourself Healthy with Your Doctor's Help

Once you've become an active participant in your own health care, it's less likely you'll need to see a doctor about illness. Good diet, enough exercise, other natural measures, an awareness of nature's plan and your spot in it will go a long way toward maintaining good health.

But there are things for which you'll need a physician's help, even if you're not sick, simply for keeping yourself as healthy as possible for as long as possible.

If you're fortunate enough to have a physician interested in preventive as well as therapeutic medicine, you'll have no trouble discussing your interests and objectives for your own health.

What if your physician isn't interested in preventive and nutritional medicine, and you can't find such a practitioner in your area to act as a consultant in these subjects? You can still get much of the help you want, but a lot depends on your physician's personality, your personality, and the way you relate. Of course, you'll have to do more of the work on your own.

It's important to get started in the right way, either with a new physician or with the one you've known all along. Possibly the best way to get started is to schedule a complete checkup. Make it clear from the beginning that a major part of your objective in doing so is to gain information about staying healthy in the future, as well as detecting any unsuspected illness.

When I say "make it clear," I don't mean that you should be aggressive or hostile. What you don't say directly may be just as important as what you do say. Pointing out that you're interested in staying healthy is a start, but a brief mention at the appropriate time of the type of exercise you're getting, or how you're watching your diet will also help to convey the idea that you're serious about being an active participant in your own care.

Show an active interest in the data of your examination and testing. Questions like "What's my blood pressure today?" as it's being taken, or other appropriately timed inquiries are not only likely to get you information but also show that you're interested in what's going on.

Some physicians may schedule a follow-up visit to go over results. Others may just say you'll be notified if anything's abnormal. Either way, you might want to ask for the actual laboratory results, along with what's considered to be that laboratory's "normal value." That is usually printed right on the laboratory slip.

Obtaining your lab test results might be more helpful to you if you're seeing a non-nutritionally oriented physician than if you are. Either way, you have a right to the information; you've paid for it.

Let's go over some of the things that might be done at the doctor's office. As good a place as any to start is with your blood pressure reading.

The upper limit of "normal" blood pressure is considered to be 140/90. For those in older age groups, a little bit higher, especially the first number, is frequently considered normal. If your blood pressure is higher than that, but not what your doctor considers immediately dangerous, there are a number of things you might try before considering drug treatment.

Why worry at all? Especially if your blood pressure is only a little bit high? Unforunately, hypertension is associated with a higher risk of strokes, heart attacks, and kidney problems. Even if your blood pressure is only a little high, it's time to work on reduction before it gets too high.

Traditionally, exercise is one of the better ways of reducing blood pressure. If you're not already exercising regularly, it'd be wise to start. But first get your doctor's approval, because some people with hypertension will get very high blood pressure during exercise and may need drug control when beginning an exercise program.

Dietary measures are numerous and have been discussed in detail earlier. Have you eliminated all sources of caffeine: coffee, regular tea, cola drinks? For many, caffeine is a blood pressure raiser. What about the sodium-potassium ratio in your diet? Do everything you can to reduce sodium; just as important, increase your intake of high-potassium foods. There's also an apparent association between consumption of vegetable source foods and lower blood pressure. If your blood pressure is high, and you're eating many animal source foods, consider trending toward a more vegetable source pattern.

Another valuable blood pressure control technique is biofeedback. This system uses medical electronics to help you get better mental control over your own blood pressure (as well as certain other body functions, if you want). Particularly if you live near or in a medium- to major-size city, there should be a biofeedback clinic available. Ask your doctor, or check the phone book.

As is often the case, a combination of all of the above means is more effective than any one of them alone.

Much attention is focused on hypertension (high blood pressure), but relatively little on hypotension (low blood pressure). Generally speaking, blood pressure of below 100/60 in an *adult* is too low, although some healthy younger adults may have lower blood pressure.

If such a blood pressure is accompanied by symptoms of dizzy spells, light-headedness, fainting spells, or definite vertigo when standing up, it's probably too low for the individual concerned.

Unfortunately, sometimes the only comment made is "Well, with blood pressure like that you won't have a stroke." That's probably so, but hypotension isn't normal either.

In my practice, I've observed that hypotension (particularly when symptomatic) is most often indicative of relatively weak function of part of the adrenal gland called the cortex. This condition is termed "hypoadrenocorticism." Lamentably, hypoadrenocorticism is another problem usually considered nonexistent in standard medical practice. I've heard all too many physicians give the opinion that if it isn't Addison's disease, then your adrenal function is normal.

Addison's disease is the term for adrenal failure, or nonfunction. Simple logic would indicate that there are degrees between nonfunction and normal. Using another endocrine gland as example, it's possible to have normal thyroid function, weak thyroid function (hypothyroidism), or nonfunction (cretinism). A single measurement of blood cortisone isn't always adequate to make a diagnosis of this problem, either. This is one area where a nutritionally oriented physician may be essential, both for diagnosis and advice about treatment.

Let's get back to helping yourself with your doctor's help, and move to two of the most common laboratory determinations, the blood count and the urinalysis.

Blood counting is done for both white and red blood cells. If the white blood cell count is too high, it usually means an infection of some sort. Occasionally it indicates other problems, but interpretation here is best left to your physician. A low white blood cell count is only rarely a serious problem, but can, of course, contribute to decreased resistance to infection.

Occasionally, a white blood cell count may be low due to an allergy, or a toxic material in the system. It doesn't hurt to look for something like that, particularly if the low white blood count is persistent.

Several tests are reported on red blood cells. These include hemoglobin (the amount of oxygen-carrying pigment material), hematocrit (the percentage of red blood cells in the total blood stream volume), and a count of the number of red blood cells per cubic millimeter of blood. If one or more of these numbers is low, the test is usually considered to indicate anemia.

There are certainly nonnutritional causes of anemia such as gastrointestinal bleeding, hemolysis (abnormally increased blood cell destruction), as well as others. However, most of these causes require professional knowledge and testing to search out. We'll cover only nutritionally related anemia here.

Anemia is most commonly due to iron deficiency, but can also be associated with a lack of copper, vitamin B_{12}, folic acid, or vitamin B_6, among the known blood-building nutrients. Excess lead or zinc can also cause anemia, although the latter can be prevented by adequate copper intake.

Unless you have a serious or dangerous anemia, when iron supplements are indicated, one of the simplest things you can do about it is to eat liver, which is probably the best single source of all the blood-building elements. If you're a vegetarian, brewer's yeast and wheat germ as well as other supplements will help.

Iron is particularly sensitive to lack of adequate stomach acid; without it, it's not well absorbed. Taking iron when it appears necessary, with no results, is sometimes a clue that this problem exists.

Urinalysis is done to check for the presence of substances not usually excreted by the kidneys, such as sugar or protein. Non-symptomatic infection can sometimes be found; a test is done (called specific gravity) for diabetes insipidus, a rare problem whose symptoms include excess urination.

If sugar is found in the urine, follow-up testing for diabetes mellitus (sugar diabetes) is usually done. Protein in the urine can be a temporary, harmless result of exercise or a possible sign of kidney disease.

Some nutritionally oriented physicians may add in a test called "Obermayer's test (urinary indican)." This is nothing new, just not always done. A positive result on this test usually indicates the presence of abnormal bacteria in the colon, or too many bad germs compared to good ones. If that is the case, normalization of the bowel bacteria with *Lactobacillus acidophilus*, *L. bul-*

garicus, bran products, and sometimes garlic can be important to future health.

Since I've mentioned diabetes mellitus, I should note a relatively new screening test for this problem. Called glycohemoglobin (Hgb Al_c), this test can help detect early or hidden diabetes mellitus even when the fasting blood sugar is normal, and the urine shows no sugar. If you have any reason to suspect diabetes, or if you're in an older age group and there's diabetes in your family, it's wise to ask to have this test done.

While on the subject of blood sugar, I wish I could tell you there was as simple a test for hypoglycemia (low blood sugar), but there isn't. A five- or preferably six-hour glucose tolerance test is the only exact way.

Hypoglycemia is another one of those controversial problems. There's a wide divergence sometimes in the interpretation of glucose tolerance tests between nutritionally oriented and non-nutritionally oriented physicians.

Unlike diabetes mellitus, which often doesn't give definite symptoms, hypoglycemia usually is suspected because of its symptoms, which may include extreme tiredness at certain times of the day, dizziness, headaches, behavioral disturbances, and symptoms which only develop when you haven't eaten for several hours or more. If you suspect it, why not put yourself on a strict antihypoglycemia program, and see what happens? It's cheaper, less hassle sometimes than persuading a physician to give you the six-hour glucose tolerance test, and less strain on your system. For details, see chapter 17, "A Case of Palpitations."

Blood fats should also be checked from time to time, particularly if you have any heart or blood vessel disease in your family. Those most frequently checked are triglycerides and cholesterol. Another new test which should be included with these two is the high-density lipoprotein test, or HDL.

Always make sure you're fasting for at least six to eight hours, or overnight, when you have these tests done. Otherwise, the results are not nearly as worthwhile.

If triglycerides are high, examine your diet for sugar, alcohol, and total carbohydrate intake, particularly refined carbohydrate.

Eliminating all these items will often help normalize triglycerides, with nothing further to be done.

Supplements that help my patients reduce triglyceride levels include essential fatty acids, particularly vegetable oils, and vitamin C. I usually recommend a tablespoon or two of vegetable oil, accompanied by 200 to 400 units of vitamin E. The vitamin C recommendation varies, but usually ranges from 1 to 6 grams daily.

Cholesterol tests can be better interpreted with the aid of the HDL test. Generally speaking, HDL is the good part of cholesterol, while its relative, low-density lipoprotein (LDL) is generally considered bad. Rather than looking at just high or normal cholesterol, it's wiser to divide the cholesterol number by the HDL number. A figure of 5 (cholesterol/HDL = 5) is considered to be average risk from the cholesterol point of view. Under 5 is less risk, over 5 is more.

If your cholesterol/HDL is too high, it's only sometimes the fault of too much dietary cholesterol.

A large number of nutrients have been found helpful in cholesterol level reduction. It's not yet proven that all of them will also alter the cholesterol/HDL ratio, but (at least in my patients) with basic good diet and some or all of the following, it usually happens.

One or 2 tablespoons of lecithin are first on the list, followed by vitamin C again, from 1 to 6 grams daily. Include 1 or 2 tablespoons of vegetable oil (for the essential fatty acids). Extra calcium, approximately 1 gram daily, can be a help; so can extra magnesium, from 150 to 500 milligrams daily. Niacin is a standby in standard medical practice. I usually recommend the time-release form, in doses of 125 to 400 milligrams twice daily, as this form produces less flushing and discomfort. Oddly enough, niacinamide usually doesn't work. Brewer's yeast also has a beneficial effect.

With all the possible metabolic and dietary alterations capable of affecting blood cholesterol levels, there should never be a need for synthetic cholesterol-lowering drugs, except in cases of severe congenital hyperlipidemia.

Almost everyone is familiar with the electrocardiogram, or EKG. The test is standard in many physician's offices. The EKG is capable of detecting heart damage from heart attack, and abnormal heart rhythm, but in itself isn't a predictive test.

Combining the electrocardiogram with the measured stress of running on a treadmill is believed to be of predictive value. The stress EKG can predict to a degree the risk of heart attack in the near future, as well as aiding in the estimation of your present and potential exercise capability.

Should you ask your doctor to have a stress EKG done for you? If you've not been exercising, and plan to start in a regular program, it's a good idea. It's a particularly good idea if you're male and past 40, or female at menopause or past. It's even more important if there are heart attacks in your family.

Putting together the results of a stress EKG, cholesterol, HDL test, and triglyceride determination, your physician can give you a better estimation of your heart attack risk.

Other common screening tests include uric acid, thyroid function tests, kidney, and liver function tests. Although these are helpful to your physician in detecting disease, they're probably going to be less helpful to you in trying to keep yourself healthy. However, there are a few points to note.

Uric acid, a breakdown product of the metabolism of nucleic acids, DNA and RNA, can cause gout symptoms if the levels are too high. Although diet can help bring down high levels slightly, extra folic acid can do much more. Some people have told me they "just feel better" if they take extra folic acid, 2 to 5 milligrams daily or more, when their uric acid levels are not abnormally high, but high within normal. I have no explanation for this, but pass it along, as it certainly can't hurt.

If your thyroid function tests are low, your physician may prescribe thyroid for you. What if they're low but within the normal range? For some, this is really not a problem. Others have taken kelp or dulse for a few months and found that not only were the results of their thyroid function tests a bit better, but that they also felt just a little better. Unless you particularly need to control salt in your diet, this can't hurt; if you do need to control salt, potassium iodide in safe nonprescription doses is also available.

Liver function tests will probably only be of use to you if you're taking very large amounts of niacinamide or niacin. With large doses, certain liver function tests go high. Whether this is dangerous or not is really not certain. Sometimes the risk involved is less than the benefit obtained from taking these vitamins. It's probably wise to keep an eye on them, and if necessary and possible, consult with a nutritionally oriented physician about it.

The common kidney function tests are called creatinine and blood urea nitrogen (BUN). If they're both too high, your physician may recommend further investigation of possible kidney disease. Not infrequently, the BUN is slightly elevated when the creatinine is well within normal. Sometimes this situation indicates only that you're not drinking enough water. Other times, it's an indicator that there's excess protein in your diet, particularly protein of animal origin. If this is a possibility, try cutting down for awhile, then have the test repeated.

If you suspect you're not making enough digestive enzymes, sometimes traditional pancreatic function tests, done on a blood specimen, can provide a clue. These aren't always done routinely, so you might have to ask specifically, but they're always available. These tests are called amylase and lipase. When low, they can contribute to a suspicion of inadequate digestive enzymes. Unfortunately, not all laboratories have a similar normal range for these tests, sometimes reporting that 0 is normal. This isn't so, but it's difficult to get more accurate information on your own.

Unless you're allergic to them, digestive enzymes are very safe. They're made from both animal (beef and pork), and vegetable (pineapple and papaya) sources. If you suspect you have a problem, perhaps gas and a little bloating or indigestion one to three hours after eating, why not just try some and see? That might avoid the need for testing.

Tests of minerals and vitamins in the bloodstream are only occasionally helpful. Calcium, phosphorus, sodium, potassium, vitamin B$_{12}$, and others frequently are reported as normal when you could actually be benefited by more of these nutrients.

Let's look at common examples of this problem. Probably the best is the fact that the vast majority of women with clear x-ray evidence of osteoporosis, with much calcium obviously lost from the bones, usually have normal calcium and phosphorus levels in the bloodstream.

Likewise, many persons with muscle weakness or cramps demonstrably helped by potassium are reported to have normal serum potassium levels.

What about hair testing for mineral levels? This is definitely more helpful in determining the need for minerals, but the interpretation of hair analysis is sometimes fairly tricky. Also, it's probably not available through a traditional physician.

Other tests mentioned in this book are those for food allergy and nutrient absorption, both very important considerations in investigating nutrition and your health. Formal tests in these categories are frequently available only through nutritionally oriented physicians, or in the case of allergy testing, through an allergist.

A word or two about testing for food allergy problems: skin tests are usually not very accurate. There are a wide variety of other tests, including the radioallergosorbent (RAST) test, cytotoxic testing, provocative testing, and other systems. But don't forget there are self-testing methods too, most notably fasting, single-food testing, and pulse testing (see chapter 46, "A Look at Food Allergy").

Quite obviously, even a routine checkup with more or less routine laboratory testing, perhaps including a stress electrocardiogram, is relatively more expensive than an average doctor visit for a particular symptom or problem. If you see a preventive or nutritionally oriented physician, some of the more specialized testing may add even more to the cost.

Is it worth the expense, particularly if you're feeling well? The argument has been made that it's a lot cheaper than a stay in the hospital, considering both the hospital expense and the possible income loss. It's also cheaper to try to stay healthy and out of the doctor's office, than to have to go numerous times for illness. On the other hand, the hospital bill is covered by insurance, even if the income loss isn't, and so are doctor visits for illness. Trying to stay healthy with preventive care often isn't covered.

There's also no guarantee it'll work. Despite the best attempts, some of us might get sick anyway.

Like anything else in life, it's a matter of weighing costs and benefits, and deciding whether it's worth it to you. It's your money, and your health.

A Resource Guide to Nutritional and Natural Therapy

49

Compiled with the help of Carol Baldwin,
Research Chief, *Prevention* magazine

It isn't easy at times to know for sure where nutritional information is coming from, and when you do, you're not sure whether it's accurate or reliable. There's just so much confusion and contradiction in the media and even from disagreeing scientists, that for the newcomer, especially, it can be a dizzying experience. To help you get a clear perspective on the field, we've prepared an annotated listing of over 175 of the key books and associations in nutrition and natural therapy.

The books that were selected—over 130 of them—each make a significant contribution to the natural health field in its own right. Most are based either on the clinical experiences of the author or on scientific medical literature. All are practical in their approach and written in an understandable style. Some are more technical than others and are better used as references. The section is organized by key subjects, which at times may seem arbitrary, since many of the books cover a wide variety of topics.

The directory of associations incorporates descriptions of over 50 lay and professional nonprofit organizations whose primary purpose is to educate the public about nutrition, orthomolecular medicine, and natural therapies through literature, publications, and/or sponsorship of seminars and workshops. They, too, are organized by key subject areas. Many provide a valuable referral service which makes available the names of physicians, dentists, pediatricians, obstetricians, psychologists, psychiatrists, etc. who are nutritionally oriented and interested in a more natural approach to the prevention and treatment of disease. When corresponding with these organizations, remember to include a self-addressed, stamped envelope.

A Selected Bibliography

AGING

Weg, Ruth B. *Nutrition and Aging: A Selected Bibliography.* Los Angeles: The University of Southern California Press, 1977.
A selected list of publications primarily focusing on the significant inadequacies of nutrition in the later years.

Weg, Ruth B. *Nutrition and the Later Years.* Los Angeles: The University of Southern California Press, 1978.
Presents scientific information relevant to the nutritional needs during the later years of life. Nutritional inadequacies are reviewed as they relate to daily life and the development of problems such as diverticulitis, diabetes, osteoporosis, etc. Attitudes and behavioral changes as they affect nutritional intake are also discussed.

Winick, Myron, ed. *Nutrition and Aging.* New York: John Wiley & Sons, 1976.
Incorporates a series of articles to document the most recent information pertaining to nutrition for the elderly. It examines the basic questions concerned with nutrition during earlier life and how these earlier requirements influence later-in-life health prob-

lems. The book is divided into three sections: effects of aging in cells, aging in normal human populations, and the nutrition-related diseases of old age, i.e., osteoporosis, periodontal disease, obesity, and atherosclerosis.

ALLERGY

Blaine, Tom R. *Goodbye Allergies.* Secaucus, N.J.: Citadel Press, 1978.
Describes the author's personal experience of being cured after a lifetime of allergic suffering, and reviews available articles from medical journals dealing with nutrition and the adrenal cortex extract treatment for allergic diseases.

Breneman, J. C. *Basics of Food Allergy.* Springfield, Ill.: Charles C Thomas, 1978.
An excellent review of the latest developments in causes and treatments of food allergies by a board-certified allergist. Thorough coverage of unusual allergies causing such problems as bed-wetting, arthritis, gallbladder disease, and mental disorders. Specific dietary advice (complete with brand names) offered for those wishing to eliminate foods including corn, beef, yeast, and soybeans extremely helpful.

Coca, Arthur F. *The Pulse Test: The Secret of Building Your Health.* New York: Lyle Stuart, 1967.
Describes in full detail how to use the pulse test to discover allergies, and sheds new light on a wide range of problems including: high blood pressure, epilepsy, diabetes, gastric ulcers, and migraine headaches, and implicates food allergies as their cause.

Crook, William Grant. *Your Allergic Child: A Pediatrician's Guide to Normal Living for Allergic Adults and Children.* New York: Medcome Press, 1973.
A very readable guide to allergies and their symptoms, diagnosis,

and treatment. Describes commonly recognizable problems of hay fever, skin rashes, and asthma along with the other, often overlooked symptoms of fatigue, irritability, headache, achy legs, etc. Practical advice on discovering and managing food allergies is offered along with how to keep new allergies from developing, planning elimination diets, how to exercise if you're asthmatic and how to work along with your doctor. Another valuable self-help guide to allergies.

Dickey, Lawrence D., ed. *Clinical Ecology.* Springfield, Ill.: Charles C Thomas, 1976.
Compiles the works of some of the most renowned researchers to explain the effects the environment (air, food, water, habitat) exerts on the human condition. The problems of individual susceptibility to such things as pesticides, herbicides, additives, chemicals, and contaminants are discussed, as are nutritional, dietary, orthomolecular, and immunological solutions.

Golos, Natalie. *Management of Complex Allergies.* HEAL, Suite 6506, 505 North Lake Shore Drive, Chicago, IL 60611, 1975.
An easy-to-read manual for anyone sensitive to foods, drugs, and/ or chemicals. Covers various aspects of living including cooking hints and recipes, household cleansers, fabric selections, insect control, cosmetics, and travel. Brand-name references very helpful. Specific references to allergies to foods in the same family complete the thorough listings.

Mackarness, Richard. *Eating Dangerously: The Hazards of Hidden Allergies.* New York: Harcourt Brace Jovanovich, 1976.
Examines allergies from the sufferer's perspective, aiding him in a practical approach to detecting food allergies that may be causing such problems as migraine headaches, colitis, asthma, sinusitis, and depression. Often the most likely candidates are sugar and processed cereals—frequently favorite foods.

Mandell, Marshall, and Scanlon, Lynne Waller. *Dr. Mandell's 5-Day Allergy Relief System*. New York: Thomas Y. Crowell, 1979.
Reviews the success Dr. Mandell has had treating hundreds of patients and reveals that physical, mental, and psychosomatic illnesses have their roots in the body's reactions to food, beverages, tap water, dust, molds, pollens, and chemicals regularly contacted. Describes in detail how to test for such sensitivities. Problems relieved using his method include: compulsive eating and drinking, depression, fatigue, arthritis, eczema, migraine, and clogged sinuses.

Randolph, Theron G. *Human Ecology and Susceptibility to the Chemical Environment*. Springfield, Ill.: Charles C Thomas, 1978.
Focuses on man and his susceptibility to his environment, drawing from the author's own clinical experiences in the field of environmental allergy. The major chemicals causing both mental and physical problems are described in detail as are ways to avoid them. The diagnostic routines to determine chemical allergies are explained along with numerous case reports.

ARTHRITIS

Broadman, Joseph. *Bee Venom: The Natural Curative for Arthritis and Rheumatism*. New York: G. P. Putnam's Sons, 1962.
A detailed description of the clinical experiences of this physician-author and his successful treatment of arthritis and rheumatism with bee venom.

Childers, Norman Franklin, and Russo, Gerard M. *The Nightshades and Health*. Somerville, N.J.: Horticultural Publications, Somerset Press, 1977.
A fascinating book describing the importance of nightshade plants—tomatoes, white potatoes, peppers, eggplant, and to-

bacco—and how they can lead to the cause and control of arthritis. The "No-Nightshades" diet is completely described, as are accounts of people on the diet who successfully alleviated their arthritic symptoms.

Kaufman, William. *The Common Form of Joint Dysfunction: Its Incidence and Treatment.* Brattleboro, Vt.: E. L. Hildreth, 1949. (Out of print; check local medical library.)
A well-researched, clinical monograph on the use of niacinamide to control the symptoms of osteoarthritis. Reviews the results compiled from hundreds of carefully documented cases of the author while in private practice of internal medicine. Also, describes four complicating syndromes of joint dysfunction that respond to niacinamide therapy.

ATMOSPHERE AND HEALTH

Burr, Harold Saxton. *The Fields of Life: Our Links with the Universe.* New York: Ballantine Books, 1972.
A Yale professor's review of what is known about electromagnetic fields and their influence on health and disease. Emphasizes how knowledge of such fields can be used to diagnose problems and provide access to the general state of the body as a whole. Complete selection of papers is included reviewing such subjects as the implications of electromagnetic tests in cancer of the female genital tract and monitoring of electromagnetic fields in hypnotic states, etc.

Llaurado, J. G.; Sances, A., Jr.; and Battocletti, J. H. *Biologic and Clinical Effects of Low-Frequency Magnetic and Electric Fields.* Springfield, Ill.: Charles C Thomas, 1974.
A technical review of current knowledge about the biological and psychological effects of electric and magnetic fields on the human system. Material in the book was contributed by 50 scientists and is written primarily for physicians, biologists, psychologists, and engineers.

Playfair, Guy L., and Hill, Scott. *The Cycles of Heaven: Cosmic Forces and What They Are Doing to You.* New York: St. Martin's Press, 1978.
Focuses on the potential for a vast range of influences the environment may have on behavior and unconscious thoughts and impulses. Covers a wide range of subjects including gravity and electromagnetism, cybernetics, the forces behind earthquakes and meteorological happenings, biorhythms, and biofeedback.

Rosen, Stephen. *Weathering: How the Atmosphere Conditions Your Body, Your Mind, Your Mood—and Your Health.* New York: M. Evans and Co., 1979.
A fascinating account of the influence atmospheric conditions have on both physiological and psychological aspects of health. Advice on what to eat, what drugs to avoid, what clothes to buy, how to plan a vacation, etc. is given on the basis of weather conditions. How to use the weather to best advantage.

Soyka, Fred, and Edmonds, Alan. *The Ion Effect: How Air Electricity Rules Your Life and Health.* New York: Bantam Books, 1977.
Reviews evidence that positive and negative ions present in the atmosphere can control moods and influence health and our sense of well-being. Information is based on the author's experiences and the scientific information he amassed in search of solutions to his own problems.

BACKACHE

Root, Leon, and Kiernan, Thomas. *Oh, My Aching Back: A Doctor's Guide to Your Back Pain and How to Control It.* New York: David McKay Co., 1973.
A prominent orthopedic surgeon describes in detail what the back is all about—how it functions and how it gets into trouble. Explains both diagnostic and treatment procedures for back

problems and provides helpful daily advice on overcoming and preventing chronic back pain.

BIOCHEMISTRY

Lehninger, Albert L. *A Short Course in Biochemistry*. New York: Worth, 1973.

A case study approach to biochemistry. Author outlines methods and approaches useful to the biochemical study of disease.

Sloane, Nathan H., and York, J. Lyndal. *Review of Biochemistry*. London, Ontario: Collier-Macmillan Canada, 1969.

A complete, yet brief textbook presenting the biochemical approach to medicine, providing a deeper understanding of disease and its diagnosis. Its outline format and 23 chapters present a survey of biochemical methods and physiological/chemical principles in a ready reference form.

BIOLOGICAL RHYTHMS

Luce, Gay Gaer. *Biological Rhythms in Psychiatry and Medicine*. Washington, D.C.: Superintendent of Documents, 1978.

Compiles the result of studies supported by the National Institute of Mental Health on the effect of biological rhythms on our daily health and well-being. Includes extensive references.

CANCER

Simonton, O. Carl; Mathews-Simonton, Stephanie; and Creighton, James. *Getting Well Again: A Step-by-Step, Self-Help Guide to Overcoming Cancer for Patients and Their Families*. Los Angeles: J. P. Tarcher, 1978.

Reviews the work of the Simontons, leading practitioners in the field of psychological causes and treatment of cancer. Using their experiences with hundreds of patients, the book helps an individual to evaluate his reaction to stress and other emotional factors that may have contributed to the onset and progress (or recurrence) of his own disease and gives detailed instructions including how to learn a positive attitude, how to relax, use of visualization, goal-setting, managing pain, exercising, and building an emotional support system to help patients recognize and deal with the problem. Provides a fascinating scientific basis for "the will to live."

CARBOHYDRATES

Cleave, T. L. *The Saccharine Disease*. New Canaan, Conn.: Keats Publishing, 1975.
Reviews the author's theory that many of the "diseases of Western civilization" (diabetes, heart disease, obesity, peptic ulcer, hemorrhoids) are the effects of consuming refined carbohydrate food like table sugar and white flour. Man's diet, Surgeon-Captain Cleave believes, has changed too rapidly for him to adapt evolutionally.

Cleave, T. L.; Campbell, G. D.; and Doll, Richard. *Diabetes, Coronary Thrombosis and the Saccharine Disease*. Bristol, England: John Wright & Sons, 1966.
Supports the idea that man's dietary change from natural, unrefined carbohydrates to refined ones was much too fast for his evolutionary adjustment. Because of his poor adaptation, problems like diabetes, obesity, and heart disease plague him. The lack of these problems among primitive cultures eating a natural, unrefined diet is convincing evidence.

Shreeve, Walton W. *Physiological Chemistry of Carbohydrates in Mammals*. Philadelphia: W. B. Saunders Co., 1974.
A thorough but brief textbook review of the important role that carbohydrates play in the dietary of mammals. Complete descriptions of the different types of carbohydrates are offered along with a discussion of their digestion and absorption.

CELLULAR THERAPY

Niehans, Paul. *Introduction to Cellular Therapy*. New York: Pageant Books, 1960.

A brief introduction to the work of the author, a Swiss physician, who theorizes that the injection of young animal or embryonic cells into human beings will revitalize worn-out cells and restore health. His successful therapies are described with people treated for various pituitary ailments, obesity, gigantism, dwarfism, angina pectoris, eczema, psoriasis, bronchial asthma, etc.

CHOLESTEROL

Pinckney, Edward R., and Pinckney, Cathey. *The Cholesterol Controversy*. Los Angeles: Sherbourne Press, 1973.

Serves to clarify some of the confusion, misconceptions, and misinformation about cholesterol and its effect on health. Written primarily for the consumer, it explains the nature of cholesterol itself and reviews the major issues, the importance of diet and physical fitness, and the effect of stress on heart disease. Its annotated bibliography and reference section completes the book.

DIABETES

Abrahamson, E. M., and Pezet, A. W. *Body, Mind, and Sugar*. New York: Avon Books, 1977.

A brief, fascinating history of the discovery and treatment of diabetes and hyperinsulinism. Detailed case reports on insulin shock, diabetic coma, and hyperinsulinism are abundant. The relationship of hyperinsulinism to allergies, asthma, alcoholism, and mental health is discussed. Also included is the Harris diet for hyperinsulinism.

DRUGS

Goodman, Louis S., and Gilman, Alfred, eds. *The Pharmacological Basis of Therapeutics*. New York: Macmillan Publishing Co., 1975.

A major reference textbook directed toward the medical professional. The whole spectrum of drug therapeutics is reviewed, ranging from drugs acting on the central nervous system all the way to a review of the major vitamins.

DRUGS AND NUTRITIONAL DEFICIENCIES

Roe, Daphne A. *Drug-Induced Nutritional Deficiencies.* Westport, Conn.: Avi Publishing, 1976.
In-depth coverage of nutritional disorders caused by such drugs as anticonvulsants, antimalarials, antibiotics, sedatives, contraceptives, cholesterol-lowering agents, and antituberculous drugs. Each of the 14 chapters includes an extensive list of references, and chapter 4 contains a detailed questionnaire for obtaining a patient's dietary and drug history.

EXERCISE

Caplow-Lindner, Erna; Harpaz, Leah; and Samberg, Sonya. *Therapeutic Dance/Movement: Expressive Activities for Older Adults.* New York: Human Sciences Press, 1979.
Provides both theoretical and practical information on dance and movement therapy for the older adult, focusing on creative and folk dance movements, yoga, and standing exercises adapted to his/her coordination and strength. Music, rhythm games, and relaxation techniques are discussed in a very clear and readable manner. A creative alternative to standard exercise practices.

Cooper, Kenneth H. *The New Aerobics.* New York: M. Evans and Co., 1970.
Details the exercise program devised by a U.S. Air Force physician which was later adopted officially by the U.S. Air Force. The reader learns what aerobics is all about, why it is important, and how much exercise is needed to develop a personal program, what kind, and how to measure the benefits.

Cooper, Mildred, and Cooper, Kenneth. *Aerobics for Women.* New York: M. Evans and Co., 1972.
Describes the pioneering program developed by Dr. Cooper, but directs it toward the needs of women. The medical, physical, emotional, and cosmetic benefits of aerobics are included along with why women have a particular need for aerobic exercise. Details aerobic exercises for such personal times as menstruation, pregnancy, and menopause replete with personal accounts from women across the country who have had success with the aerobics program.

FASTING

Cott, Allan. *Fasting: The Ultimate Diet.* New York: Bantam Books, 1975.
A complete guide to fasting and its health benefits. Provides practical advice which will be of help to anyone interested in exploring the subject of fasting.

FATIGUE

Graham, M. F. *Inner Energy: How to Overcome Fatigue.* New York: Sterling Publishing Co., 1979.
Chronic fatigue and its relationship to drug and alcohol abuse, physical illness (cancer, high blood pressure, diabetes), tension, stress, and improper nutrition is explained by a physician with a strong interest in physical fitness and preventive medicine. Anecdotes and brief case histories help to illustrate the problems.

FATTY ACIDS

Mead, James F., and Fulco, Armand J. *The Unsaturated and Polyunsaturated Fatty Acids in Health and Disease.* Springfield, Ill.: Charles C Thomas, 1976.
Details the roles that unsaturated and polyunsaturated fatty acids play in membrane structure and function as precursors to prostaglandin hormones and as essential dietary factors. The clinical and

medical aspects of deficiency diseases in certain polyunsaturated acids are discussed as are laboratory analyses.

FEMALE PROBLEMS

Fredericks, Carlton. *Breast Cancer: A Nutritional Approach.* New York: Grosset & Dunlap, 1977.
Marshalls evidence that the typical American diet increases the risk of menstrual disturbances, cystic mastitis, uterine fibroid tumors, and susceptibility to breast and uterine cancer. Intriguing links are made between the female hormone estrogen and cancer along with advice on how all these problems can be eliminated through dietary change.

FIBER

Burkitt, Denis P., and Trowell, Hugh C. *Refined Carbohydrate Foods and Disease: Some Implications of Dietary Fiber.* New York: Academic Press, 1975.
An extensively documented book providing very convincing scientific support for diseases of Western civilization—heart disease, diverticular disease, gallstones, appendicitis, varicose veins, hemorrhoids, obesity, and diabetes—and their relationship to the lack of fiber in the diet.

Fredericks, Carlton. *Carlton Fredericks' High-Fiber Way to Total Health.* New York: Pocket Books, 1976.
Describes the important role fiber plays in the network of diseases of civilization such as colitis, diverticulosis, ulcers, and heart disease. A special section on high-fiber, low carbohydrate reducing plans.

Reuben, David. *The Save-Your-Life Diet: High-Fiber Protection from Six of the Most Serious Diseases of Civilization.* New York: Random House, 1975.

A scientifically based review of the medical literature on the value of high-fiber diets by a physician in clinical practice with a keen interest in spreading the word that major "diseases of civilization" (heart attacks, diverticular disease, varicose veins, appendicitis, obesity, constipation, hemorrhoids) can practically be eliminated by following a high-fiber diet. A complete recipe selection on high-fiber foods as well as the selected bibliography are very helpful.

FOOD

Goldbeck, Nikki, and Goldbeck, David. *The Supermarket Handbook: Access to Whole Foods.* New York: Signet, 1976.

An extremely helpful guide for anyone interested in whole foods. The reader is guided down the supermarket aisles and shown how to select the best whole, natural, and unadulterated foods. All information is brought out in the open including brand-name references, additive ingredients, nutritional values, etc.

FOOD (HISTORICAL)

Cohen, Mark Nathan. *The Food Crisis in Prehistory: Overpopulation and the Origins of Agriculture.* New Haven, Conn.: Yale University Press, 1977.

Traces the development of agriculture in different population groups. Explains the emergence of agriculture on a worldwide scale through the existence of population pressure.

Heiser, Charles B., Jr. *Seed to Civilization: The Story of Man's Food.* San Francisco: W. H. Freeman and Co., 1973.

A historical perspective written in somewhat of a textbook style which reviews man's relationship with basic food plants and describes the origin of agriculture. Historical perspectives on individual foods like legumes, potatoes, cereal grains, beverages, and spices make for very interesting reading.

FOOD (INSTITUTIONAL)

Moyer, Anne. *Better Food for Public Places: A Guide for Improving Institutional Food.* Emmaus, Pa.: Rodale Press, 1977.

Addresses the food-service problems of day care and Head Start centers, elementary and high schools, colleges, hospitals and government feeding programs, and tells what pioneering people in each of these areas are doing to incorporate more natural foods into their menus, and generally to raise the quality of the food they serve. It also examines the concrete problems involved in serving more whole, natural foods to large numbers of people.

FOOD ADULTERATION

Jacobson, Michael. *Eater's Digest: The Consumer's Factbook of Food Additives.* Garden City, N.Y.: Doubleday & Co., 1972.

A very informative study that provides the answers to the most frequently asked questions consumers have about food additives. It describes over 100 commonly used additives, such as EDTA, monoglycerides and diglycerides, benzoate, propylene glycol, artificial flavoring and coloring, etc.

Turner, James S. *The Chemical Feast.* New York: Grossman Publishers, 1970.

Examines in great detail how the quality of the American diet has deteriorated. It calls to task the Food and Drug Administration which sets food standards that promote dishonesty in the marketplace and attempts to deceive consumers and conceal important information. A review of cyclamates, food-borne diseases, hidden ingredients, and governmental regulatory practices.

Verrett, Jacqueline, and Carper, Jean. *Eating May Be Hazardous to Your Health: How Your Government Fails to Protect You from the Dangers in Your Food.* New York: Simon and Schuster, 1974.

Written by a Food and Drug Administration scientist and a consumer writer, this book explains how the FDA's bureaucracy appears almost to endorse and promote the use of additive-laden chemical food. The scope of the problem is reviewed along with a listing of the dangers from specific additives that are found in foods that we eat every day. Practical advice for positive action that each consumer can take to protect his or her own health is very valuable.

FOOD COMPOSITION

Adams, Catherine F. *Nutritive Value of American Foods in Common Units.* Handbook No. 456. Washington, D.C.: Superintendent of Documents, 1975.

Provides a guide to values for calories and nutrients supplied by various household measures and market units of foods. Nutritional information on approximately 1,500 foods including menu items, snacks, and market products, ready-to-eat foods, and some that require preparation or are used as ingredients can be found on its pages.

Kraus, Barbara. *The Barbara Kraus 1979 Calorie Guide to Brand Names and Basic Foods.* New York: Signet, 1978.

A handy pocket guide to calories in foods.

Kraus, Barbara. *The Barbara Kraus 1979 Carbohydrate Guide to Brand Names and Basic Foods.* New York: Signet, 1978.

A handy pocket guide to counting carbohydrates contained in commonly eaten foods.

Orr, Martha Louise. *Pantothenic Acid, Vitamin B_6 and Vitamin B_{12} in Foods.* Home Economics Research Report No. 36. Washington, D.C.: Superintendent of Documents, 1969.

Data on three important vitamins—pantothenic acid, vitamin B_6, and vitamin B_{12}—are summarized based on data reported from scientific investigations in many laboratories. Values are selected based on their suitability for estimating content of these vitamins in foods, diets, and food supplies.

FOOD PROCESSING

Harris, Robert S., and Karmas, Endel, eds. *Nutritional Evaluation of Food Processing.* Westport, Conn.: The Avi Publishing Co., 1975.

Presents a collection of works by 30 authors competent in the fields of nutrition, food science, and food technology, who are interested in the nutritional effects of food processing from garden to table. It includes such interesting areas as nutrients in raw foods, the effects of commercial processing and storage on nutrients, the effects of preparation and service of food on nutrients, and the enrichment of foods.

HAIR ANALYSIS

Valkovic, Vlado. *Trace Elements in Human Hair.* New York: Garland STPM Press, 1977.

A complete summary of current studies about trace element analysis of human hair, including descriptions of the growth and structure of hair and how trace element values vary according to sex, age, health, and environmental exposure. Interesting reading for anyone looking for an up-to-date account of whether hair analysis is a valuable diagnostic tool.

HEADACHE

Evans, Peter. *Mastering Your Migraine.* New York: Granada Publishing, 1978.

A brief survey of the whole spectrum of present knowledge on treatment of migraine headaches written by a medical journalist. Lists addresses of migraine clinics and foundations along with further reading material.

Kurland, Howard D. *Quick Headache Relief without Drugs: How to Relieve Your Headache in Seconds: A Physician's Do-It-Yourself Technique.* New York: William Morrow & Co., 1977. Describes the auto-acupressure technique developed by the author, a physician, used to relieve all types of tension headaches, migraines, and sinus headaches. The author locates various pressure points that he believes directly relate to headache pain and shows how to obtain quick relief by using pressure exerted by the thumb.

HEART DISEASE

Farquhar, John W. *The American Way of Life Need Not Be Hazardous to Your Health.* New York: W. W. Norton & Co., 1978. A cardiologist's presentation that poor diet, too much stress, lack of exercise, and smoking can lead to premature strokes and heart attacks. He points out that once man takes an active role in eliminating the major cardiovascular risk factors, he can effectively achieve health. Practical advice is offered to help the reader change habits, relieve stress, develop a personalized exercise program, change diet, and lose weight.

Levy, Robert I. et al. *Nutrition, Lipids, and Coronary Heart Disease: A Global View.* New York: Raven Press, 1979. A very thorough and comprehensive textbook review of the current knowledge relating nutrition to coronary heart disease prepared by four scientists. Subject areas covered are: epidemiology of diets, lipids, and heart disease; effect of dietary components on lipids and lipoproteins; use of nutrients in preserving health; behavior; food supply and patterns; and nutrition in relationship to other risk factors.

Price, Joseph M. *Coronaries/Cholesterol/Chlorine.* New York: Pyramid Communications, 1971.

Presents the author's controversial theory that chlorine in our drinking water—not cholesterol in our food—is the major cause of coronary disease.

HOLISTIC HEALTH

Ardell, Donald B. *High Level Wellness: An Alternative to Doctors, Drugs, and Disease.* Emmaus, Pa.: Rodale Press, 1977.
Approaches lifestyle in a very holistic way with an emphasis on integrating nutritional awareness, physical fitness, stress management, environmental sensitivity, and self-responsibility to achieve a feeling of optimal well-being. The reader is guided to accept responsibility for his/her own health and offered practical ways to evaluate his/her current health status and to make necessary changes.

Benson, Herbert. *The Mind/Body Effect: How Behavioral Medicine Can Show You the Way to Better Health.* New York: Simon and Schuster, 1979.
Explores the intricate relationship the mind and body share and points out in depth that the mind has a great bearing on our state of physical health. This physician-author makes a very convincing argument for the practice of behavioral medicine which incorporates the principles of medicine, physiology, psychiatry, and psychology.

Rodale, Robert. *The Best Health Ideas I Know: Including My Personal Plan for Living.* Emmaus, Pa.: Rodale Press, 1974.
Reviews the author's personal plan for healthful living, including the vitamins he takes, the foods he seeks out and avoids, how he controls his weight, how he motivates himself to exercise, and many other ways that he has devised to maintain good health. Provides discussions on some of the most important of these measures, including herb therapy, hair analysis, the role of meat in a

diet, trace elements, and advice on how the energy crisis can be turned into a healthful advantage. A helpful book to anyone just getting started.

HYPERACTIVITY

Crook, William G. *Can Your Child Read? Is He Hyperactive?* Jackson, Tenn.: Professional Books, 1977.

A helpful, informative book on the causes and treatment of hyperactivity, learning disorders, and allergies, and their interrelationships. It describes case studies based on the personal experiences of the author working with approximately 200 children with hyperactive and learning problems, as well as thousands of children with allergies over nearly two decades. It emphasizes the key role that diet plays in a successful treatment outcome and provides a ready reference to books, pamphlets, articles, and organizations providing help on the subject.

Feingold, Ben F. *Why Your Child Is Hyperactive.* New York: Random House, 1975.

An easy-to-read presentation of the development of the Feingold diet (K-P) for hyperactive children. Using case histories as examples, the author, a well-known pediatrician, discusses problems in long-term drug management of the hyperactive child and shows how hyperactivity can often be treated with the K-P diet. The diet with instructions for its use, sample menus, and tasty recipes are included.

Smith, Lendon H. *Improving Your Child's Behavior Chemistry.* Englewood Cliffs, N.J.: Prentice-Hall, 1976.

Written by a pediatrician, this book contains many vivid descriptions of behaviorally disturbed children. Dietary suggestions as well as other suggestions for dealing with problem children are practical and based on experience. Charts enable the reader to determine a child's susceptibility to behavior problems.

HYPOGLYCEMIA

Airola, Paavo. *Hypoglycemia: A Better Approach.* Phoenix, Ariz.: Health Plus, 1977.

A complete account of a unique new approach to hypoglycemia including a review of its causes, symptoms, and cure. Includes a special description of Dr. Airola's "Optimum Diet" which focuses on complex carbohydrates like grains, nuts, seeds, and many raw vegetables and fruits. A discussion of case studies and helpful recipes are included.

Fredericks, Carlton, and Goodman, Herman. *Low Blood Sugar and You.* New York: Constellation International, 1969.

A complete review of hypoglycemia, its causes and treatments, with primary emphasis on the high-protein, low-carbohydrate diet as an aid to relieving a variety of physical and emotional problems caused by low blood sugar.

HYPOTHYROIDISM

Barnes, Broda O., and Galton, Lawrence. *Hypothyroidism: The Unsuspected Illness.* New York: Thomas Y. Crowell Co., 1976.

Provides a full explanation of what low thyroid function is and how it may be responsible for causing constant fatigue, chronic headaches, repeated infections, unyielding skin problems, circulatory difficulties, and many emotional disturbances. Written by a physician, this book offers advice on how to find out if such a problem exists and how to correct it.

LABORATORY TESTING

Sauberlich, H. E.; Skala, J. H.; and Dowdy, R. P. *Laboratory Tests for the Assessment of Nutritional Status.* Cleveland, Ohio: CRC Press, 1977.

A scientific summary of the major laboratory methods currently available for the evaluation of nutritional status along with a criticism of their usefulness and limitations.

LIGHT

Ott, John N. *Health and Light: The Effects of Natural and Artificial Light on Man and Other Living Things.* Old Greenwich, Conn.: The Devin-Adair Co., 1973.

Reviews the discovery of the author, a pioneer in time-lapse photography, that light is of great importance to plants, animals, and man. The author demonstrates that the full spectrum of daylight is needed to stimulate man's endocrine system and that without it he suffers.

MAGNESIUM

Aikawa, Jerry K. *The Role of Magnesium in Biologic Processes.* Springfield, Ill.: Charles C Thomas, 1963.

Reviews not only the history of magnesium and early biological studies, but surveys its use in veterinary medicine and its role in human disease.

MAN (HISTORICAL)

Fagan, Brian M. *People of the Earth: An Introduction to World Prehistory.* Boston, Mass.: Little, Brown and Co., 1977.

Provides a general look at the "life history" of the human species from the origin of mankind to the beginnings of literate civilization. Includes special sections on food and diet.

MEDICINE (HISTORY)

Martin, Wayne. *Medical Heroes and Heretics.* Old Greenwich, Conn.: The Devin-Adair Co., 1977.

A historical account of the agony of famous scientists as they proceed on the path to scientific discovery. Emphasis is on the resistance to scientific discovery that they experienced from orthodox medicine. Louis Pasteur, Frederick Banting, Jonas Salk, Ernst Krebs, Jr., Evan Shute, and Denis Burkitt are just a few of the people described.

MENTAL HEALTH

Cheraskin, Emanuel, and Ringsdorf, W. Marshall, Jr. with Brecher, Arline. *Psychodietetics: Food as the Key to Emotional Health.* New York: Stein & Day, 1974.
An interesting variation on the mind-body problem. Underscores the close relationship between diet and emotional health, discussing such varied topics as crash dieting, alcoholism, schizophrenia, hypoglycemia, drug addiction, sexual inadequacy, allergy, and hyperactivity. Dietary solutions with special attention to an "optimum diet" are included.

Fredericks, Carlton. *Psycho-Nutrition.* New York: Grosset & Dunlap, 1976.
Explains the intricate connection between the psyche and nutrition for the benefit of those suffering from neurosis, schizophrenia, alcoholism, hyperactivity, autism, and learning disabilities and extends a way to achieve the highest potential. It puts to final rest the old cliché "It's all in your mind."

Moody, Raymond A. *Laugh After Laugh: The Healing Power of Humor.* Jacksonville, Fla.: Headwaters Press, 1978.
Describes an overlooked avenue of healing—laughter and a sense of humor. Traces the history of the idea of humor and relates it to health. The author's message: "We can utilize our sense of humor to achieve a cosmic perspective on the world and ourselves, and thereby harness the positive power of a sense of humor to help cope with the uptight world we live in."

Newbold, H. L. *Mega-Nutrients for Your Nerves.* New York: Peter H. Wyden, 1975.
A thorough account of how to achieve "total nutrition" written by a psychiatrist with both a personal and clinical interest in nutrition. Practical descriptions of how individuals can determine their own vitamin and mineral needs as well as overcome specific

health problems (especially emotional) ranging from allergies and hypoglycemia to the inherent problems of aging. Included is a very helpful section on the hypoglycemia controversy and appropriate interpretation of glucose tolerance test results.

Watson, George. *Nutrition and Your Mind: The Psychochemical Response.* New York: Harper & Row, 1972.

A fascinating book that puts the psychological and physiological side by side. It warns that the wrong nutrition and health habits over a period of years may deplete the body's tissues to the point where they're incapable of utilizing proper nutrients. It relates in case-history style the complete restoration of mental health to several hundred patients, all of whom had exhausted the possibilities of psychotherapy and standard medical treatment. These "hopeless" cases were found to respond to simple vitamin and mineral therapy, or to findings that household poisons such as moth balls were causing a problem. A test for determining psychochemical types, suggested diets, and vitamin and mineral programs along with how to discover personal requirements for optimal mental and physical health are explored.

MULTIPLE SCLEROSIS

Swank, Roy L., and Pullen, Mary-Helen. *The Multiple Sclerosis Diet Book: A Low-Fat Diet for the Treatment of M.S., Heart Disease and Stroke.* Garden City, N.Y.: Doubleday & Co., 1977.

Reviews the work of the author, a neurologist, who has been successfully treating patients with a diet low in saturated fats and relatively high in polyunsaturated oils. Incorporates the results of his own findings primarily in the treatment of multiple sclerosis. Recipes following the Swank Low-Fat Diet are included.

NATURAL HEALING

Bricklin, Mark. *The Practical Encyclopedia of Natural Healing.* Emmaus, Pa.: Rodale Press, 1976.

A comprehensive, easy-to-understand guide to natural health care, providing detailed, documented information on preventing and treating over 140 health problems from acne and arthritis to warts and yeast infections. By the Executive Editor of *Prevention* magazine.

NIACIN

Altschul, Rudolf, ed. *Niacin in Vascular Disorders and Hyperlipemia.* Springfield, Ill.: Charles C Thomas, 1964.
Surveys the work of scientists supporting the effects of large doses of nicotinic acid on lipid metabolism in general and cholesterolemia in particular and on the course of atherosclerosis.

Kaufman, William. *The Common Form of Niacin Amide Deficiency Disease: Aniacinamidosis.* Bridgeport, Conn.: Yale University Press, 1943. (Out of print; check local medical library.)
A report based on a clinical study of more than 150 patients seen by the author with a variety of symptoms including memory impairment, tenseness, irritability, lack of humor, no interest in work, etc. and their eventual cure with niacinamide therapy.

NUTRITION

Altschule, Mark D. *Nutritional Factors in General Medicine: Effects of Stress and Distorted Diets.* Springfield, Ill.: Charles C Thomas, 1978.
Provides current scientific support for nutrition's place in medical practice. Includes separate reviews of major and minor nutrients with special emphasis on recommended daily allowances and food processing effects on nutritive values. Practical recommendations and complete, up-to-date references most valuable. Although directed toward medical clinicians, anyone interested in nutrition's practical application would find this book helpful.

Burton, Benjamin T. *Human Nutrition.* New York: McGraw-Hill Book Co., 1976.

A basic textbook presenting scientific and clinical thought on the subjects of nutrition and diet and their relationship to health and disease. It covers all areas of nutrition, from basic physiology and biochemistry of food intake and utilization, through the clinical application of therapeutic diets. Some of the topics covered include: infant nutrition, nutrition and diet in pregnancy and lactation, obesity, postoperative diets, and psychological aspects of food and appetite. Written in a very clear manner which enables it to be used as a ready reference for many people who do not have a strong background in the subject area.

Cheraskin, Emanuel; Ringsdorf, W. Marshall, Jr.; and Clark, J. W. *Diet and Disease*. Emmaus, Pa.: Rodale Press, 1968.
Suggests a parallel between diet and disease and recommends that the role of diet in the development of diseases anywhere from early obstetrical complications and birth defects to later development of heart disease and cancer have been grossly underestimated. A comprehensive referencing system is incorporated after each chapter's discussion.

Goodhart, Robert S., and Shils, Maurice E. *Modern Nutrition in Health and Disease: Dietotherapy*. Philadelphia, Pa.: Lea & Febiger, 1973.
A major textbook on all aspects of nutrition requirements during health and disease. A ready reference for students and practitioners in the fields of nutrition, medicine, and public health.

Guthrie, Helen Andrews. *Introductory Nutrition*. Saint Louis, Mo.: C. V. Mosby Co., 1975.
An introductory textbook written by a professor of nutrition describing the basics of nutrition and its importance to health throughout life. Easily understood by the student with no college background. A helpful ready reference.

Kaldor, George. *Physiological Chemistry of Proteins and Nucleic Acids in Mammals.* Philadelphia, Pa.: W. B. Saunders Co., 1969.
One of a series of monographs discussing the important physiological roles that proteins and nucleic acids play in health. Primarily directed toward the physician interested in detailed explanations, it describes the important functions of antigens and antibody structures and reactions, coagulation of blood, and the chemistry of muscular contractions.

Pfeiffer, Carl C. *Mental and Elemental Nutrients: A Physician's Guide to Nutrition and Health Care.* New Canaan, Conn.: Keats Publishing, 1975.
A discussion of the role and function of all known nutrients from proteins and vitamins to trace elements. The author's own research and clinical practice works as a supporting framework. While emphasizing the important mental aspects of nutrients, the health of the whole body is considered. The value of nutritional treatment in skin conditions, sleep problems, headaches, arthritis, and other problems are reviewed along with practical advice on how to avoid them.

Price, Weston A. *Nutrition and Physical Degeneration: A Comparison of Primitive and Modern Diets and Their Effects.* Santa Monica, Calif.: The Price-Pottenger Foundation, 1972.
A fascinating cross-cultural account of the health status of both isolated and modernized primitive people. The Swiss, Eskimo, Indian, Aborigine, Peruvian, Maori and other peoples are discussed in light of the devastating effect a "civilized" dietary change has had on their health.

Schneider, Howard A.; Anderson, Carl E.; and Coursin, David B., eds. *Nutritional Support of Medical Practice.* New York: Harper & Row, 1977.

A thoroughly documented text that discusses the importance of nutrition in various health areas such as burns, alcoholism, diabetes, obstetrics, psychiatry, pediatrics, surgery, and obesity. Material is contributed by more than 45 physicians and scientists and is excellent reading for both the professional and nonprofessional.

Seelig, Mildred S., ed. *Nutritional Imbalances in Infant and Adult Disease: Mineral, Vitamin D and Cholesterol.* New York: Spectrum Publications, 1977.
A collection of scientific works presented at the Sixteenth Annual Meeting of the American College of Nutrition, detailing how nutritional and metabolic imbalances in infancy and childhood can contribute to heart disease and other chronic disorders later in life. Epidemiological data on hard and soft water and elevated vitamin D intake and the incidence of heart disease and kidney stones is included, along with reviews of the importance of other nutrients like vitamin D, calcium, magnesium, and unsaturated and saturated fats.

Smith, Lendon. *Feed Your Kids Right: Dr. Smith's Program for Your Child's Total Health.* New York: McGraw-Hill, 1979.
A pediatrician's nutritional approach to the problems of childhood. It identifies "five levels of health," each providing parents with what they need to know to recognize fluctuations in the well-being of their child and a special nutritional need for each level. Allergies, junk food, hyperactivity, acne, skin rash, bedwetting, depression, and hives are just a few of the many subjects covered.

Spies, Tom D. *Rehabilitation Through Better Nutrition.* Philadelphia, Pa.: W. B. Saunders Co., 1947. (Out of print; check local medical library.)

One of the classics in the field, written by a physician attempting to help other colleagues use nutritional therapy in their day-to-day practice. Special advice is given suggesting the physician is responsible for treating a patient until "good health is regained and maintained."

Williams, Roger J. *Nutrition in a Nutshell.* Garden City, N.Y.: Doubleday & Co., 1962.
Written by a well-known nutritionist—a scientist in his own right, this book describes what nutrition is all about: where nutrition starts, what nourishing food is, what vitamins are and what they can do. Provides a perspective on the many theories of nutrition and advice on nutritional supplementation.

Williams, Roger J. *Nutrition Against Disease: Environmental Prevention.* New York: Pitman Publishing Corp., 1971.
A summary of the available scientific evidence relating nutrition to the prevention of nine major health problems from tooth decay to cancer. Written by a scientist who was the first to identify, isolate, and synthesize pantothenic acid, an important B vitamin, and who is a pioneer worker with folic acid.

Williams, Roger J. *Physicians' Handbook of Nutritional Science.* Springfield, Ill.: Charles C Thomas, 1975.
Primarily designed for the physician who wants to stay on top of the subject of nutrition and to understand its meaning and importance in medical practice.

Williams, Roger J. *The Wonderful World Within You.* New York: Bantam Books, 1977.
A good book to introduce the reader to the basics of nutrition from the inside of the human body to the factors affecting it outside.

NUTRITION AND SURGERY

American College of Surgeons. *Manual of Surgical Nutrition.*
Philadelphia, Pa.: W. B. Saunders Co., 1975.
A manual prepared under the direction of the committee on pre-
operative and postoperative care of the American College of Surgeons. It describes the history of nutrition as a science and
reviews the basic principles underlying clinical nutrition and currently available methods of management, with specific reference
to surgical patients.

NUTRITIONAL DEFICIENCIES

Somogyi, J. C., and Tashev, T., eds. *Early Signs of Nutritional
Deficiencies.* New York: S. Karger, 1976.
Presents an in-depth survey of the latest findings in the fields of
nutrition and the most advanced methods for assessing early signs
of malnutrition. It approaches the problem that minor vitamin or
nutritional deficiencies produce subclinical symptoms which
makes diagnosis difficult. Basically a collection of lectures presented at the thirteenth symposium of European nutritionists.

ORTHOMOLECULAR MEDICINE

Hawkins, David, and Pauling, Linus. *Orthomolecular Psychiatry:
Treatment of Schizophrenia.* San Francisco: W. H. Freeman
and Co., 1973.
Explains orthomolecular psychiatry as applied to the treatment of
schizophrenia, alcoholism, and the mental disorders of drug
abuse. The authors have compiled the works of 37 medical and
scientific authorities interested not only in theories of orthomolecular psychiatry but clinical laboratory research and the application of the theory in research findings to everyday clinical
practice. Written so that patients and their families can use it as a
handbook for the application of orthomolecular psychiatry.

Williams, Roger J., and Kalita, Dwight K. *A Physician's Handbook on Orthomolecular Medicine.* New York: Pergamon Press,
1977.

A collection of works prepared by some of the most renowned orthomolecular professionals in the field. The most complete handbook for any professional interested in understanding and utilizing the principles of orthomolecular medicine.

OSTEOPOROSIS

Albanese, Anthony A. *Bone Loss: Causes, Detection, and Therapy.* New York: Alan R. Liss, 1977.
Reviews one of the major health problems of the elderly—skeletal bone loss—and details the available knowledge on bone formation and calcium metabolism, analyzing the epidemiology, etiology, diagnosis, treatment, and management of osteoporosis.

POLLUTION

Calabrese, Edward J. *Pollutants and High-Risk Groups: The Biological Basis of Increased Human Susceptibility to Environmental and Occupational Pollutants.* New York: John Wiley & Sons, 1978.
Defines the effects pollutants have on high-risk groups by presenting reviews of the available scientific literature on the subject. Susceptibility of different age groups is reviewed along with attention to genetic disorders, nutritional deficiencies, heart-lung diseases, smoking, and alcohol and drug abuse. Screening methods to detect high-risk groups and practical solutions round out the approach.

PREGNANCY

Brewer, Gail Sforza with Brewer, Tom. *What Every Pregnant Woman Should Know: The Truth About Diets and Drugs in Pregnancy.* New York: Random House, 1977.
An excellent book advising the pregnant mother that diet and nutrition have a profound influence on the development of toxemia and can increase or decrease the risk of having a healthy baby. The author warns against restricting food at the risk of nutritional inadequacy, to be careful about taking drugs—espe-

cially diuretics—and not to restrict salt intake. An entire section is devoted to showing her exactly what to eat to have a healthy baby, complete with recipes and menus for high-protein, high-nutrition foods.

Brewer, Thomas H. *Metabolic Toxemia of Late Pregnancy: A Disease of Malnutrition.* Springfield, Ill.: Charles C Thomas, 1966.

Describes the author's experiences in clinical obstetrical practice treating hundreds of women with toxemia of pregnancy. His view—for which he provides much support—is that nutritional deficiencies caused by poor diet can simply be prevented by proper diet, with a strong emphasis on protein, adequate salt, and restraint in the use of drugs.

RELAXATION

Benson, Herbert. *The Relaxation Response.* New York: William Morrow and Co., 1975.

If you want to learn how to relax, don't let this book get past you. Written by a physician, it shows you how a simple, meditative technique can help you relieve inner tensions, deal more effectively with stress, lower blood pressure, and improve your general physical and emotional health.

SLEEP

Goldberg, Philip, and Kaufman, Daniel. *Natural Sleep: How to Get Your Share.* Emmaus, Pa.: Rodale Press, 1978.

A well-written, practical handbook for the prevention and treatment of insomnia. Reviews both the orthodox and unorthodox treatments of insomnia and provides very useful information on evaluating personal sleep needs, and how such factors as diet, work, stress, exercise, bedding, and noise can affect sleep. It provides specific direction for using what many have found to be effective natural methods for regaining normal sleep, including what to eat, what to avoid, exercises, breathing and relaxation techniques, massage, herbal remedies, and simple changes in attitude, habit, behavior, and environment.

STRESS

Pelletier, Kenneth R. *Mind as Healer, Mind as Slayer: A Holistic Approach to Preventing Stress Disorders.* New York: Dell Publishing Co., 1977.
A psychologist's survey of the nature of stress and how it relates to the development of illnesses such as cardiovascular disease, cancer, arthritis, and respiratory disease. It provides guidelines for helping to evaluate one's own stress level and practical information on how to prevent stress problems using such techniques as meditation and biofeedback.

Selye, Hans. *The Stress of Life.* New York: McGraw-Hill Book Co., 1976.
Probably one of the most definitive books on the subject of stress, written by the man who formulated the entire theoretical concept. Introduces the reader to stress, both the mental and physical components, and provides practical solutions to relieving stress in tense situations.

SUGAR

Dufty, William. *Sugar Blues.* New York: Warner Books, 1975.
A fascinating exposure of the health hazards of sugar and how the author cured his "sugar addiction." Helpful solutions for kicking the habit are included along with sugar-free recipes.

Yudkin, John. *Sweet and Dangerous: The New Facts About the Sugar You Eat as a Cause of Heart Disease, Diabetes, and Other Killers.* New York: Peter H. Wyden, 1972.
A fascinating explanation in lay language of Dr. Yudkin's discov-

eries that ordinary table sugar is a principal cause of heart disease, diabetes, and other killers.

TRACE ELEMENTS

Brewer, George J., and Prasad, Ananda S. *Zinc Metabolism: Current Aspects in Health and Disease.* New York: Alan R. Liss, 1977.
Reviews the recent advances in the role zinc plays in health and disease. Topics include dietary sources of zinc, dietary factors which inhibit zinc absorption, the relationship of zinc with vitamin A, and the relationship zinc deficiency has to protein. Particular reference is made to zinc's role in infection and immunity. Incorporates the work of the major scientists in the field of zinc metabolism.

Hambridge, K. Michael, and Nichols, Buford L., eds. *Zinc and Copper in Clinical Medicine.* New York: SP Medical and Scientific Books, 1978.
A collection of ten scholarly articles on the roles of zinc and copper in human nutrition. Contributed by research scientists and physicians, the articles describe deficiencies, metabolism, and biochemistry for both zinc and copper. Throughout the book, references to scientific material on the trace elements in nutrition are given.

Hemphill, Delbert D., *Trace Substances in Environmental Health,* vols. 1 & 2. Proceedings of the University of Missouri's eleventh annual conference on trace substances in environmental health. Columbia, Mo.: University of Missouri, 1966–1977.
Brings together the works of scientists worldwide who are interested in sharing what is known about the beneficial and the deleterious roles trace elements play in the quality of our environment and health of man. Trace elements are discussed in terms of their roles in epidemiology, geochemistry, health, and environmental pollutants, along with methods of analysis. This

series is valuable to any person interested in a detailed, technical study of trace elements and their influences on man's health.

Mills, C. S., ed. *Trace Element Metabolism in Animals.* Proceedings of WAAP/IBP International Symposium, Aberdeen, Scotland, July 1969. Teviot Place, Edinburgh, Scotland: E. & S. Livingstone, 1970.

Presents the published results of a professional meeting on the metabolism and functional roles of trace elements and their application to the field of nutrition and human or veterinary medicine. A few of the topics discussed include: the metabolism, pathology, and clinical consequences of specific trace element deficiencies and excesses; the distribution, storage, absorption, transport, and excretion of various trace elements; the experimental methods of analysis; and the availability of trace elements.

Pfeiffer, Carl C. *Zinc and Other Micro-Nutrients.* New Canaan, Conn.: Keats Publishing, 1978.

Reviews information on the roles of 22 minerals in the human body from essential ones like zinc, iron, sulphur, and phosphorus, to potentially toxic minerals like copper, mercury, and lead. It points out foods and other sources of trace elements along with the body's reactions to them and provides practical information on how to regulate them for good health.

Prasad, Ananda S., and Oberleas, Donald, eds. *Trace Elements in Human Health and Disease*, vol. 1, *Zinc and Copper*, vol. 2, *Essential and Toxic Elements.* New York: Academic Press, 1976.

Volume 1 is a comprehensive examination of the effects of trace elements on human health and disease, encompassing advances in the field of trace element research over the past decade. This volume covers the role of zinc and copper in human metabolism, with an in-depth discussion of clinical, biochemical, nutritional, and toxicological aspects.

Volume 2 is an extremely helpful textbook of the major contributions in the field of trace elements to human health and disease by two very well known researchers. Chromium, selenium, magnesium, fluoride, manganese, cadmium, and mercury are included in this review.

Schroeder, Henry A. *The Trace Elements and Man: Some Positive and Negative Aspects*. Old Greenwich, Conn.: The Devin-Adair Co., 1973.

An easy-to-read book on the importance of trace elements in a diet. The major emphasis is placed on food processing and how the various techniques used remove essential minerals. The author reviews chromium, iodine, copper, cobalt, zinc, and manganese and talks about the hazards of cadmium and lead to health. An excellent review of trace element nutrition.

Underwood, Eric J. *Trace Elements in Human and Animal Nutrition*. New York: Academic Press, 1977.

Explains in detail the physiological role of the trace elements, their needs, tolerances, and interactions with each other and with other nutrients and the biochemical and pathological changes that result from deficient, toxic, or imbalanced mineral intakes by animals and man. Includes separate sections on: iron, copper, molybdenum, cobalt, nickel, manganese, zinc, cadmium, chromium, iodine, selenium, fluorine, mercury, vanadium, silicon, lead, and arsenic, as well as other elements including aluminum and strontium. A special section is devoted to soil, plant, and animal interrelations. Complete citations of major works in the field of trace elements are helpful especially to those with specialized interest in the subject.

VEGETARIANISM

Lappé, Frances Moore. *Diet for a Small Planet*. New York: Ballantine Books, 1975.

A very excellent and complete account of how to insure proper protein balances from nonmeat foods to produce high-grade protein nutrition at least equivalent to meat proteins. An extensive recipe section provides deliciously clear examples of just what foods complement each other to achieve protein richness. A very helpful *must* for anyone getting into vegetarianism.

VITAMIN B_6

Ellis, John M. *The Doctor Who Looked at Hands*. New York: Vantage Press, 1966.
Explores the fascinating critical effects of vitamin B_6 deficiency as seen through the eyes of the clinician who first made the discovery. Numerous case histories and an easy-to-understand style make for intriguing reading.

Ellis, John M., and Presley, James. *Vitamin B_6: The Doctor's Report*. New York: Harper & Row, 1973.
A thorough presentation on the history and importance of vitamin B_6 carefully documented with numerous case histories of patients improving during vitamin B_6 therapy. Successes were achieved with problems such as arthritis, certain forms of heart disease, diabetes, edema, and those encountered by pregnant women and women on the Pill.

VITAMIN B_{12}

Merck & Co., Inc., publisher. *Vitamin B_{12}: Merck Service Bulletin*. Rahway, N.J.: Merck & Co., 1958. (Out of print; check local medical library.)
Presents comprehensive information on vitamin B_{12}, including chemical, pharmaceutical, and analytical information and the roles it plays in human nutrition and metabolism. A selected, annotated bibliography of scientific studies establishing the clinical use of vitamin B_{12} along with its therapeutic or nutritional use is included.

VITAMIN C

Kalokerinos, Archie. *Every Second Child*. Sidney, Australia: Thomas Nelson, 1974.

Every second child born to the Australian aborigines is doomed to die in infancy, or at least that was the case until Dr. Kalokerinos discovered what their problem was. This book reports the amazing discovery of a physician's search for the cause of this high infant mortality and his findings—that these infants suffered from a vitamin C deficiency disease. His discovery and later treatment has led to the amazing, rapid fall in their death rate.

Pauling, Linus. *Vitamin C and the Common Cold*. San Francisco: W. H. Freeman and Co., 1970.

Reviews the evidence that led the author to his conclusion—that vitamin C taken in proper amounts can both prevent and alleviate the common cold and related diseases. It discusses in detail man's needs for ascorbic acid and the specifics of the "anticold" regimen.

Pauling, Linus. *Vitamin C, the Common Cold and the Flu*. San Francisco: W. H. Freeman and Co., 1976.

A fascinating, well-referenced presentation on how vitamin C can prevent both the common cold and the flu supported by Dr. Pauling's research as well as others. Exactly how ascorbic acid does this is discussed along with its side effects, and the attitude of the medical profession toward it. Practical information on how to buy and take ascorbic acid very helpful.

Stone, Irwin. *The Healing Factor: "Vitamin C" Against Disease*. New York: Grosset & Dunlap, 1972.

Summarizes the evidence that man, because of a genetic mutation, is completely dependent on outside sources for ascorbic acid and has suffered both mental and physical diseases as a result. The role ascorbic acid plays in health problems like cancer, allergies, stress, heart and eye disease, diabetes, poisoning, eye problems, etc. are discussed and fully referenced. Extremely well documented with over 500 scientific references.

VITAMIN E

Shute, Wilfrid E., with Taub, Harald J. *Vitamin E for Ailing and Healthy Hearts.* New York: Pyramid House, 1969.
Asserts that heart disease is directly tied to the lack of vitamin E in our diet. In over three decades (at the time of writing) this noted heart specialist believed that modern milling processes had eliminated vitamin E from our flour and unmistakably influenced the development of heart disease. He describes case after case in which the administration of alpha tocopherol has brought relief and in some cases eliminated the need for heart surgery. Topics include: angina and ischemic heart disease, rheumatic fever, high blood pressure, vascular disease, peripheral vascular disease, varicose veins, diabetes, burns, estrogens, etc.

Shute, Wilfrid E. *Dr. Wilfrid E. Shute's Complete Updated Vitamin E Book.* New Canaan, Conn.: Keats Publishing, 1975.
A follow-up to Dr. Shute's earlier work, *Vitamin E for Ailing and Healthy Hearts.* It combines not only the clinical experiences this Canadian physician has had in treating and preventing cardiovascular disease, but also includes the work of other physicians and references to many publications and other bibliographical references. The author draws heavily on his experience in treating over 35 thousand cases of cardiovascular disease and presents it in a very readable style. The conditions he has found responsive to vitamin E include not only heart disease but diabetes and other circulatory diseases—even burns.

Shute, Wilfrid E. *Health Preserver: Defining the Versatility of Vitamin E.* Emmaus, Pa.: Rodale Press, 1977.
A review of the amazing versatility vitamin E has in the treatment

of a wide range of human conditions from the healing of burns to the prevention of heart attacks. Dr. Shute's experiences treating thousands of patients with vitamin E are incorporated, along with the works of other scientists to provide convincing evidence for vitamin E's usefulness.

VITAMINS

Gerras, Charles, ed. *The Complete Book of Vitamins.* Emmaus, Pa.: Rodale Press, 1977.

A relatively complete guide to individual vitamins, providing details on their historical backgrounds, their interaction with other food elements, and their current application and potential for preventing and curing disease. Charts listing the daily allowances, primary food sources, major body activities, clinical deficiency signs, and prevention and/or therapeutic applications are most helpful.

Rosenberg, Harold, and Feldzamen, A. N. *The Doctor's Book of Vitamin Therapy: Megavitamins for Health.* New York: G. P. Putnam's Sons, 1974.

Negates the concept that the current typical American diet is the "key" to health. Describes in detail avenues of vitamin therapy and the essential role both vitamins and minerals play in maximizing long-ranging health and in preventing disease. Guides the reader on what vitamins and minerals to take, how much, and when, and reviews the value of each major vitamin and mineral and how it works to achieve maximum benefit.

Sebrell, W. H., Jr., and Harris, Robert S. *The Vitamins: Chemistry, Physiology, Pathology, Methods,* vols. 1–5. New York: Academic Press, 1967–1971.

A series of textbooks presenting current knowledge of the chemistry, industrial production, biochemistry, deficiency effects, requirements, pharmacology, and pathology of each of the vitamins with bibliographical material noting major reference works. The vitamins reviewed include: vitamin A, ascorbic acid, vitamin B_6, vitamin B_{12}, biotin, niacin, pantothenic acid, riboflavin, tocopherol, thiamine, choline, vitamin D, essential fatty acids, inositol, and vitamin K.

X-RAYS

Laws, Priscilla W. *X-Rays: More Harm Than Good?* Emmaus, Pa.: Rodale Press, 1977.

Reviews the uses, benefits, costs, and risks of diagnostic x-rays. Describes and discusses the common problems encountered by x-ray users with the hope of helping others avoid some of the same pitfalls, and to understand and evaluate currently accepted x-ray practices. The author offers an unbiased consideration of the problems associated with the use of diagnostic x-rays, from the perspective of both patients and health-care professionals.

A Directory of Associations

AGING

Association for Humanistic Gerontology
1711 Solano Avenue
Berkeley, CA 94707
(415) 525-3128

Founded in response to a growing need to develop a positive and healthy image for the aging and for the services to the elderly, this organization serves simultaneously as a professional society and as an international resource clearing house for information related to programs for the elderly. It sponsors nationwide seminars and programs for professionals interested in gerontology, psychology, health, and counseling fields. A particular area of involvement is in preventive and innovative programs for the elderly. It publishes a quarterly newsletter and a journal, *Journal of Humanistic Gerontology*. A referral service is available to active members only.

ALLERGY

Human Ecology Action League (HEAL)
505 North Lake Shore Drive
Chicago, IL 60611
(312) 329-9097

An organization representing the aims and programs of patients, physicians, and others interested in environmental health. It promotes and finances research into allergies from an environmental perspective, collects and disseminates information on clinical ecology, and works to eliminate the use of chemicals and other substances and any conditions in the environment which are hazardous to human health. It provides specific information on foods, drugs, air, water, and other elements and how they affect health, through their publications, including the newsletter *Human Ecologist,* and sponsors a yearly meeting.

Society for Clinical Ecology
4045 Wadsworth Boulevard
Wheat Ridge, CO 80033
(303) 424-5515

This society acts as a forum for both professionals and lay persons interested in the principles and practice of ecologic medicine. It focuses on individual susceptibility to specific environmental contaminants and publishes a newsletter. Continuing medical education credits are also offered. It also provides a referral service to its membership.

BIOFEEDBACK

Biofeedback Society of America (BSA)
U.C.M.C. C268
4200 East Ninth Avenue
Denver, CO 80262
(303) 394-7054

An open forum for the exchange of ideas, methods, and results of biofeedback and related studies. Serves to advance biofeedback as a means of human welfare through the encouragement of scientific research and to improve both research and clinical methods through meetings, workshops, and literature. The official publications of the society are *Biofeedback and Self-Regulation* and a quarterly newsletter, *Biofeedback*. A membership directory is made available to anyone interested in locating a biofeedback therapy center in their particular local area.

BREAST-FEEDING

La Leche League International, Inc.
  9616 Minneapolis Avenue
  Franklin Park, IL 60131
  (312) 455-7730

An organization founded to give help and encouragement primarily through personal instruction to those mothers who want to nurse their babies. Provides information on the location of local chapters and publishes material on breast-feeding including their manual *The Womanly Art of Breastfeeding*, cookbook *Mother's in the Kitchen*, and bimonthly newsletter *La Leche League News*. A board of professional advisors is available to the league for consultation. It sponsors annual medical seminars for physicians and nurses and biannual conferences for parents. They also have many books and films about childbirth, breast-feeding, and parenting. Key publications have been translated into a number of foreign languages. Maintains a 24-hour hot line answering service.

CANCER

Foundation for Alternative Cancer Therapies, Ltd.
  Box HH
  Old Chelsea Station
  New York, NY 10011
  (212) 741-2790

Encourages the testing of all viable, biological cancer treatments through sponsorship of research, annual conventions, seminars, and the publication of *Cancer Forum*. Information is provided on nontoxic cancer treatments, and a referral service to clinics, centers, and/or doctors using a biological and nutritional approach to the restoration of body chemistry is available.

Northwest Cancer Association
  P.O. Box 3216
  Bellevue, WA 98009
  (206) 883-0171
Disseminates information on nontoxic cancer treatments. A book and tape library is open to the public and a yearly convention is sponsored on nontoxic cancer treatments. Information on alternative cancer treatments, including the names of doctors and clinics using such treatments, is available to anyone.

CHILDBIRTH

American Society for Psychoprophylaxis in Obstetrics
  1411 K Street, NW
  Washington, DC 20005
  (202) 783-7050
Devoted to the promotion and teaching of the Lamaze method of childbirth and to the training of teachers in this method. Membership is open to physicians, professionals, and consumers. It sponsors an annual national conference and teacher-training seminars and publishes a newsletter, brochures about the training programs, and a handbook for physicians. All questions are individually answered and a directory which includes the names of physicians, chapters, and other associations providing information on childbirth and breast-feeding is also available.

Association for Childbirth at Home, International (ACHI)
  P.O. Box 1219
  Cerritos, CA 90701
  (213) 802-1020

Gives support and encouragement to women and their families interested in giving birth at home. Makes information available through parent-oriented classes and counseling and collects and disseminates "accurate, up-to-date information" concerning childbirth at home. Information on classes, a teacher-training course, conferences, books, and reprints is provided to the interested public. Referrals to competent birth attendants in varying areas of the country are provided as is information on what hospital policies are regarding home birth practices, what doctors are doing home births, and what prenatal care is being made available in specific areas.

Home Oriented Maternity Experience (HOME)
511 New York Avenue
Takoma Park, Washington, DC 20012
(301) 587-4664

An educational association providing information and support to couples desiring a safe home or home-oriented birth experience. Publishes *Home Oriented Maternity Experience: A Comprehensive Guide to Homebirth*, and a newsletter, *News from H.O.M.E.* Names of resources and sources of community help all over the U.S. and Canada are available to those interested, as is information on speakers and childbirth classes.

International Childbirth Education Association (ICEA)
P.O. Box 20852
Milwaukee, WI 53220
(612) 881-9194

An interdisciplinary, primarily volunteer organization representing groups and individuals who share a genuine interest in the goals of family-centered maternity care, infant care, and parenting. Offers international conventions, regional conferences, province/state meetings and sharing days, four newsletters, books, and member counseling through teacher services, outreach, and parent education. A network of province/state coordinators has been established to provide up-to-date information regarding prepared childbirth classes, birthing alternatives, and options within each province/state.

National Association of Parents and Professionals for Safe Alternatives in Childbirth (NAPSAC)
P.O. Box 267
Marble Hill, MO 63764
(314) 238-2010
Functions as a consumer advocate organization which provides information on natural childbirth, family-centered maternity care in hospitals, and safe home birth programs. Activities include: international conferences, publishing of books and a quarterly newsletter, and a speaking and consulting service. A referral service provides names of physicians and midwives doing home births, birth centers, and nutritional professionals.

CHIROPRACTIC

American Chiropractic Association
2200 Grand Avenue
Des Moines, IA 50312
(515) 243-1121
An official organization serving representatives of the chiropractic profession. Aside from its involvement in the public service area of radio and television, this association coordinates educational conferences and seminars and publishes a journal, *Journal of Chiropractic* and *Healthways* magazine. Referrals are made to nearest members.

HEALING

American Healers Association
P.O. Box 213
Princeton, NJ 08540
Provides the public with literature and research information

about nonmedical healers—what they can and cannot do. Its purpose is to upgrade the status of healers, to screen and certify them, to provide training courses where needed, to educate the public that reliable healers are available, to help reduce the risk of legal difficulties of healers, and to sponsor scientific research in healing. A referral list of certified healers willing to work with physicians and clergy is available on request.

HOLISTIC MEDICINE

American Holistic Medical Association
  Route 2, Welsh Coulee
  La Crosse, WI 54601
  (608) 786-0611
Educates physicians and other health professionals on the principles of the "medicine of the whole person." Primary objectives include: experiencing holistic health, evaluating and expanding scientific medicine, establishing standards for new concepts of therapy, and providing new tools for physicians and other health professionals. Sponsors continuing medical education credits through its three programs a year and publishes a monthly newsletter. An official quarterly journal, *American Holistic Medicine,* is scheduled for future publication. Referrals are made to physicians in a given area.

International Academy of Biological Medicine, Inc.
  P.O. Box 31313
  Phoenix, AZ 85046
A professional corporation aimed at educating its members as well as the public in general in the philosophy and working principles of biological medicine. Interested in all types of healing systems including nutritional, naturopathic, preventive, molecular, holistic, spiritual, chiropractic, and osteopathic. Major emphasis is on the treatment of the whole man, to restore his health and to prevent disease. This professional organization sponsors seminars several times a year and makes available to the public a list of its membership for referral.

HYPERACTIVITY

Feingold Association of the United States
  Drawer A-G
  Holtsville, NY 11742
Devoted to helping children, their parents, and other persons interested in behavioral and learning problems. The hyperactive child is of special interest. Information on local chapter groups is available. Information on the detailed investigations of products containing food additives that could be harmful to the hyperactive child, and on the Feingold diet, is available to members. Publishes a newsletter as do most local associations for their members.

The New York Institute for Child Development, Inc.
  205 Lexington Avenue
  New York, NY 10016
  (212) 686-3630
The institute is a private center specializing in the diagnosis and treatment of learning-disabled, hyperactive, and underachieving children. Emphasizes physical instead of the psychological or academic causes of learning disabilities. In the course of treatment, nutrition management and sensory motor therapy is used. A diagnostic service is available as well as audiovisual aids, a speaker program, and workshops on the above subjects. Publishes a monthly newsletter called *Reaching Children.*

HYPNOSIS

The American Society of Clinical Hypnosis
  2400 East Devon Avenue, Suite 218
  Des Plaines, IL 60018
  (312) 297-3317
An educational organization of professionals in the fields of medicine, dentistry, and psychology who share scientific and clinical interests in hypnosis. It has been developed to encourage educational programs and to further research in the field of hypnosis.

Membership is limited to professionals with advanced degrees such as M.D., D.D.S., D.M.D., D.O., or Ph.D. To help keep members abreast of what's happening in clinical hypnosis, it publishes the *American Journal of Clinical Hypnosis*, a quarterly scientific journal, and a biquarterly newsletter for members only. Annual workshops and scientific meetings limited to qualified professionals are also a part of the society's activities. It will make referrals to members by geographical area.

HYPOGLYCEMIA

Adrenal Metabolic Research Society of the Hypoglycemia Foundation, Inc.
153 Pawling Avenue
Troy, NY 12180
(518) 272-7154

An association interested in furthering scientific investigation into the knowledge of metabolic aspects of hypoglycemia and hyperinsulinism through laboratory research and publication. Attempts are made to apply such knowledge to the prevention and treatment of these problems. Information from medical literature is provided about hypoglycemia, allergies, addiction, alcoholism, etc. A quarterly newsletter entitled *Homeostasis* and information on the work of John Tintera, M.D., is also available. Referrals are made to physicians throughout the U.S. supporting the foundation's philosophies.

JOGGING

American Medical Joggers Association
P.O. Box 4704
North Hollywood, CA 91607
(213) 985-0079

An organization fostering jogging and running among physicians in the U.S. Provides educational material on running and jogging, and sponsors meetings and marathons and continuing medical education credits. Publishes a quarterly newsletter and will provide the names of physicians who are members and who practice running or jogging in local areas.

National Jogging Association
    919 Eighteenth Street, NW, Suite 830
    Washington, DC 20006
    (202) 785-8050
Encourages and fosters individual, family, and club jogging and running among all people in the belief that such a program can lead to improved health and a greater sense of well-being. Publishes a monthly newsletter, the *Jogger*, and provides information on all aspects of the sport to interested persons. Referrals are made to podiatrists interested in sports medicine, running, and jogging.

LEARNING DISABILITIES

Academic Therapy Publications
    20 Commercial Boulevard
    Novato, CA 94947
    (415) 883-3314
Publishes material dealing with the education of children, youth, and adults with learning and language dysfunctions. It publishes a journal, *Academic Therapy*, plus books and materials on the identification, diagnosis, and the remediation of learning difficulties. A directory listing over 400 centers in North America treating the learning disabled is available for 35¢ to cover postage, as is information on the scheduled workshops and seminars.

Association for Children with Learning Disabilities
    4156 Library Road
    Pittsburgh, PA 15234
    (412) 341-1515

Interested in advancing the education and general well-being of children and adults with learning disabilities. It's holistic in its approach and attempts to increase public understanding, and to improve school and community relationships. Publishes a newsletter entitled *ACLD Newsbriefs* six times a year. Nutrition is a part of its total program.

MASSAGE

American Massage & Therapy Association
P.O. Box 1270
Kingsport, TN 37660
(615) 245-8071

A national association with state chapters interested in organizing all professional and ethical massage therapists; to upgrade the image of massage through legislation, educational standardization, and professionalism; and to inform the general public about certified massage therapists. Holds regional and national conferences, provides literature describing massage and the association, and provides a referral to its members.

Potomac Massage Therapy Institute
421 Butternut Street, NW
Washington, DC 20012
(202) 829-4201

An institute which trains professionals and interested lay persons in the art and science of therapeutic massage and promotes therapeutic massage in holistic health concepts and practices. As primarily an educational organization, it offers a five-month training program, weekend workshops, and individual massage sessions. Involved in publishing a local directory of holistic health, preventive medicine, and alternative therapy practitioners entitled *Baltimore-Washington Healing Resources*. Referrals are made to massage therapists and other professionals.

MATERNAL AND CHILD HEALTH

American Foundation for Maternal and Child Health
  30 Beekman Place
  New York, NY 10022
  (212) 759-5510

A health research foundation which focuses attention on obstetric management during the perinatal period and its effect on infant outcome and child development. Acts as a clearing house for information from various national and international medical and social disciplines concerned with the perinatal period and sponsors educational programs and medical research designed to shed light on the effects of that period. Extremely interested in patients' rights and will provide a copy of "Pregnant Patients' Bill of Rights." An exchange-of-ideas conference is sponsored for health professionals.

MEDICAL INFORMATION

Center for Medical Consumers
  and Health Care Information, Inc.
  237 Thompson Street (Greenwich Village)
  New York, NY 10012
  (212) 674-7105

An association serving the medical and health-care information needs of the consumer. It encourages individuals to check and critically evaluate information they receive from physicians. To help consumers, this organization has its own library with medical texts and other backup material. *Health Facts* is its newsletter, published six times a year. The library facilities are available to both members and nonmembers.

MENTAL HEALTH

The Huxley Institute for Biosocial Research
  1114 First Avenue
  New York, NY 10021
  (212) 759-9554

Devoted to informing professionals and lay persons about schizophrenia, learning disabilities, alcoholism, drug abuse, childhood disorders, and hypoglycemia with a special focus on nutrition and diet. Sponsors training programs for physicians interested in learning more about orthomolecular medicine and publishes a newsletter. A referral service is available which provides the names of both psychiatric and nonpsychiatric professionals interested in the preventive medicine fields.

NUTRITION

Consumers for Nutrition Action, Inc. (CNA)
   3404 Saint Paul Street, Suite 1-B
   Baltimore, MD 21218
   (301) 235-9039
This educational center primarily serves as a food and nutrition action organization for the state of Maryland. Very much involved in legislative advocacy and interacts with such agencies as the FDA, USDA, and FTC on food and nutrition issues. Involved in improving school lunches and breakfasts and educating senior citizens about nutrition. A variety of publications is available including a newsletter and a listing of natural food sources in the Baltimore metropolitan area. Referrals are made to nutritionally aware medical and chiropractic physicians along with other organizations involved in food and nutrition issues. Cosponsors Food Day and other nutrition conferences each year.

Cooking for Survival Consciousness
   Box 26762
   Elkins Park, PA 19117
   (215) 635-1022
The creation of a "nutrition consciousness" is the purpose of this organization which provides information on health cookery. Among the pages of its publications, including a journal and a newsletter, you'll find references to diet and its value in preventive health care, on the health values of reducing meat, and on

the ill effects of chemical food additives and preservatives. Classroom demonstrations—slide and cassette programs on sprouts, for example—are available to those interested. Speakers are available and a referral service to doctors, clinics, and exercise programs is currently being established.

Foundation for the Study and Treatment of Nutrigenic Diseases
    2235 Castillo Street
    Santa Barbara, CA 93105
    (805) 682-2682

Interested in the education and research of disease as it relates to tolerances and intolerances to food. Sponsors nutritional programs and guidance through its affiliation with the Kaslow Medical Center. Special interest areas include: acupuncture, hearing rehabilitation through electroacupuncture without needles, and the Metabolic Rejectivity Syndrome. Makes referrals to both the center and to medical professionals who have trained through the foundation.

Health and Nutrition Resources, Inc.
    P.O. Box 258
    Syosset, Long Island, NY 11791
    (516) 938-2883

With nutrition education its primary goal, this organization conducts periodic seminars and workshops by qualified professionals interested in preventive medicine, as well as teaches an ongoing course in nutrition. The public is provided information on all aspects of nutrition, health, and the environment, and may participate in its yearly health and nutrition fair activities.

International College of Applied Nutrition (ICAN)
    P.O. Box 386
    La Habra, CA 90631
    (213) 697-4576

A society of qualified physicians, dentists, veterinarians, and others with doctoral degrees engaged in the practical application and/or research of nutrition. Primarily concerned with continuing postgraduate education through scientific meetings, symposia, and conferences. Publishes a quarterly journal, *Journal of Applied Nutrition*, and a handbook, *Nutrition—Applied Personally* along with newsletters. Referrals are made to members in local areas interested in preventive and nutrition-oriented health care.

Northwest Academy of Preventive Medicine
  15650 North East Twenty-Fourth Street
  Bellevue, WA 98008
  (206) 747-9660
The primary purpose of this organization is to educate professionals in the nutritional and nontoxic treatment of disease. Membership is open to professionals with degrees in the healing arts, health administrators, and students. It provides cassette and video tapes of seminars and publishes the *Northwest Academy of Preventive Medicine Journal* and a newsletter. A list of doctors throughout the U.S. and Canada is maintained for referral.

Parents for Better Nutrition, Inc.
  33 North Central, Room 200
  Medford, OR 97501
  (503) 772-8020
An organization devoting itself to stimulating an interest in better nutrition in the home, the school, and the community. Maintains an educational resource center to make nutritional information available to members in the community through books, tapes and films, lectures and workshops. Publishes a monthly newsletter and works to improve the quality of school lunches by encouraging the use of whole grains, sprouts, natural sweeteners, and fresh fruits and vegetables, and by placing fresh fruits, nuts, seeds, and cheese in school vending machines in place of soft drinks and candy.

Price-Pottenger Nutrition Foundation
P.O. Box 2614
La Mesa, CA 92041
(714) 582-4168

An educational association conducting programs to increase the awareness of the medical and dental professions and the public of the importance of good nutrition. Believes in the benefits of whole foods without additives and conducts research programs to supplement and improve modern food. Nutrition exhibits are maintained as well as bibliographical archives and a library. Publishes Dr. Weston Price's book *Nutrition and Physical Degeneration* and his famous cat studies entitled, *The Effect of Heat Processed Foods and Metabolized Vitamin D Milk on the Dentofacial Structures of Experimental Animals.* Films and slides also available.

Southern Academy of Clinical Nutrition
1045 East Atlantic Avenue
Delray Beach, FL 33444
(305) 278-1213

An educational association whose purpose is to define health— how to attain it and keep it. It sponsors two yearly conferences and publishes numerous articles and a cookbook.

NUTRITION (PRENATAL)

Society for the Protection of the Unborn through Nutrition (SPUN)
17 North Wabash Avenue, Suite 603
Chicago, IL 60602
(312) 332-2334

Provides educational services to health-care professionals (especially obstetricians), social service agencies, and individuals on a holistic approach to the prevention of complications of pregnancy. Special emphasis on encouraging the medical profession to adopt nutritional standards for pregnant women and to discourage low-salt, low-calorie regimens, weight-control programs, and the use of drugs during pregnancy. Publishes a bimonthly newsletter *Pregnant Issue: Medicate or Educate* and a scientific bibliography along with other reports on all aspects of prenatal nutrition. The organization also conducts seminars and maintains a speakers' bureau. Referrals are made to nutrition-oriented obstetricians, midwives, and childbirth educators in the U.S.

NUTRITION (SCHOOL)
School Nutrition Awareness Council (SNAC)
  8106 Subet Road
  Baltimore, MD 21207
  (301) 922-4967
Committed to raising the community's nutritional awareness with the hope of convincing local schools to remove all nonnutritious and imitation foods from vending machines and school lunches, and to replace them with foods which build health. Provides nutrition education to students, teachers, parents, principals, school boards, advisory councils, and food service staff, and acts as a resource center. Also offers recipes on the how-to's of sprouts, bread-making, and yogurt-making.

ORTHOMOLECULAR MEDICINE
Academy of Orthomolecular Psychiatry
  1691 Northern Boulevard
  Manhasset, NY 11030
  (516) 627-7535
A professional organization interested in disseminating scientific knowledge in the field of orthomolecular psychiatry and in serving as a meeting ground for professionals interested in extending their own knowledge for the alleviation of mental disorders and related conditions. Publishes *Journal of Orthomolecular Psychiatry*. Membership is limited to practicing professionals in orthomolecular psychiatry, to those who have made a contribution to the development of this field, and to distinguished scientists with

a special interest. Holds an annual scientific symposiums and makes referrals to members practicing in specific geographic locations.

Canadian Association for Preventive
  and Orthomolecular Medicine
  2177 Park Crescent
  Coquitlam, British Columbia, Canada V3J 6T1
  (604) 461-9383

This organization promotes preventive and orthomolecular medicine and encourages the improvement and quality of all food as well as the elimination of all harmful additives and adulterants. It educates the public in regard to these objectives by conducting meetings, seminars, and public lectures and through the pages of its publications. Referrals are made to physicians interested in its philosophies.

Canadian Schizophrenia Foundation
  2229 Broad Street
  Regina, Saskatchewan, Canada S4P 1Y7
  (306) 527-7969

This foundation dedicates itself to reducing the suffering and the social and economic problems caused by schizophrenia and related illnesses. Interested in diagnosis, treatment, and prevention of these various problems—especially by nutritional means. Numerous meetings and other public information programs, seminars, workshops, and conferences are conducted and a library is maintained. A quarterly newsletter and a journal, *Journal of Orthomolecular Psychiatry* are also published by this group. Pamphlets, brochures, etc. are provided on the areas of learning disability, schizophrenia, megavitamin therapy, orthomolecular psychiatry, alcoholism, aging, and the importance of nutritional therapy.

Orthomolecular Medical Society
2698 Pacific Avenue
San Francisco, CA 94115
(415) 346-5692

A scientific research organization of health-care professionals interested in the subject of orthomolecular medicine. Holds annual meetings, and acts as a clearing house for information on the subject. A referral booklet of physicians and other clinicians in the U.S. using an orthomolecular medical approach in their treatment is provided to members.

PREVENTIVE MEDICINE

American Academy of Medical Preventics
2811 L Street
Sacramento, CA 95816
(916) 456-3378

An educational society for health-care professionals and the public interested in the prevention and/or treatment of chronic degenerative diseases. Its goals are to insure public awareness of alternative, holistic methods of prevention and treatment. Conferences, symposiums, and workshops are sponsored and extensive bibliographic and clinical information on chelation therapy is provided to interested professionals. Information is also available to the public regarding new alternatives, and nonsurgical therapy employed for the treatment and prevention of atherosclerosis. Referrals to members of the academy who offer such approaches are made.

Integral Health Services
245 School Street
Putnam, CT 06260
(203) 928-7729

A preventive medicine and holistic health-care facility interested in promoting health by educating and encouraging each individual to accept responsibility for improving their own health. A healthy person is believed to be conscious of how the physical, nutritional, emotional, and environmental aspects of life can affect him/her. The focus of this organization is on prevention, correction, and education, by providing services including individual medical and chiropractic care, massage, yoga, and exercise therapy, nutritional counseling, psychotherapy, and a combination of comprehensive diagnostic evaluations.

International Academy of Preventive Medicine (IAPM)
 10409 Town & Country Way, Suite 200
 Houston, TX 77024
 (713) 468-7851
Pursues professional education and research in the field of preventive medicine and the applications of medical nutrition. Sponsors national meetings and seminars on the subject of preventive medicine and dentistry, medical nutrition and holistic health, psychiatry and podiatry. The *Journal of the International Academy of Preventive Medicine* is its professional journal. Provides copies of membership directory at no charge to assist in locating professionals interested in preventive medicine.

Linus Pauling Institute of Science and Medicine
 2700 Sand Hill Road
 Menlo Park, CA 94025
 (415) 854-0843
Engages in research in the sciences of biology and medicine conducive to the increase in the value of human life and reduction in the amount of human suffering. Research areas include vitamin C and cancer, the effects of aging, orthomolecular medicine, and preventive medicine. It provides bibliographical information to both professionals and laypersons and publishes a quarterly newsletter.

RAW FOOD

Hippocrates Health Institute
  25 Exeter Street
  Boston, MA 02116
  (617) 267-9525
An organization whose purpose is to teach the health virtues of a vegetarian health program featuring 100 percent raw food (including sprouts). Many publications available on sprouting.

SOIL AND HEALTH

Soil and Health Foundation
  33 East Minor Street
  Emmaus, PA 18049
  (215) 967-5171
A nonprofit foundation which promotes research—professional and lay—into natural systems, both environmental and medical. Sponsors and conducts scientific research, education, and training programs concerning the soil, foods, and the health of man and their relationship to each other. Studies the effects of natural and chemical substances on soil, plants, animals, water, and man in order to help its members safely grow more of their own food, upgrade their drinking water, better their nutrition, and improve their health. Publishes a quarterly newsletter and provides a trace mineral and heavy metal analysis of hair and water samples to interested persons.

VEGETARIANISM

Vegetarian Information Service, Inc.
  P.O. Box 5888
  Washington, DC 20014
  (301) 530-1737
An organization formed to collect, organize, and disseminate information on all aspects of vegetarianism. Advises public officials and mass media representatives on the benefits of a vegetarian

way of life through testimonies, conferences, and letters. Currently is in the process of compiling a medical bibliography of scientific information on vegetarianism.

VITAMIN E
The Shute Institute for Clinical and Laboratory Medicine
  10 Grand Avenue
  London, Ontario, Canada N6C 1K9
  (519) 432-1884

This foundation sees itself as the "world headquarters" for the therapeutic use of vitamin E based on the pioneering work of Drs. Evan and Wilfrid Shute. Primary focus is on the treatment of coronary artery disease and problems of poor circulation, burns, and diabetes. Nutrition, exercise, and orthomolecular medicine play a prominent role in the clinic's treatment methods. Inquiries are answered from both professionals and laypersons interested in obtaining information on any aspect of vitamin E research.

Best Food Sources of Vitamins and Minerals

VITAMINS

Biotin

brewer's yeast

cauliflower

eggs

legumes°

liver

milk

nuts

Choline

lamb

oats

organ meats†

soybeans

veal

wheat germ

°Such as peas, beans, peanuts, lentils.
†Such as liver, heart, kidneys.

Folacin (folic acid)

asparagus	onions (green)
brewer's yeast	parsley
broccoli	tempeh
legumes	vegetables (dark green, leafy)*
liver	wheat germ
nuts	whole-grain products

Inositol

barley	oranges
beef	organ meats
cantaloupe	peanuts
grapefruit	peas
molasses (blackstrap)	wheat germ
oats	whole wheat products

Pantothenic Acid

avocado	mushrooms
brewer's yeast	organ meats
broccoli	peanuts
cashews	pecans
cauliflower	poultry (dark meat)
filberts	trout

Vitamin A

apricots	sweet potatoes
broccoli	vegetables (dark green, leafy)
carrots	winter squash (butternut,
fish-liver oils	hubbard)
liver	

Vitamin B₁ (thiamine)

brewer's yeast	sunflower seeds
legumes	vegetables (dark green, leafy)
nuts	wheat germ
organ meats	whole-grain products

*Such as beet, collard, mustard, and turnip greens; kale, parsley, watercress.

Vitamin B₂ (riboflavin)

almonds
asparagus
broccoli
cheese
eggs

milk
organ meats
rice (wild)
wheat germ
whole-grain products

Vitamin B₃ (niacin)

brewer's yeast
legumes
nuts
organ meats

poultry
seafoods
veal
whole-grain products

Vitamin B₆ (pyridoxine)

bananas
brewer's yeast
buckwheat flour (dark)
filberts
organ meats
peanuts
poultry

rice (brown)
salmon
sunflower seeds
tomatoes
wheat germ
whole-grain products

Vitamin B₁₂ (cyanocobalamin)

eggs
meat
milk

organ meats
seafoods

Vitamin C

amaranth
broccoli
brussels sprouts
cabbage
cantaloupe
cauliflower
citrus fruits
currants (black European)
green and red peppers (sweet)

guavas
honeydew
kohlrabi
papaya
persimmon
pimientos
strawberries
tomatoes
vegetables (dark green, leafy)

Vitamin D

fish-liver oils
herring
mackerel

salmon
sardines
tuna

Vitamin E (alpha tocopherol)

almonds
corn oil
filberts
olive oil
peanut oil
peanuts

safflower oil
sesame oil
soybean oil
sunflower oil (and seeds)
wheat germ
wheat germ oil

Vitamin K

alfalfa
asparagus
broccoli
cabbage
cauliflower

green beans
liver (beef)
peas
soybeans
vegetables (dark green, leafy)

MINERALS

Calcium

brewer's yeast
broccoli
herring
mackerel
milk products
salmon

sardines
soybeans
tempeh
tofu
vegetables (dark green, leafy)

Chromium

beef
brewer's yeast
chicken
chili peppers (fresh)

cornmeal
liver (calf)
whole wheat products

Iron

brewer's yeast
dried fruits
fish
legumes
meat
molasses (blackstrap)

organ meats
potatoes
vegetables (dark green, leafy)
wheat germ
whole-grain products

Magnesium

molasses (blackstrap)
nuts
peas
rice (brown)

soybeans
vegetables (dark green, leafy)
whole-grain products

Manganese

bananas
beans
beets
corn
kale
lettuce
liver
nuts
oatmeal

peas
prunes
rice (brown)
rye (whole grain)
snap beans
spinach
sweet potatoes
whole wheat products

Phosphorus

almonds
Brazil nuts
brewer's yeast
cereal products
cheese
cod
egg
English walnuts
halibut
liver
meat

milk
peanuts
peas
poultry
salmon
sardines
sunflower seeds
sweetbreads
wheat germ
whole wheat products

Potassium

apples	oranges
apricots	peanut butter
avocados	potatoes
bananas	raisins
beef	salmon
brewer's yeast	sesame seeds
broccoli	sunflower seeds
carrots	tomatoes
chicken	tuna
molasses (blackstrap)	wheat germ

Zinc

cheese	nuts
eggs	pumpkin seeds
green beans	seafoods
lamb	sunflower seeds
lima beans	wheat germ
meat	whole-grain products

FURTHER READING

Adams, Catherine F. *Nutritive Value of American Foods in Common Units,* Handbook No. 456. (Washington, D.C.: Superintendent of Documents, 1975).

Burton, Benjamin T. *Human Nutrition* (New York: McGraw-Hill, 1976).

Freeland, Jeanne H., and Cousins, Robert J. "Zinc Content of Selected Foods," *Journal of the American Dietetic Association,* vol. 68, no. 6, June 1976, pp. 526–30.

Guthrie, Helen Andrews, *Introductory Nutrition* (St. Louis, Mo.: C. V. Mosby, 1975).

Herting, David C., and Drury, Emma-Jane E. "Vitamin E Content of Vegetable Oils and Fats." *The Journal of Nutrition,* vol. 81, no. 4, December 1963, pp. 335–42.

Monsen, Elaine et al. "Estimation of Available Dietary

Iron." *The American Journal of Clinical Nutrition,* vol. 31, January 1978, pp. 134-41.

Murphy, Elizabeth W.; Willis, Barbara Wells; and Watt, Bernice K. "Provisional Tables on the Zinc Content of Foods," *Journal of the American Dietetic Association,* vol. 66, April 1975, pp. 345-55.

National Academy of Sciences, *Recommended Dietary Allowances* (Washington, D.C.: National Academy of Sciences, 1974).

Orr, Martha Louise. *Pantothenic Acid, Vitamin B_6 and Vitamin B_{12} in Foods,* Handbook No. 36 (Washington, D.C.: Superintendent of Documents, 1969).

Perloff, Betty P., and Butrum, Ruva R. "Folacin in Selected Foods." *Journal of the American Dietetic Association,* vol. 70, no. 2, February 1977, pp. 161-72.

Sebrell, W. H., Jr., and Harris, Robert S. *The Vitamins: Chemistry, Physiology, Pathology, Methods,* vols. 2, 3, and 5 (New York: Academic Press, 1968, 1971, and 1972).

Toepfer, Edward W. "Chromium in Foods in Relation to Biological Activity," *Journal of Agricultural and Food Chemistry,* vol. 21, no. 1, 1973, pp. 69-73.

Index